Say It in
SPANISH

Say It in SPANISH

SECOND EDITION

A Guide for Health Care Professionals

Esperanza Villanueva Joyce, Ed.D., CNS, RN
Professor
Texas A&M University—Corpus Christi
School of Nursing and Health Sciences
Corpus Christi, Texas

Maria Elena Villanueva, M.D.
Mexico, D.F.

W.B. SAUNDERS COMPANY
A Harcourt Health Sciences Company

Philadelphia London New York St. Louis Sydney Toronto

W.B. Saunders Company
A Harcourt Health Sciences Company

The Curtis Center
Independence Square West
Philadelphia, Pennsylvania 19106

Library of Congress Cataloging-in-Publication Data

Joyce, Esperanza Villanueva.
Say it in Spanish : a guide for health care professionals / Esperanza Villanueva Joyce, Maria Elena Villanueva — 2nd ed.
p. cm.
Includes bibliographical references and indexes.
ISBN 0-7216-8613-3
1. Spanish language—Conversation and phrase books (for medical personnel)
I. Villanueva, Maria Elena. II. Title.
[DNLM: 1. Medicine—Phrases—English. 2. Medicine—Phrases—Spanish.]
PC4120.M3 J68 2000
468.3'42102461—dc21

99-051713

SAY IT IN SPANISH ISBN 0-7216-8613-3

Printed in the United States of America

Last digit is the print number: 9 8 7 6 5 4 3 2 1

I want to thank my husband Raymond, for preserving his sense of humor, even after retyping the same chapters many, many times. He also carefully edited each chapter and provided feedback that was not only useful but very practical. My special thanks to my daughter Leslie Ann, who understood why I was not able to attend so many of her golf tournaments.

E.V. Joyce

Special thanks to my daughter Claudia who helped with the translations and José, my husband, who contributed with his support.

M.E. Villanueva

Preface

I am pleased to present you with the second edition of *Say It in Spanish: A Guide for Health Care Professionals*. The idea for this text grew from multiple observations in clinical settings where the frustrations of non–Spanish-speaking providers are evident. These frustrations stem from the lack of control providers feel when they are not in command of the language of their patients and must depend on translators for data collection. My bicultural background and my bilingualism have afforded me the opportunity to translate for many Spanish-speaking patients. This has allowed me to understand the predicament that Spanish-speaking patients find themselves in when they require medical care. The communication of simple facts can be difficult, and miscommunication can have lethal consequences.

As a faculty member in nursing schools I was often amused by my students' comments: "Don't assign me a Spanish-speaking patient," or "I don't know how to speak Spanish." I had little choice because 46 percent of our large medical center patient population was Hispanic. For many years I have taught a Spanish course for nurses in academic and clinical centers. Evaluations confirmed that the course helped students provide better care to their Spanish-speaking patients. Students were able to interact with families, collect data, and make meaningful contributions to their patients' care. In these settings, it was clear that the opportunities gained by knowledge of a second language were innumerable!

Approach

Say It in Spanish is designed primarily to meet the needs of health care professionals and students who anticipate contact with Spanish-speaking patients. Health providers in hospitals, clinics, physician's offices, outpatient and community centers, as well as students in nursing and allied health schools, can benefit from the use of this textbook. This text can also be used as a self-instructional program for those whose occupations bring them into daily contact with patients whose primary language is Spanish. To facilitate the self-instructional approach, translations are accompanied by their pronunciations.

Over the past decade there has been a growing recognition in health care settings of the importance of communicating directly with Spanish-speaking patients. Clinicians who can communicate directly with their patients are able to assess more effectively the success of the treatment they are providing. The Spanish expressions used in this book are primarily those used in Spanish-speaking countries close to the United States and Spanish communities within the United States. This text provides an introduction to the Spanish language, but it is not a comprehensive grammar textbook. The intent is to present practical language that can be used in clinical settings in which interaction with a Spanish-speaking patient may be short term or long term. Those who use this text will be able to express in simple Spanish what they need to say. Special emphasis is placed on the use of meaningful medical vocabulary. Medical situations mentioned in the text are those experienced in everyday life.

New to This Edition

Much of the content from the first edition has been rearranged, some chapters have been combined, and seven new chapters have been added.

- Chapter 2, "Pre-Hospital Care," was added at the request of emergency medical technicians and emergency personnel, to provide basic communication knowledge of the nature of assessing and transporting a patient.
- Chapter 7, "A Visit to the Family Doctor," deals specifically with a patient with AIDS. Its dialogues assist the clinician in explaining the disease to his or her patients.
- Chapter 9, "A Visit to the Cardiologist," helps explain heart problems and hypertension to the patient, in addition to focusing on questions that relate to cardiac symptoms.
- Chapter 10, "A Visit to the Endocrinologist," discusses diabetes, its symptoms, appropriate laboratory exams, and recommendations to assist the clinician in the implementation of discharge planning. This chapter was added at the request of students and hospital personnel who encounter a high incidence of diabetes in Hispanic patients.

- Chapter 12, "Amputations," helps the clinician explain to the patient the pre-operative procedure as well as the medical–surgical care of the amputated limb.
- Chapter 13, "A Visit to the Surgeon," focuses on the symptoms and diagnosis of appendicitis.
- Chapter 14, "A Visit to the Psychologist," explores factors that threaten the mental health of patients. The dialogues help the clinician in asking pertinent questions related to depression and suicide.
- Chapter 15, "A Visit to the Dentist," has been updated to reflect the current trends in dental care.

In addition, a 90-minute audiotape is included. The audiotape allows the clinician to listen to Chapter 22, "Physical Exam," and Chapter 23, "Greetings and Common Expressions." Each phrase is introduced in English and then in Spanish. The Spanish is repeated twice to increase familiarity with the pronounciation.

Features of the Text

For the convenience of the health provider, Chapters 1–38 include English–Spanish usage. This bilingual text eliminates the time-consuming process of looking up words in the dictionary.

The questioning techniques presented have been selected to elicit "yes" or "no" answers. These will assist those providers who have a limited knowledge of Spanish.

Dialogues are presented as situations with corresponding appropriate basic vocabulary. The dialogues deal with familiar situations in the medical setting. And they are simple and interesting, so the provider has the opportunity to use repetition that will enhance retention.

Scenes are illustrated using basic vocabulary. This will help health providers to link the object with its Spanish equivalent without reference to English.

English phrases are not always translated literally; instead, the most common Spanish words have been selected and presented.

Tables throughout the text help the provider review key words, ideas, and concepts.

A cultural perspective that increases the awareness of the health care provider for the needs of the Spanish-speaking population is also included.

Organization

The text is comprised of chapters organized to present a patient's usual movement from the community to the hospital setting. Chapters 1–3 focus on practical language skills that are used in first aid and pre-hospital care, as well as in emergency situations. The use of short dialogues that will elicit "yes" and "no" answers will facilitate data collection essential for immediate care. Chapters 5 and 6 provide essential information needed to admit and interview a patient. Chapters 7–15 focus on specialties reflecting current health care emphasis. Chapter 16 assists home health-care workers in asking pertinent questions related to the health status of family members. Chapters 17–21 emphasize the most common vocabulary used in various hospital departments such as pharmacy, laboratory, and X-ray. The health provider can refer quickly to the appropriate chapter, thus increasing his or her communication skills and not delaying treatment while waiting for a translator.

The discussion of physical assessment (chapter 22) specifically relates to internal and external parts of the body. Chapters 23–25 and Chapter 27 provide specific content related to greetings and common expressions that will assist in creating a welcoming environment for the patient. The chapters on phrases and commands facilitate the completion of a physical assessment.

Chapters 28–31 present the terminology of numbers, time, colors, and members of the family. These sections have been selected to enhance the health provider's knowledge of everyday terms that will be useful in the clinical setting.

Chapters 32–38 present an overview of the most essential grammatical concepts. The pronunciation and spelling of Spanish sounds are explained in detail. Most of the Spanish sounds are similar to sounds in English and therefore are easy to learn. These chapters provide the basis for appropriate use of the language and also serve as a quick reference.

The last two chapters, 39 and 40, describe cultural variations among Spanish-speaking groups as well as the common health beliefs and popular health cures practiced by each group. The intent in this unit is to increase the health provider's awareness of cultural differences in the health perceptions of Spanish-speaking patients.

The English–Spanish index is divided into two sections: a Phrase and Sentence index and a Word index. The unique phrase and sentence index is a useful tool that will save the health care worker time when determining which question to ask.

Difficult terms, important terms, and useful vocabulary are highlighted in tables that appear throughout the book.

Esperanza Villanueva Joyce

Contents

Unit 1—Unidad 1 1

1 First Aid—*Primeros auxilios* 3

2 Pre-Hospital Care—*Cuidados pre-hospitalarios* 14

3 Emergency Care—*Cuidado de urgencia (emergencia)* 27

4 In the Hospital—*En el hospital* 40

5 Admitting a Patient—*Admitiendo al paciente* 52

6 The Clerical Staff—*Las secretarias* 64

Unit 2—Unidad 2 73

7 A Visit to the Family Doctor—*Una visita al médico familiar* 75

8 A Visit to the Pediatrician—*Una visita a la pediatra* 83

9 A Visit to the Cardiologist—*Una visita al cardiólogo* 97

10 A Visit to the Endocrinologist—*Una visita al endocrinólogo* 101

11 A Visit to the OB-GYN—*Una visita al gineco-obstetra* 106

12 Amputations—*Amputaciones* 115

13 A Visit to the Surgeon—*Una visita al cirujano* 128

14 A Visit to the Psychologist—*Una visita al psicólogo* 133

15 A Visit to the Dentist—*Una visita al dentista* 145

16 A Home Visit—*Una visita al hogar* 157

Unit 3—Unidad 3 163

17 The Patient's Room—*El cuarto del paciente* 165

18 The Laboratory—*El laboratorio* 174

19 The Pharmacy—*La farmacia* 182

20 The X-Ray Department—*El departamento de rayos X* 195

21 The Meals—*Las comidas* 206

Unit 4—Unidad 4 221

22 Physical Exam—*Examen físico* 223

23 Greetings and Common Expressions—*Saludos y expresiones comunes* 239

24 Commands—*Órdenes o mandatos* 242

25 Phrases—*Frases* 246

Unit 5—Unidad 5 251

26 Useful Vocabulary at Home—*Vocabulario útil sobre la vivienda* 253

27 Cognates—*Cognados* 257

28 Numbers—*Números* 265

29 Time—*La hora* 270

30 The Colors, the Seasons, the Months, the Days—*Los colores, las estaciones del año, los meses, los días* 273

31 The Members of the Family—*Los miembros de la familia* 277

Unit 6—Unidad 6 281

32 The Alphabet—*El abecedario* 283

33 Accents—*Acentos* 286

34 Gender of Nouns—*Género de los sustantivos* 287

35 Adjectives and Pronouns—*Adjetivos y pronombres* 292

36 Simple Questions, Interrogatives, Exclamations—*Preguntas sencillas, interrogativas, exclamaciones* 298

37 Negatives, Affirmatives—*Negativos, afirmativos* 301

38 Verbs—*Verbos* 303

Unit 7—Unidad 7 313

39 A Cultural Perspective 315

40 Home Cures and Popular Beliefs 320

Phrase and Sentence Index 327

Word Index 391

Say It in

SPANISH

Unit 1 — Unidad 1

Chapter One | **Capítulo uno**

First Aid

Primeros auxilios

Injury or sudden illness becomes an emergency when life is threatened. Injured persons depend on others for their well-being. Health providers must communicate accurately and in a language a patient can understand. In an emergency, there is no time for lengthy conversation. Use short phrases that elicit either a "yes" or "no" response.

Una herida o enfermedad repentina se convierte en una emergencia cuando la vida corre peligro. Las personas que han sufrido daños de-

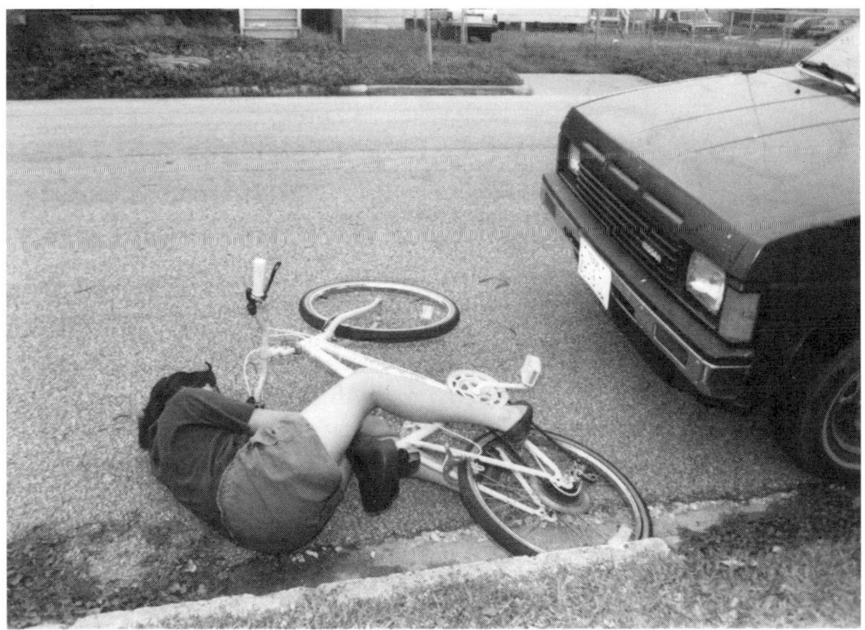

Figure 1–1 Injury or sudden illness becomes an emergency when life is threatened. Health providers must communicate accurately and in a language a person can understand.

penden de otros para sobrevivir. Los proveedores de la salud deben comunicarse con exactitud para darse a entender por el paciente. En un caso de emergencia, no hay tiempo para conversar. Use frases cortas para que las respuestas sean "sí" o "no".

Excuse me.	**Con permiso.** *(Kohn pehr-mee-soh)*
Let me go through.	**Déjeme pasar.** *(Deh-heh-meh pah-sahr)*
I need to see the injured.	**Necesito ver al accidentado.** *(Neh-seh-see-toh vehr ahl ahk-see-dehn-tah-doh)*
Make some room!	**¡Haga lugar!** *(Ah-gah loo-gahr)*
Stay away!	**¡Hágase a un lado!** *(Ah-gah-seh ah uhn la-doh)*
Don't touch anything!	**¡No toque nada!** *(Noh toh-keh nah-dah)*
Do not move the patient!	**¡No mueva al paciente!** *(Noh moo-eh-bah ahl pah-see-ehn-teh)*
I have to assess first.	**Necesito evaluar primero.** *(Neh-seh-see-toh eh-bah-loo-ahr pree-meh-roh)*

Other EMS staff ask questions if there are witnesses.

Otros empleados de servicios de emergencia hacen preguntas si hay testigos.

Who saw the accident?	**¿Quién vió el accidente?** *(Kee-ehn bee-oh ehl ahk-see-dehn-teh)*
What kind of accident?	**¿Qué tipo de accidente?** *(Keh tee-poh deh ahk-see-dehn-teh)*
How many cars crashed?	**¿Cuántos carros chocaron?** *(Koo-ahn-tohs kah-rohs choh-kah-rohn)*
How many people were in the car/bus/truck?	**¿Cuántas personas estaban en el carro/el autobús/la camioneta?** *(Koo-ahn-tahs pehr-soh-nahs ehs-tah-bahn ehn ehl kah-roh/ehl ah-oo-toh-buhs/lah kah-mee-oh-neh-tah)*
Was the victim on the road?	**¿Estaba la víctima en el camino?** *(Ehs-tah-bah lah beek-tee-mah ehn ehl kah-mee-noh)*

How did you move the victim?	**¿Cómo movió a la víctima?** *(Koh-moh moh-bee-oh ah lah beek-tee-mah)*
Was the victim alive/dead?	**¿Estaba la víctima con vida/muerta?** *(Ehs-tah-bah lah beek-tee-mah kohn bee-dah/moo-ehr-tah)*
Was the victim unconscious?	**¿Estaba la víctima inconsciente?** *(Ehs-tah-bah lah beek-tee-mah een-kohn-see-ehn-teh)*

Use your hands when talking, pantomime, point, use facial expressions! There are several expressions you can use to get someone's attention. Table 1–1.

Use las manos al hablar, haga pantomimas, apunte, ¡use expresiones faciales! Hay varias expresiones que puede usar para atraer la atención. Tabla 1–1.

Miss	**señorita** *(seh-nyoh-ree-tah)*
Mrs.	**señora** *(seh-nyoh-rah)*
Mr.	**señor** *(seh-nyohr)*
Hello!	**¡Hola!** *(Oh-lah)*
Can you hear me?	**¿Puede oírme?** *(Poo-eh-deh oh-eer-meh)*
Can you talk?	**¿Puede hablar?** *(Poo-eh-deh ah-blahr)*

TABLE 1–1
Attention-Getting Phrases

TABLA 1–1
Frases para atraer atención

English	Spanish	Pronunciation
Mr.	**señor**	*(seh-nyohr)*
Mrs.	**señora**	*(seh-nyoh-rah)*
Miss	**señorita**	*(seh-nyoh-ree-tah)*
young man/woman	**joven**	*(hoh-behn)*
boy/girl	**muchacho(a)**	*(moo-chah-choh)/(moo-chah-chah)*
boy/girl	**niño(a)**	*(nee-nyoh)/(nee-nyah)*
Listen!	**¡Oiga!**	*(Oh-ee-gah)*
Excuse me!	**¡Perdón!**	*(Pehr-dohn)*

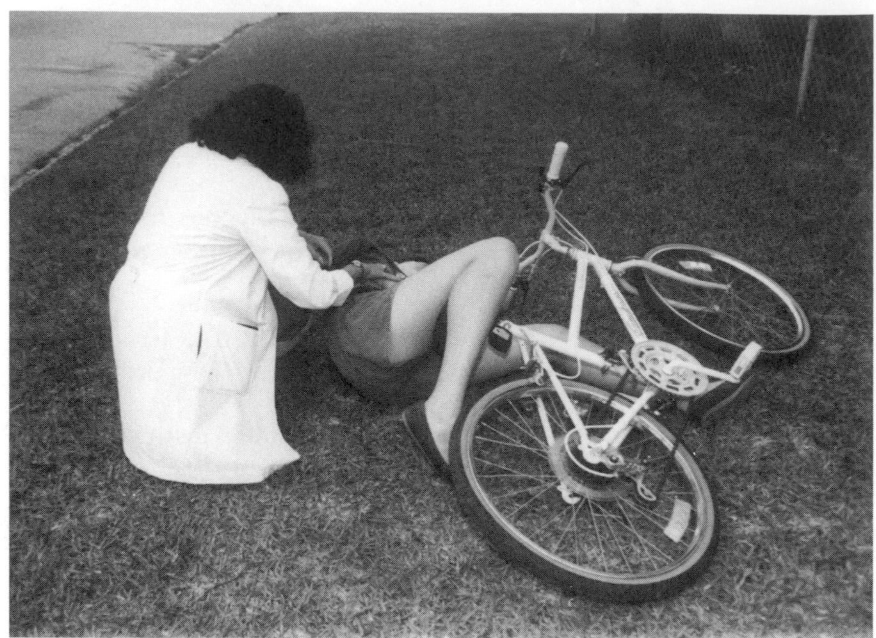

Figure 1–2 In an emergency, tell the patient to speak slowly, remind him/her to respond with "yes" or "no" as much as possible.

Can you breathe?	**¿Puede respirar?** ***(Poo-eh-deh rehs-pee-rahr)***
What is your name?	**¿Cómo se llama?** ***(Koh-moh seh yah-mah)***
Do you know where you are?	**¿Sabe dónde está?** ***(Sah-beh dohn-deh ehs-tah)***
Do you know the day?	**¿Qué día es hoy?** ***(Keh dee-ah ehs oh-ee)***
Please don't move.	**Por favor, no se mueva.** ***(Pohr fah-bohr noh seh moo-eh-bah)***
I need to see if you are hurt.	**Necesito ver si está lastimado.** ***(Neh-seh-see-toh behr see ehs-tah lahs-tee-mah-doh)***

Unless an emergency is life threatening, a person needs to participate in his/her own care to maintain a sense of control. Ask the patient to speak slowly when speaking Spanish and remind him/her to respond with "yes" or "no" as much as possible. Table 1–2 shows a list of common commands you can use.

A menos que esté en peligro la vida, una persona necesita participar en su cuidado para mantener el sentido de control. Pídale al paciente que hable despacio cuando hable en español y recuérdele que responda "sí" o "no" lo más posible. La Tabla 1–2 le muestra una lista de mandatos comunes que puede usar.

Open your eyes.	**Abra los ojos.** *(Ah-brah lohs oh-hos)*
Don't turn.	**No voltee.** *(Noh bohl-teh-eh)*
Where does it hurt?	**¿Dónde le duele?** *(Don-deh leh doo-eh-leh)*
Point.	**Apunte./Señale.** *(Ah-poon-teh/Seh-nyah-leh)*
Did you fall?	**¿Se cayó?** *(Seh kah-yoh)*
Were you hit by a car?	**¿Le golpeó un carro?** *(Leh gohl-peh-oh oon kah-roh)*
Did you lose consciousness?	**¿Perdió el conocimiento?** *(Pehr-dee-oh ehl koh-noh-see-mee-ehn-toh)*
Where do you live?	**¿Dónde vive?** *(Dohn-deh bee-beh)*
Do you remember the street?	**¿Recuerda la calle?** *(Reh-koo-ehr-dah lah kah-yeh)*

TABLE 1–2
Pronunciation of Commands

TABLA 1–2
Pronunciación de mandatos

English	Spanish	Pronunciation
Be still!	¡Quieto!	*(Kee-eh-toh)*
Bend!	¡Doble!	*(Doh-bleh)*
Breathe!	¡Respire!	*(Rehs-pee-reh)*
Don't move!	¡No se mueva!	*(Noh seh moo-eh-bah)*
Move!	¡Muevase!	*(Moo-eh-bah-say)*
Open!	¡Abra!	*(Ah-brah)*
Point!	¡Apunte!	*(Ah-poon-teh)*
	¡Señale!	*(Seh-nyah-leh)*
Sit!	¡Siéntese!	*(See-ehn-teh-seh)*
Speak!	¡Hable!	*(Ah-bleh)*
Turn!	¡Voltee!	*(Bohl-teh-eh)*

Where were you going?	**¿A dónde iba?** *(Ah dohn-deh ee-bah)*
Your leg is broken.	**Tiene la pierna quebrada/fracturada.** *(Tee-eh-neh lah pee-ehr-nah keh-brah-dah/frahk-too-rah-dah)*
I need to cut the pants.	**Necesito cortar el pantalón.** *(Neh-seh-see-toh kohr-tahr ehl pahn-tah-lohn)*
I am going to put a splint on the leg.	**Voy a ponerle una tablilla en la pierna.** *(Boy ah poh-nehr-leh oo-nah tah-blee-yah ehn lah pee-ehr-nah)*
Do not bend your leg!	**¡No doble la pierna!** *(Noh doh-bleh lah pee-ehr-nah)*
Keep the leg straight.	**Mantenga la pierna derecha.** *(Mahn-tehn-gah lah pee-ehr-nah deh-reh-chah)*
I am going to cover you.	**Lo voy a cubrir.** *(Loh boy ah koo-breer)*
I will put you on the stretcher.	**Voy a ponerlo en la camilla.** *(Boy ah poh-nehr-loh ehn lah kah-mee-yah)*
We are going to the hospital.	**Vamos al hospital.** *(Bah-mohs ahl ohs-pee-tahl)*
We are going in the ambulance.	**Vamos en la ambulancia.** *(Bah-mohs ehn lah ahm-boo-lahn-see-ah)*
It takes 10 minutes.	**Se toma diez minutos.** *(Seh toh-mah dee-ehs mee-noo-tohs)*
Have you been a patient before?	**¿Ha sido un paciente antes?** *(Ah see-doh oon pah-see-ehn-teh ahn-tehs)*
Have you had any accidents?	**¿Ha tenido algún accidente?** *(Ah teh-nee-doh ahl-goon ahk-see-dehn-teh)*

While traveling to the Emergency Room—and if the patient's condition is stable—ask for more information. This helps the staff to complete forms and decrease delays in calling family or friends (Table 1–3).

Mientras que viaja al cuarto de emergencias —y si la condición del paciente es estable—haga más preguntas. Esto ayuda a los empleados a completar las formas y disminuye la demora en llamar a la familia o a los amigos (Tabla 1–3).

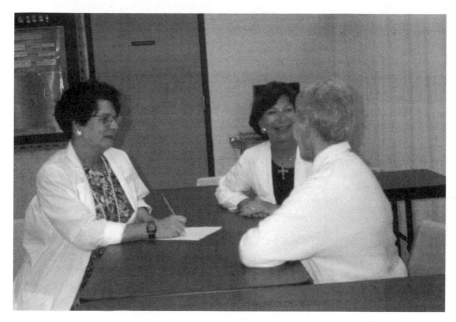

Figure 1–3 Gather as much information as possible after the accident.

What kind?	**¿Qué clase?** *(Keh klah-seh)*
Have you had anything broken?	**¿Ha tenido algo quebrado?** *(Ah teh nee-doh ahl-goh keh-brah-doh)*
How long ago?	**¿Hace cuánto tiempo?** *(Ah-seh koo-ahn-toh tee-ehm-poh)*
Were you hospitalized?	**¿Lo hospitalizaron?** *(Loh ohs-pee-tah-lee-sah-rohn)*
Do you know the hospital name?	**¿Sabe el nombre del hospital?** *(Sah-beh ehl nohm-breh dehl ohs-pee-tahl)*
The doctor will see you in the Emergency Room.	**Lo verá el doctor en el cuarto de emergencia.** *(Loh beh-rah ehl dohk-tohr ehn ehl koo-ahr-toh deh eh-mehr-hehn-see-ah)*
The doctor will give you something for the pain.	**El doctor le dará algo para el dolor.** *(Ehl dohk-tohr leh dah-rah ahl-goh pah-rah ehl doh-lohr)*
The nurse will ask how you feel.	**La enfermera le preguntará cómo se siente.** *(Lah ehn-fehr-meh-rah leh preh-goon-tah-rah koh-moh seh see-ehn-teh)*

TABLE 1–3
Other Important Questions

TABLA 1–3
Otras preguntas importantes

English	Spanish	Pronunciation
Did you faint?	**¿Se desmayó?**	*(Seh dehs-mah-yoh)*
Do you feel nauseated?	**¿Siente náuseas?**	*(Seh-ehn-teh nah-oo-seh-ahs)*
Do you feel weak?	**¿Se siente débil?**	*(Seh see-ehn-teh deh-beel)*
Do you feel dizzy?	**¿Se siente mareado?**	*(Seh see-ehn-teh mah-reh-ah-doh)*
Are you cold?	**¿Tiene frío?**	*(Tee-eh-neh free-oh)*
Are you hot?	**¿Tiene calor?**	*(Tee-eh-neh kah-lohr)*

They will let you talk to your family.
Le dejarán hablar con su familia.
(Leh deh-hah-rahn ah-blahr kohn soo fah-mee-lee-ah)

Do you have a phone?
¿Tiene teléfono?
(Tee-eh-neh teh-leh-foh-noh)

Give it to the clerk.
Déselo a la secretaria.
(Deh-seh-loh ah lah seh-kreh-tah-ree-ah)

Is your family in town?
¿Está su familia en la ciudad?
(Ehs-tah soo fah-mee-lee-ah ehn lah see-oo-dahd)

Add *es* to a singular noun that ends in a consonant to make it a plural. In words ending in *z*, change the *z* to *c* before adding *es*. Add *s* to a singular noun that ends in a vowel to make it a plural noun. Table 1–4 lists examples of singular and plural nouns and articles.

Añada *es* al nombre singular que termina en una consonante para hacerlo plural. Si la palabra termina en *z*, cambie la *z* a *c* antes de agregrar *es*. Añada *s* al nombre singular que termina en una vocal para hacerlo plural. La Tabla 1–4 da una lista de ejemplos de nombres y artículos singulares y plurales.

Do you have any children?
¿Tiene niños?
(Tee-eh-neh nee-nyohs)

How many?
¿Cuántos?
(Koo-ahn-tohs)

How many boys/girls?
¿Cuántos niños?/¿Cuántas niñas?
(Koo-ahn-tohs nee-nyohs/Koo-ahn-tahs nee-nyahs)

TABLE 1–4
Singular and Plural

TABLA 1–4
Singular y plural

Singular		Plural	
the girl	**la niña** *(lah nee-nyah)*	the girls	**las niñas** *(lahs nee-nyahs)*
the boy	**el niño** *(ehl nee-nyoh)*	the boys	**los niños** *(lohs nee-nyohs)*
the doctor	**el doctor** *(ehl dohk-tohr)*	the doctors	**los doctores** *(lohs dohk-toh-rehs)*
the hospital	**el hospital** *(ehl ohs-pee-tahl)*	the hopitals	**los hospitales** *(lohs ohs-pee-tah-lehs)*
a heart	**un corazón** *(oon koh-rah-sohn)*	some hearts	**unos corazones** *(oo-nohs koh-rah-sohn-ehs)*
a table	**una mesa** *(oo-nah meh-sah)*	some tables	**unas mesas** *(oo-nahs meh-sahs)*
a pencil	**un lápiz** *(oon lah-pees)*	some pencils	**unos lápices** *(oo-nohs lah-pee-sehs)*

How old are they? **¿Cuántos años tienen?** *(Koo-ahn-tohs ah-nyohs tee-eh-nehn)*

Do all go to school? **¿Todos van a la escuela?** *(Toh-dohs bahn ah lah ehs-koo-eh-lah)*

What is the name of the school? **¿Cómo se llama la escuela?** *(Koh-moh seh yah-mah lah ehs-koo-eh-lah)*

Do you have a husband/wife? **¿Tiene esposo/esposa?** *(Tee-eh-neh ehs-poh-soh/ehs-poh-sah)*

Is he/she at work? **¿Está trabajando?** *(Ehs-tah trah-bah-hahn-doh)*

Do you know his/her phone number? **¿Sabe su teléfono?** *(Sah-beh soo teh-leh-foh-noh)*

Do you have brothers/sisters? **¿Tiene hermanos/hermanas?** *(Tee-eh-neh ehr-mah-nohs/ehr-mah-nahs)*

Do they live close to you? **¿Viven cerca de usted?** *(Bee-behn sehr-kah deh oos-tehd)*

What do you do? **¿Qué hace usted?** *(Keh ah-seh oos-tehd)*

Are you employed? **¿Trabaja usted?** *(Trah-bah-hah oos-tehd)*

Where do you work?	**¿Dónde trabaja?** *(Dohn-deh trah-bah-hah)*
Do you know the street name?	**¿Sabe el nombre de la calle?** *(Sah-beh ehl nohm-breh deh lah kah-yeh)*
Do you work every day?	**¿Trabaja todos los días?** *(Trah-bah-hah toh-dohs lohs dee-ahs)*
How many hours do you work?	**¿Cuántas horas trabaja?** *(Koo-ahn-tahs oh-rahs trah-bah-hah)*
Who can take care of the children?	**¿Quién puede cuidar a los niños?** *(Kee-ehn poo-eh-deh koo-ee-dahr ah lohs nee-nyohs)*
You will need a cast.	**Necesitará un yeso.** *(Neh-seh-see-tah-rah oon yeh-soh)*
You can walk on crutches.	**Puede caminar con muletas.** *(Poo-eh-deh kah-mee-nahr kohn moo-leh-tahs)*
Keep your leg elevated.	**Mantenga la pierna elevada.** *(Mahn-tehn-gah lah pee-ehr-nah eh-leh-bah-dah)*
Can you take off work?	**¿Puede faltar al trabajo?** *(Poo-eh-deh fahl-tahr ahl trah-bah-hoh)*
Are you on vacation?	**¿Está de vacaciones?** *(Ehs-tah deh bah-kah-see-ohn-ehs)*
Can you take vacation?	**¿Puede tomar vacaciones?** *(Poo-eh-deh toh-mahr bah-kah-see-ohn-ehs)*
Do you have another car?	**¿Tiene otro carro?** *(Tee-eh-neh oh-troh kah-roh)*
Do you have car insurance?	**¿Tiene seguro de carro?** *(Tee-eh-neh seh-goo-roh deh kah-roh)*
Do you have hospital insurance?	**¿Tiene seguro de hospital?** *(Tee-eh-neh seh-goo-roh deh ohs-pee-tahl)*
Do you have help at home?	**¿Tiene ayuda en casa?** *(Tee-eh-neh ah-yoo-dah ehn kah-sah)*
Will you need help?	**¿Va a necesitar ayuda?** *(Bah ah neh-seh-see-tahr ah-yoo-dah)*
Call your friends.	**Llame a sus amigos.** *(Yah-meh ah soos ah-mee-gohs)*

They can help clean.	**Pueden ayudar a limpiar.** *(Poo-eh-dehn ah-yoo-dahr ah leem-pee-ahr)*
Try to calm down.	**Trate de calmarse.** *(Trah-teh deh kahl-mahr-seh)*
You will get help.	**Se le ayudará.** *(Seh leh ah-yoo-dah-rah)*

We know the gender of a Spanish word by its ending. If the word ends in *a* usually it is feminine. If the word ends in *o* usually it is masculine. Table 1–5.

Se determina el género de la palabra en español al ver su terminación. Si la palabra termina en *a* es femenina. Si la palabra termina en *o* es masculina. Tabla 1–5.

TABLE 1–5
Nouns and Articles

TABLA 1–5
Sustantivos y artículos

Nouns ending in *a, d, ión,* or *z* are generally feminine. Female nouns are feminine.		**Nouns ending in *o, or, al,* or *ador* are masculine. Male nouns are masculine even though the noun may end in *a*.**	
the	**la** (feminine) *(lah)*	the	**el** (masculine) *(ehl)*
a/an	**una** (feminine) *(oo-nah)*	a/an	**un** (masculine) *(oon)*
the house	**la casa** *(lah kah-sah)*	the man	**el hombre** *(ehl ohm-breh)*
a door	**una puerta** *(oo-nah poo-ehr-tah)*	an author	**un autor** *(oon ah-oo-tohr)*
the daughter	**la hija** *(lah ee-hah)*	the son	**el hijo** *(ehl ee-hoh)*
the friend	**la amiga** *(lah ah-mee-gah)*	the friend	**el amigo** *(ehl ah-mee-goh)*
the woman	**la mujer** *(lah moo-hehr)*	the hospital	**el hospital** *(ehl ohs-pee-tahl)*
the health	**la salud** *(lah sah-lood)*	the month	**el mes** *(ehl mehs)*

Important exception: the hand → **la mano** ***(lah mah-noh)***. Note the ending *o;* yet **la mano** is feminine.

The days of the week, months of the year, and the names of a language are masculine.

Chapter Two	Capítulo dos

Pre-Hospital Care

Cuidados pre-hospitalarios

Emergency Medical Technicians are trained to provide efficient and immediate care to persons who have sustained injuries or trauma.

Los técnicos de Cuidados de Emergencia están entrenados para proveer cuidado inmediato y eficiente a personas que han sufrido daño o trauma.

Typical EMT questions when the patient is conscious may include:

Preguntas típicas que hacen los técnicos cuando el paciente está consciente pueden incluir:

Are you from this area?	**¿Es usted de esta área?** *(Ehs oos-tehd deh ehs-tah ah-reh-ah)*
Are you under a doctor's care?	**¿Está bajo el cuidado de un doctor?** *(Ehs-tah bah-hoh ehl koo-ee-dah-doh deh uhn dohk-tohr)*
At what hospital have you been treated?	**¿En qué hospital lo han tratado?** *(Ehn keh ohs-pee-tahl loh ahn trah-tah-doh)*
Did you take medications today?	**¿Tomó sus medicinas hoy?** *(Toh-moh soos meh-dee-see-nahs oh-ee)*
when?	**¿cuándo?** *(koo-ahn-doh)*
Do you have any symptoms: nausea, dizziness, other unusual feelings?	**¿Tiene algún síntoma como náuseas, vértigo, otra sensación rara?** *(Tee-eh-neh ahl-goon seen-toh-mah koh-moh nah-oo-seh-ahs, behr-tee-goh, oh-trah sehn-sah-see-ohn rah-rah)*

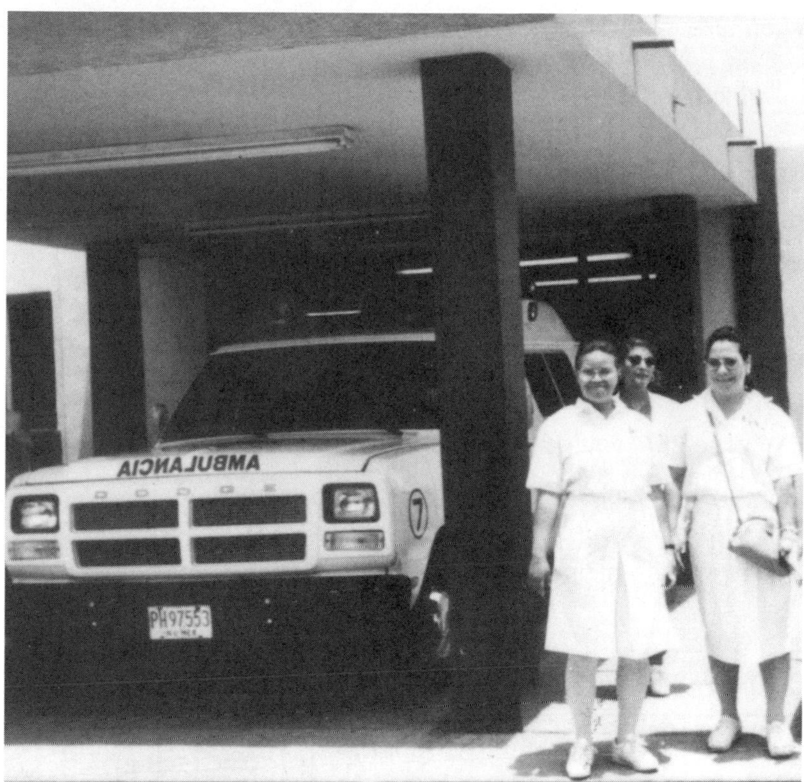

Figure 2–1 Emergency personnel are trained to provide efficient care.

Do you have allergies?	**¿Tiene alergias?** *(Tee-eh-neh ah-lehr-gee-ahs)*
Do you have medical problems:	**¿Tiene problemas médicos:** *(Tee-eh-neh proh-bleh-mahs meh-dee-kohs)*
cardiac problems,	**problemas cardíacos,** *(proh-bleh-mahs kahr-dee-ah-kohs)*
respiratory problems,	**problemas respiratorios,** *(proh-bleh-mahs rehs-pee-rah-toh-ree-ohs)*
renal problems?	**problemas renales?** *(proh-bleh-mahs reh-nah-lehs)*
Do you live here?	**¿Vive aquí?** *(Bee-beh ah-kee)*

Do you take medications?	**¿Toma medicinas?** *(Toh-mah meh-dee-see-nahs)*
what (which ones)?	**¿cuáles?** *(koo-ah-lehs)*
Does the pain move from one place to another?	**¿El dolor se mueve de un lugar a otro?** *(Ehl doh-lohr seh moo-eh-beh deh oon loo-gahr ah oh-troh)*
Does the pain get better if you stop and rest?	**¿Se mejora el dolor si se detiene y descansa?** *(Seh meh-hoh-rah ehl doh-lohr see seh deh-tee-eh-neh ee dehs-kahn-sah)*
Did anyone treat you prior to our arrival?	**¿Lo trató alguien antes de nuestra llegada?** *(Loh trah-toh ahl-gee-ehn ahn-tehs deh noo-ehs-trah yeh-gah-dah)*
Has this problem happened before?	**¿Le ha pasado antes este problema?** *(Leh ah pah-sah-doh ahn-tehs ehs-teh proh-bleh-mah)*

TABLE 2–1
Typical Questions

TABLA 2–1
Preguntas típicas

English	Spanish	Pronunciation
Do you have a doctor?	**¿Tiene un doctor?**	*Tee-eh-neh oon dohk-tohr?*
What hospital do you go to?	**¿A qué hospital va?**	*Ah keh ohs-pee-tahl bah?*
Do you take medicines?	**¿Toma medicinas?**	*Toh-mah meh-dee-see-nahs?*
What do you feel?	**¿Qué siente?**	*Keh see-ehn-teh?*
Do you have pain?	**¿Tiene dolor?**	*Tee-eh-neh doh-lohr?*
Are you nauseated?	**¿Está nauseado?**	*Ehs-tah nah-oo-seh-ah-doh?*
Do you have medical problems?	**¿Tiene problemas médicos?**	*Tee-eh-neh proh-bleh-mahs meh-dee-kohs?*
Has this happened to you before?	**¿Le ha pasado esto antes?**	*Leh ah pah-sah-doh ehs-toh ahn-tehs?*
What were you doing?	**¿Qué estaba haciendo?**	*Keh ehs-tah-bah ah-see-ehn-doh?*
What caused the accident?	**¿Qué causó el accidente?**	*Keh kah-oo-soh ehl ahk-see-dehn-teh?*

Has the pain gotten worse or gotten better?
¿Se ha puesto el dolor peor o mejor?
(Seh ah poo-ehs-toh ehl doh-lohr peh-ohr oh meh-hohr)

Did you take drugs or alcohol in the last 3 hours?
¿Tomó drogas o alcohol en las últimas tres horas?
(Toh-moh droh-gahs oh ahl-kohl ehn lahs ool-tee-mahs trehs oh-rahs)

How much medicine did you take?
¿Cuánta medicina tomó?
(Koo-ahn-tah meh-dee-see-nah toh-moh)

How old are you?
¿Cuántos años tiene?
(Koo-ahn-tohs ahn-yohs tee-eh-ney)

How often do you have the pain?
¿Qué tan seguido tiene el dolor?
(Keh tahn seh-gee-doh tee-eh-neh ehl doh-lohr)

How severe is the pain?
¿Qué tan severo es el dolor?
(Keh tahn seh-beh-roh ehs ehl doh-lohr)

On a scale from 1 [insignificant] to 10 [unbearable]:
En una escala del 1 [insignificante] al 10 [intolerable]:
(Ehn oo-nah ehs-kah-lah dehl oo-noh [een-seeg-nee-fee-kahn-teh] ahl dee-ehs [een-toh-leh-rah-bleh])

Is the pain there all the time, or does it come and go?
¿Está el dolor allí todo el tiempo, o va y viene?
(Ehs-tah ehl doh-lohr ah-yee toh-doh ehl tee-ehm-poh, oh bah ee bee-ehn-eh?)

Tell me, have you ever had a heart attack?
Dígame, ¿ha tenido alguna vez un ataque cardíaco?
(Dee-gah-meh, ah teh-nee-doh ahl-goo-nah behs oon ah-tah-keh kahr-dee-ah-koh)

What is bothering you the most?
¿Qué es lo que más le molesta?
(Keh ehs loh keh mahs leh moh-lehs-tah)

What caused the pain?
¿Qué causó el dolor?
(Keh kah-oo-soh ehl doh-lohr)

What did you do that caused the pain?
¿Qué hacía cuando apareció el dolor?
(Keh ah-see-ah koo-ahn-doh ah-pah-reh-see-oh ehl doh-lohr)

What makes the pain better?
¿Qué hace mejorar el dolor?
(Keh ah-seh meh-hoh-rahr ehl doh-lohr)

Get close to the patient if he is responsive and appears to be alert. It will help ease his fear. Ask questions clearly and at a normal rate. Do not say such things as, "Everything will be okay," or "Take it easy." The patient knows differently. He may have little confidence in you if you use such phrases.

Acérquese al paciente si responde y parece estar alerta. Esto ayuda a disminuir el miedo. Haga preguntas claras y de manera normal. No le diga cosas como "Todo estará bien" o "Tómelo con calma". El paciente sabe lo contrario y tendrá menos confianza en usted si usa frases semejantes.

Were you knocked down, did you fall, or were you thrown?

¿Se golpeó, se cayó o lo lanzó el impacto?
(Seh gohl-peh-oh, seh kah-yoh oh loh lahn-soh ehl eem-pahk-toh)

Did you hit the windshield/steering wheel?

¿Se pegó contra el parabrisas/volante?
(Seh peh-goh kohn-trah ehl pah-rah-bree-sahs/boh-lahn-teh)

TABLE 2–2 Typical Questions to Witnesses

TABLA 2–2 Preguntas típicas a testigos

English	Spanish	Pronunciation
Did you see how the accident happened?	**¿Vió cómo pasó el accidente?**	*Bee-oh koh-moh pah-soh ehl ahk-see-dehn-te?*
Are you related?	**¿Es pariente?**	*Ehs pah-ree-ehn-teh?*
Do you know him/her?	**¿Lo/la conoce?**	*Loh/lah koh-noh-seh?*
Who moved him/her?	**¿Quién lo/la movió?**	*Kee-ehn loh/lah moh-bee-oh?*
Was the car burning?	**¿Estaba el carro en llamas?**	*Ehs-tah-bah ehl kah-roh ehn yah-mahs?*
Was he/she conscious?	**¿Estaba conciente?***	*Ehs-tah-bah kohn-see-ehn-teh?*
How did he/she fall?	**¿Cómo se cayó?***	*Koh-moh seh kah-yoh?*
From what height did he/she fall?	**¿De qué altura cayó?***	*Deh keh ahl-too-rah kah-yoh?*

*Note that there is no need to repeat the article for the person (he/she) in Spanish. It is understood.

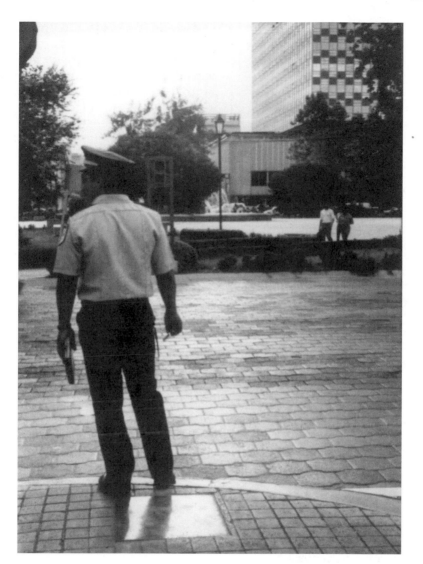

Figure 2–2 Look for bystanders or witnesses who may be able to provide important information.

Has this happened before?	**¿Pasó esto antes?** *(Pah-soh ehs-toh ahn-tehs)*
How did this injury happen?	**¿Cómo ocurrió esta lesión?** *(Koh-moh oh-koo-ree-oh ehs-tah leh-see-ohn)*

Were you thrown forward/backward?	**¿Fué lanzado hacia adelante/hacia atrás?** *(Foo-eh lahn-sah-doh ah-see-ah ah-dehl-ahn-teh/ah-see-ah ah-trahs)*
How old are you?	**¿Cuántos años tiene?** *(Koo-ahn-tohs ah-nyohs tee-eh-neh)*
I have to call your parents.	**Tengo que llamar a sus padres.** *(Tehn-goh keh yah-mahr ah soos pah-drehs)*
Is there numbness/a tingling sensation/burning in your leg/arm/foot/hand?	**¿Está entumecido/adormecido/tiene ardor en su pierna/brazo/pie/mano?** *(Ehs-tah ehn-too-meh-see-doh/ah-dohr-meh-see-do/tee-eh-neh ahr-dohr ehn soo pee-ehr-nah/brah-soh/pee-eh/mah-noh)*
Were you thrown from the car?	**¿Fué lanzado fuera del carro?** *(Foo-eh lahn-sah-doh foo-eh-rah dehl kah-roh)*
What is wrong?	**¿Qué pasa?** *(Keh pah-sah)*
Is there any pain?	**¿Tiene algún dolor?** *(Tee-eh-neh ahl-goon doh-lohr)*
What problems do you have?	**¿Qué problema tiene?** *(Keh proh-bleh-mah tee-eh-neh)*
Where can I reach your mother or father?	**¿Dónde puedo localizar a su mamá o su papá?** *(Dohn-deh poo-eh-doh loh-kah-lee-sahr ah soo mah-mah oh soo pah-pah)*

As part of the assessment, EMTs must frequently give commands to the patients.

Como parte de la evaluación, los Técnicos de Emergencia dan órdenes a los pacientes.

The following are typical commands.

Las siguientes son órdenes comunes.

Breathe in.	**Respire.** *(Rehs-pee-reh)*
Breathe out.	**Saque el aire.** *(Sah-keh ehl ah-ee-reh)*
Hold your breath.	**Sostenga la respiración.** *(Sohs-tehn-gah la rehs-pee-rah-see-ohn)*

Open your mouth.	**Abra la boca.** *(Ah-brah lah boh-kah)*
Open your eyes.	**Abra los ojos.** *(Ah-brah lohs oh-hohs)*
Follow my finger.	**Siga mi dedo.** *(See-gah mee deh-doh)*
Don't move.	**No se mueva.** *(Noh seh moo-eh-bah)*
Push down with your feet against my hands.	**Empuje los pies contra mis manos.** *(Ehm-poo-heh lohs pee-ehs kohn-trah mees mah-nohs)*
Relax your leg.	**Relaje la pierna.** *(Reh-lah-heh lah pee-ehr-nah)*
Relax your arm.	**Relaje el brazo.** *(Reh-lah-heh ehl brah-soh)*
Squeeze my hand.	**Apriete mi mano.** *(Ah-pree-eh-teh mee mah-noh)*
Squeeze the fingers of each of my hands.	**Apriete los dedos de cada una de mis manos.** *(Ah-pree-eh-teh lohs deh-dohs deh kah-dah oo-nah deh mees mah-nohs)*
Stick your tongue out.	**Saque la lengua.** *(Sah-keh lah lehn-goo-ah)*
Tell me if this hurts.	**Dígame si esto le duele.** *(Dee-gah-meh see ehs-toh leh doo-eh-leh)*

TABLE 2–3
Typical Commands

TABLA 2–3
Mandatos típicos

English	Spanish	Pronunciation
Do not move!	¡No se mueva!	*Noh seh moo-eh-bah*
Keep moving!	¡Siga moviéndose!	*See-gah moh-bee-ehn-doh-seh!*
Listen!	¡Escuche!	*Ehs-koo-cheh!*
	¡Oiga!	*Oh-ee-gah!*
Move carefully!	¡Muévase con cuidado!	*Moo-eh-bah-seh kohn koo-ee-dah-doh*
Open your mouth!	¡Abra la boca!	*Ah-brah lah boh-kah*
Open your eyes!	¡Abra los ojos!	*Ah-brah lohs oh-hohs*
Push!	¡Empuje!	*Ehm-poo-heh!*
Squeeze my hand!	¡Apriete mi mano!	*Ah-pree-eh-teh mee mah-noh*

Patients have a variety of responses when questions are asked about their condition or accident.

Los pacientes dan una variedad de respuestas cuando se les pregunta acerca de su condición o su accidente.

The following are some examples of responses.

Los siguientes son unos ejemplos de respuestas.

I was just sitting, watching television when the pain started.	**Sólo estaba sentado, viendo televisión cuando comenzó el dolor.** *(Soh-loh ehs-tah-bah sehn-tah-doh, bee-ehn-doh teh-leh-bee-see-ohn koo-ahn-doh koh-mehn-soh ehl doh-lohr)*
I was doing nothing.	**No estaba haciendo nada.** *(Noh ehs-tah-bah ah-see-ehn-doh nah-dah)*
Nothing seems to make it better or worse.	**Nada parece hacerlo peor o mejor.** *(Nah-dah pah-reh-seh ah-sehr-loh peh-ohr oh meh-hohr)*
The pain is sharp.	**El dolor es agudo.** *(Ehl doh-lohr ehs ah-goo-doh*
The pain starts here [beneath the sternum] and goes to my jaw.	**El dolor comienza aquí [abajo del esternón] y se va a la mandíbula.** *(Ehl doh-lohr koh-mee-ehn-sah ah-kee [ah-bah-joh dehl ehs-tehr-nohn] ee seh bah ah lah mahn-dee-boo-lah)*
The pain is constant.	**El dolor es constante.** *(Ehl doh-lohr ehs kohns-tahn-teh)*
The pain has gotten worse.	**El dolor ha empeorado.** *(Ehl doh-lohr ah ehm-peh-ohr-ah-doh)*
The pain starts here and travels down my left arm.	**El dolor comienza aquí y se recorre por el brazo izquierdo.** *(Ehl doh-lohr koh-mee-ehn-sah ah-kee ee seh reh-koh-reh pohr ehl brah-soh ees-kee-ehr-doh)*
The pain is cutting.	**El dolor es cortante.** *(Ehl doh-lohr ehs kohr-tahn-teh)*
The pain started two hours ago.	**El dolor comenzó hace dos horas.** *(Ehl doh-lohr koh-mehn-soh ah-seh dohs oh-rahs)*
The pain is throbbing.	**El dolor es punzante.** *(Ehl doh-lohr ehs poon-sahn-teh)*

Dialogue between a paramedic and a patient.
Diálogo entre un paramédico y un paciente.

Paramedic:	**Paramédico:** *(Pahr-ah-meh-dee-koh)*
Hello, I'm John Goodguy.	**Hola, soy John Goodguy.** *(Oh-lah, soh-ee John Goodguy)*
I'm a paramedic.	**Soy paramédico.** *(Soh-ee pahr-ah-meh-dee-koh)*
What happened here?	**¿Qué pasó aquí?** *(Keh pah-soh ah-kee)*
Patient:	**Paciente:** *(Pah-see-ehn-teh)*
The kids left their skates on the stairs and I fell over them.	**Los niños dejaron los patines en las escaleras y me tropecé.** *(Lohs nee-nyohs deh-hah-rohn lohs pah-tee-nehs ehn lahs ehs-kah-leh-rahs ee meh troh-peh-seh)*
Paramedic:	**Paramédico:** *(Pahr-ah-meh-dee-koh)*
I guess this wasn't a planned activity for today!	**¡Supongo que esta actividad no estaba planeada para hoy!** *(Soo-pohn-goh keh ehs-tah ahk-tee-bee-dahd noh ehs-tah-bah plah-neh-ah-dah pah-rah oh-ee)*
Patient:	**Paciente:** *(Pah-see-ehn-teh)*
That is for sure!	**¡Délo por seguro!** *(Deh-loh pohr seh-goo-roh)*
Paramedic:	**Paramédico:** *(Pahr-ah-meh-dee-koh)*
Tell me your name.	**Dígame su nombre.** *(Dee-gah-meh soo nohm-breh)*
How old are you?	**¿Cuántos años tiene?** *(Koo-ahn-tohs ah-nyohs tee-eh-neh)*
Patient:	**Paciente:** *(Pah-see-ehn-teh)*
My name is Mr. Badluck.	**Mi nombre es señor Badluck.** *(Mee nohm-breh ehs seh-nyohr Bad-luck)*
I'm 53.	**Tengo cincuenta y tres años.** *(Tehn-goh seen-koo-ehn-tah ee trehs ah-nyos)*
Paramedic:	**Paramédico:** *(Pahr-ah-meh-dee-koh)*
Tell me where it hurts, Mr. Badluck.	**Dígame dónde le duele, señor Bad-luck.** *(Dee-gah-meh dohn-deh leh doo-eh-leh, seh-nyohr Badluck)*

Patient:	**Paciente:** *(Pah-see-ehn-teh)*
My left leg hurts.	**Me duele la pierna izquierda.** *(Meh doo-eh-leh lah pee-ehr-nah ees-kee-ehr-dah)*
I think it is broken.	**Creo que está rota.** *(Kreh-oh keh ehs-tah roh-tah)*
Paramedic:	**Paramédico:** *(Pahr-ah-meh-dee-koh)*
Well, it is possible.	**Pues, es posible.** *(Poo-ehs ehs poh-see-bleh)*
What is the pain like?	**¿Qué tipo de dolor tiene?** *(Keh tee-poh deh doh-lohr tee-eh-neh)*
Patient:	**Paciente:** *(Pah-see-ehn-teh)*
Right now it is throbbing like a bad toothache.	**Ahora está punzando, como un mal dolor de muelas.** *(Ah-oh-rah ehs-tah poon-sahn-doh, koh-moh oon mahl doh-lohr deh moo-eh-lahs)*
Paramedic:	**Paramédico:** *(Pahr-ah-meh-dee-koh)*
How bad is it?	**¿Qué tan mal está?** *(Keh tahn mahl ehs-tah)*
Patient:	**Paciente:** *(Pah-see-ehn-teh)*
It is not as bad when I stay still, but it hurts a lot if I try to move the leg.	**No está tan mal cuando estoy quieto, pero me duele mucho si trato de mover la pierna.** *(Noh ehs-tah tahn mahl koo-ahn-doh ehs-toh-ee kee-eh-toh, peh-roh meh doo-eh-leh moo-choh see trah-toh deh moh-behr lah pee-ehr-nah)*
Paramedic:	**Paramédico:** *(Pahr-ah-meh-dee-koh)*
Is there anything else bothering you?	**Hay otra cosa que le moleste?** *(Ah-ee oh-trah koh-sah keh leh moh-lehs-teh)*
Patient:	**Paciente:** *(Pah-see-ehn-teh)*
No, not that I know of.	**No, que yo sepa.** *(Noh, keh yoh seh-pah)*
Well, I do have a tingling feeling in my left foot. It must have gone to sleep.	**Pues, tengo picazón en el pie izquierdo. Se me durmió.** *(Poo-ehs, tehn-goh pee-kah-sohn ehn ehl pee-eh ees-kee-ehr-doh. Seh meh duhr-mee-oh)*
Paramedic:	**Paramédico:** *(Pahr-ah-meh-dee-koh)*
I see.	**Ya veo.** *(Yah beh-oh)*

Patient:
Also, I have a headache.

Paciente: *(Pah-see-ehn-teh)*
También, tengo dolor de cabeza.
(Tahm-bee-ehn, tehn-goh doh-lohr deh kah-beh-sah)

I never have headaches!

¡Nunca tengo dolor de cabeza!
(Noon-kah tehn-goh doh-lohr deh kah-beh-sah)

Paramedic:
Are you under a doctor's care, Mr. Badluck?

Paramédico: *(Pahr-ah-meh-dee-koh)*
¿Está bajo el cuidado de un doctor, señor Badluck?
(Ehs-tah bah-hoh ehl koo-ee-dah-doh deh oon dohk-tohr, seh-nyohr Badluck)

Patient:
Yes, Dr. Fellow at Juan Sealy General. He keeps track of my cholesterol.

Paciente: *(Pah-see-ehn-teh)*
Sí, el doctor Fellow en Juan Sealy General. Él me controla el colesterol.
(See. Ehl dohk-tohr Fellow ehn Juan Sealy General. Ehl meh kohn-troh-lah ehl koh-lehs-teh-rohl)

Paramedic:
Besides your cholesterol, are there any other medical problems?

Paramédico: *(Pahr-ah-meh-dee-koh)*
Además de su colesterol, ¿tiene otros problemas médicos? *(Ah-deh-mahs deh soo koh-lehs-teh-rohl, tee-eh-neh oh-throhs proh-bleh-mahs meh-dee-kohs)*

Patient:
None.

Paciente: *(Pah-see-ehn-teh)*
Ninguno.
(Neen-goo-noh)

Paramedic:
Do you take any medication?

Paramédico: *(Pahr-ah-meh-dee-koh)*
¿Toma alguna medicina?
(Toh-mah ahl-goo-nah meh-dee-see-nah?

Patient:
Lescol for the cholesterol and naproxin for my aches.

Paciente: *(Pah-see-ehn-teh)*
Lescol para el colesterol y naproxeno para mis dolores.
(Lehs-kohl pah-rah ehl koh-lehs-teh-rohl ee nah-prohx-eh-noh pah-rah mees doh-loh-rehs)

Paramedic:
Are you allergic to anything?

Paramédico: *(Pahr-ah-meh-dee-koh)*
¿Es alérgico a alguna cosa?
(Ehs ah-lehr-hee-koh ah ahl-goo-nah koh-sah)

Patient:
Nothing that I have ever known of.

Paciente: *(Pah-see-ehn-teh)*
A nada que yo sepa.
(Ah nah-dah keh yoh seh-pah)

Paramedic:
OK, Mr. Badluck, my partner and I are going to put the leg in a splint to keep it from moving around on the way to the hospital.

Paramédico: *(Pahr-ah-meh-dee-koh)*
OK, señor Badluck, mi compañero y yo vamos a entablillar la pierna para no moverla mucho en el viaje al hospital.
(OK, seh-nyohr Badluck, mee kohm-pah nyeh-roh ee yoh bah-mohs ah ehn-tah-blee-yahr lah pee-ehr-nah pah-rah noh moh-behr-lah moo-choh ehn ehl bee-ah-heh ahl ohs-pee-tahl)

Chapter Three

Capítulo tres

Emergency Care

Cuidado de urgencia (emergencia)

Emergency rooms are frequently very busy. There is a tendency to rush through procedures. When possible, take a few extra minutes to attempt to communicate so your diagnosis is accurate. This saves time in the long run.

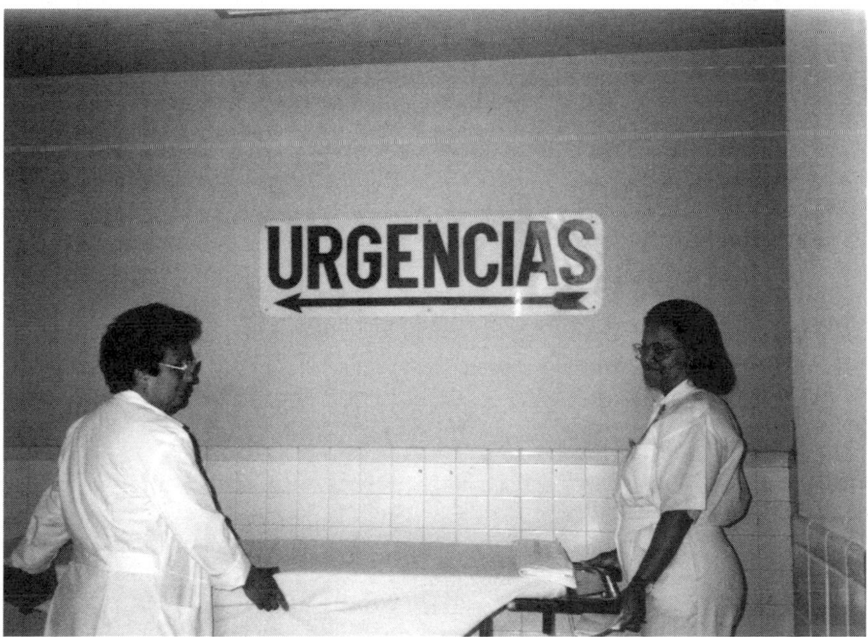

Figure 3–1 Emergency rooms are often busy places. Signs become very important.

Los cuartos de urgencia (emergencia) frecuentemente están ocupados. Hay una tendencia a apurarse en los procedimientos. Cuando le sea posible, tome unos minutos adicionales para intentar la comunicación para que su diagnóstico sea exacto. Esto ahorra tiempo a la larga.

While taking the vital signs, the triage nurse observes the patient's breathing. She checks the carotid and peripheral pulses. She next checks for uncontrolled bleeding and shock. Finding no immediate problems, she begins a systematic assessment.

Mientras toma los signos vitales, la enfermera del área del triage observa la respiración del paciente. Ella revisa los pulsos de la carótida y los periféricos. Después verifica si hay sangrados y choque. Al no encontrar problemas inmediatos, inicia una evaluación sistemática.

May I help you?	**¿Puedo ayudarlo?** *(Poo-eh-doh ah-yoo-dahr-loh?*
—I have been sick all morning.	**—Me he sentido mal toda la mañana.** *(Meh eh sehn-tee-doh mahl toh-dah lah mah-nyah-nah)*
Are you having problems breathing?	**¿Tiene problemas al respirar?** *(Tee-eh-neh proh-bleh-mahs ahl rehs-pee-rahr)*
—I have noticed some difficulty for the last two days.	**—Me he dado cuenta de alguna dificultad para respirar en los últimos dos días.** *(Meh eh dah-doh koo-ehn-tah deh ahl-goo-nah dee-fee-kuhl-tahd pah-rah rehs-pee-rahr ehn lohs ool-tee-mohs dohs dee-ahs)*
Have you had any hard blows to your head or chest?	**¿Se ha golpeado fuerte la cabeza o el tórax?** *(Seh ah gohl-peh-ah-doh foo-ehr-teh lah kah-beh-zah oh ehl toh-rahx)*
—No.	**—No.** *(Noh)*
Have you had any bleeding, swelling, or bruising?	**¿Ha tenido sangrados, hinchazón o moretones?** *(Ah teh-nee-doh sahn-grah-dohs, een-chah-sohn oh moh-reh-toh-nehs)*
—No, I have not noticed any.	**—No, no me he dado cuenta de ninguna cosa.** *(Noh, noh meh eh dah-doh koo-ehn-tah deh neen-goo-nah koh-sah)*

Your skin color looks good.	**El color de su piel es normal.** *(Ehl koh-lohr deh soo pee-ehl ehs nohr-mahl)*
Fever?	**¿Fiebre?** *(Fee-eh-breh)*
—About 99 degrees today.	**—Cerca de noventa y nueve grados hoy.** *(Sehr-kah deh noh-behn-tah ee noo-eh-beh grah-dohs oh-ee)*
—I feel dizzy.	**—Me siento mareado.** *(Meh see-ehn-toh mah-reh-ah-doh)*
Have you had neck pain?	**¿Ha tenido dolor en el cuello?** *(Ah teh-nee-doh doh-lohr ehn ehl koo-eh-yoh)*
—Once in a while.	**—De vez en cuando.** *(Deh behs ehn koo-ahn-doh)*
Stay sitting here.	**Quédese sentado aquí.** *(Keh-deh-seh sehn-tah-doh ah-kee)*
I am going to get a wheelchair.	**Voy a traer una silla de ruedas.** *(Boy ah trah-ehr oo-nah see-yah deh roo-eh-dahs)*

TABLE 3–1
Pronunciation of Selected Words

TABLA 3–1
Pronunciación de palabras selectas

English	Spanish	Pronunciation
airway	**vía aérea**	*(bee-ah ah-eh-reh-ah)*
anaphylactic shock	**choque anafilático**	*(choh-keh ah-nah-fee-lah-tee-koh)*
arrest	**arresto**	*(ah-rehs-toh)*
cardiopulmonary	**cardiopulmonar**	*(kahr-dee-oh-pool-moh-nahr)*
choking	**ahogar**	*(ah-oh-gahr)*
dizzy	**mareado**	*(mah-reh-ah-doh)*
hyperthermia	**hipertermia**	*(ee-pehr-tehr-mee-ah)*
obstruction	**obstrucción**	*(ohb-strook-see-ohn)*
respiratory arrest	**paro respiratorio**	*(pah-roh rehs-pee-rah-toh-ree-oh)*
swelling	**hinchazón**	*(een-chah-sohn)*
swollen	**hinchado**	*(een-chah-doh)*
temperature	**temperatura**	*(tehm-peh-rah-too-rah)*
traumatic	**traumático**	*(trah-oo-mah-tee-koh)*

Mrs. Vargas, a pregnant 30-year-old woman, was involved in a car accident. She just arrived at the emergency room.

La señora Vargas, una mujer embarazada que tiene 30 años de edad, estuvo en un accidente automovilístico. Acaba de llegar al cuarto de urgencias (emergencias).

Hello, Mrs. Vargas.	**Hola, señora Vargas.** *(Oh-lah, seh-nyoh-rah Bahr-gahs)*
I am going to ask you questions.	**Voy a hacerle preguntas.** *(Boy ah ah-sehr-leh preh-goon-tahs)*
What is your name?	**¿Cómo se llama?** *(Koh-moh seh yah-mah)*
What is your last name?	**¿Cuál es su apellido?** *(Koo-ahl ehs soo ah-peh-yee-doh)*
Answer "yes" or "no".	**Conteste "sí" o "no".** *(Kohn-tehs-teh "see" oh "noh")*
Did you lose consciousness?	**¿Perdió el conocimiento?/¿Se desmayó?** *(Pehr-dee-oh ehl koh-noh-see-mee-ehn-toh/Seh dehs-mah-yoh)*

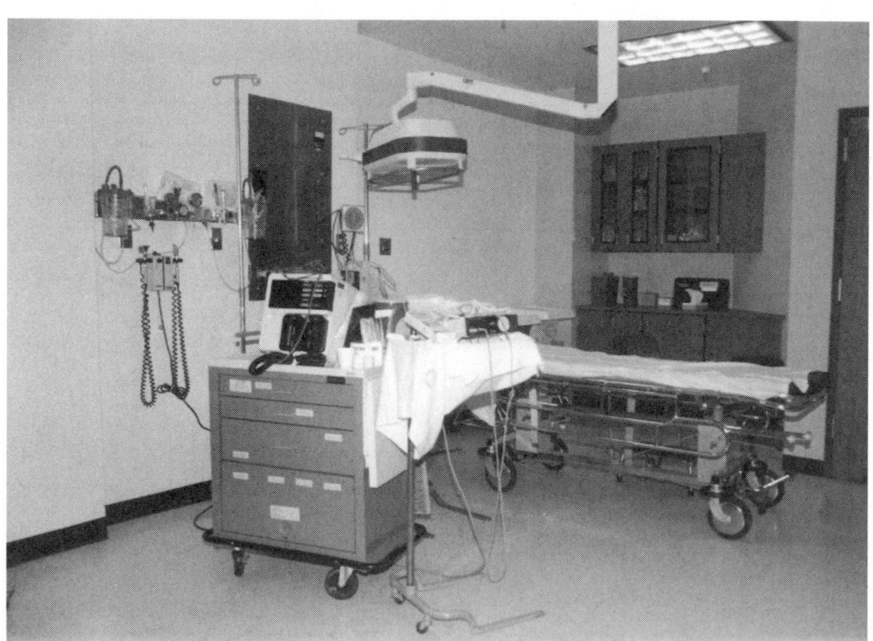

Figure 3–2 Emergency rooms are often impersonal and may frighten the patient. Ensure privacy and accept reactions to fear and pain.

Do you know where you are?	**¿Sabe dónde está?** *(Sah-beh dohn-deh ehs-tah)*
Do you know the day of the week?	**¿Sabe el día de la semana?** *(Sah-beh ehl dee-ah deh lah seh-mah-nah)*
Are you nauseated?	**¿Tiene náuseas?** *(Tee-eh-neh nah-oo-seh-ahs)*
Are you bleeding?	**¿Está sangrando?** *(Ehs-tah sahn-grahn-doh)*
How many months pregnant?	**¿Cuántos meses tiene de embarazo?** *(Koo-ahn-tohs meh-sehs tee-eh-neh deh ehm-bah-rah-soh)*
When was your last normal period?	**¿Cuándo tuvo su última menstruación normal?** *(Koo-ahn-doh too-boh soo ool-tee-mah mehns-troo-ah-see-ohn nohr-mahl)*
Is your water bag broken?	**¿Se reventó su bolsa de agua?** *(Seh reh-behn-toh soo bohl-sah deh ah-goo-ah)*
When?	**¿Cuándo?** *(Koo-ahn-doh)*
Did you feel warm water run out of your vagina?	**¿Sintió que salió agua tibia de su vagina?** *(Seen-tee-oh keh sah-lee-oh ah-goo-ah tee-bee-ah deh soo bah-hee-nah)*

In an emergency situation, the objective is to obtain as much information as correctly as possible. Get to the point!

En una situación urgente, el objetivo es obtener información lo más correcta posible. ¡Sea breve!

Have you eaten?	**¿Ha comido?** *(Ah koh-mee-doh)*
At what time?	**¿A qué hora?** *(Ah keh oh-rah)*
What did you eat?	**¿Qué comió?** *(Keh koh-mee-oh)*
Mrs. Vargas, I need to help you change clothes.	**Señora Vargas, necesito ayudarle a cambiarse la ropa.** *(Seh-nyoh-rah Bahr-gahs, neh-seh-see-toh ah-yoo-dahr-leh ah kahm-bee-ahr-say lah roh-pah)*
I have a gown.	**Tengo una bata.** *(Tehn-goh oo-nah bah-tah)*
I am going to examine you.	**Voy a examinarla.** *(Boy ah ehx-ah-mee-nahr-lah)*

Some words are difficult to pronounce because they are too long. Don't hurry, make a pause. Table 3–2.

Algunas palabras son difíciles de pronunciar porque son muy largas. Tome su tiempo, haga una pausa. Tabla 3–2.

How far apart are your contractions?	**¿Cada cuánto tiempo tiene las contracciones?** *(Kah-dah koo-ahn-toh tee-ehm-poh tee-eh-neh lahs kohn-trahk-see-ohn-ehs)*
Tell me when you feel a contraction!	**¡Dígame cuando sienta una contracción!** *(Dee-gah-meh koo-ahn-doh see-ehn-tah oo-nah kohn-trahk-see-ohn)*
We need to count them.	**Tenemos que contarlas.** *(Teh-neh-mohs keh kohn-tahr-lahs)*
Are you cold?	**¿Tiene frío?** *(Tee-eh-neh free-oh)*
Are you hot?	**¿Tiene calor?** *(Tee-eh-neh kah-lohr)*
Where were you hit?	**¿Dónde se golpeó?** *(Dohn-deh seh gohl-peh-oh)*
Point!	**¡Apunte!/¡Señale!** *(Ah-poon-teh/Seh-nyah-leh)*
Do you have pain?	**¿Tiene dolor?** *(Tee-eh-neh doh-lohr)*
Where?	**¿Dónde?** *(Dohn-deh)*

TABLE 3–2
Pronunciation of Selected Words

TABLA 3–2
Pronunciación de palabras selectas

English	**Spanish**	**Pronunciation**
ambulance	**ambulancia**	*(ahm-boo-lahn-see-ah)*
bleeding	**sangrando**	*(sahn-grahn-doh)*
consciousness	**conocimiento**	*(koh-noh-see-mee-ehn-toh)*
contractions	**contracciones**	*(kohn-trahk-see-ohn-ehs)*
examine her, you (*f.*)	**examinarla**	*(ehx-ah-mee-nahr-lah)*
examine him, you (*m.*)	**examinarlo**	*(ehx-ah-mee-nahr-loh)*
pregnant	**embarazada**	*(ehm-bah-rah-sah-dah)*
receptionist	**recepcionista**	*(reh-sehp-see-ohn-ees-tah)*
temperature	**temperatura**	*(tehm-peh-rah-too-rah)*

Pain at the waist?	**¿Dolor en la cintura?** *(Doh-lohr ehn lah seen-too-rah)*
Back pain?	**¿Dolor de espalda?** *(Doh-lohr deh ehs-pahl-dah)*
Is the pain sharp?	**¿El dolor es agudo?** *(Ehl doh-lohr ehs ah-goo-doh)*
Is the pain in one place?	**¿El dolor es fijo?** *(Ehl doh-lohr ehs fee-hoh)*
Does it come and go?	**¿Va y viene?** *(Bah eeh bee-eh-neh)*
Are you feeling a contaction?	**¿Está sintiendo una contracción?** *(Ehs-tah seen-tee-ehn-doh oo-nah kohn-trahk-see-ohn)*
Tell me when!	**¡Dígame cuándo!** *(Dee-gah-meh koo-ahn-doh)*
I am going to listen to the baby's heartbeat.	**Voy a escuchar el latido de corazón del bebé.** *(Boy ah ehs-koo-chahr ehl lah-tee-doh deh koh-rah-sohn dehl beh-beh)*
Please breathe normally.	**Por favor, respire normal.** *(Pohr fah-bohr, rehs-pee-reh nohr-mahl)*
It sounds good.	**Se oye bien.** *(Seh oh-yeh bee-ehn)*
Do you have allergies?	**¿Tiene alergias?** *(Tee-eh-neh ah-lehr-hee-ahs)*
To foods/dust/medicines?	**¿A comidas/polvo/medicinas?** *(Ah koh-mee-dahs/pohl-boh/meh-dee-see-nahs)*
How old are you?	**¿Cuántos años tiene?** *(Koo-ahn-tohs ah-nyohs tee-eh-neh)*
How many pregnancies have you had?	**¿Cuántos embarazos ha tenido?** *(Koo-ahn-tohs ehm-bah-rah-sohs ah teh-nee-doh)*
How many children do you have?	**¿Cuántos niños tiene?** *(Koo-ahn-tohs nee-nyohs tee-eh-neh)*
Have you had an abortion?	**¿Ha tenido abortos?** *(Ah teh-nee-doh ah-bohr-tohs)*
How many?	**¿Cuántos?** *(Koo-ahn-tohs)*
When was the last one?	**¿Cuándo fue el último?** *(Koo-ahn-doh foo-eh ehl ool-tee-moh)*
Did you have a miscarriage?	**¿Tuvo un niño nacido muerto?** *(Too-boh oon nee-nyoh nah-see-doh moo-ehr-toh)*

Did you have an ectopic (tubal) pregnancy?	**¿Tuvo un embarazo fuera de la matriz o en las trompas?** *(Too-boh oon ehm-bah-rah-soh foo-eh-rah deh lah mah-trees oh ehn lahs trohm-pahs)*
Are you working also?	**¿Trabaja también?** *(Trah-bah-hah tahm-bee-ehn)*
Are you a housewife?	**¿Es ama de casa?** *(Ehs ah-mah deh kah-sah)*
What kind of work do you do?	**¿Qué clase de trabajo hace?** *(Keh klah-seh deh trah-bah-hoh ah- seh)*
How many pounds have you gained?	**¿Cuántas libras ha aumentado?** *(Koo-ahn-tahs lee-brahs ah ah-oo-mehn-tah-doh)*
Do you smoke?	**¿Fuma usted?** *(Foo-mah oos-tehd)*
Do you drink alcohol?	**¿Toma bebidas alcohólicas?** *(Toh-mah beh-bee-dahs ahl-koh-lee-kahs)*
Do you drink coffee?	**¿Toma café?** *(Toh-mah kah-feh)*
Do you take any medicines?	**¿Toma algunas medicinas?** *(Toh-mah ahl-goo-nahs meh-dee-see-nahs)*
What medicines do you take?	**¿Qué medicinas toma?** *(Keh meh-dee-see-nahs toh-mah)*
For what reason?	**¿Cuál es la razón?** *(Koo-ahl ehs lah rah-sohn)*
Do you take any narcotics?	**¿Toma narcóticos?** *(Toh-mah nahr-koh-tee-kohs)*
Do you take drugs from habit?	**¿Tiene vicio de tomar drogas?** *(Tee-eh-neh bee-see-oh deh toh-mahr droh-gahs)*
Are you married/single?	**¿Está casada o es soltera?** *(Ehs-tah kah-sah-dah oh ehs sohl-teh-rah)*
Do you live with your husband?	**¿Vive con su esposo?** *(Bee-beh kohn soo ehs-poh-soh)*
Where is your husband?	**¿Dónde está su esposo?** *(Dohn-deh ehs-tah soo ehs-poh-soh)*
Do you have relatives/friends?	**¿Tiene parientes/amigos?** *(Tee-eh-neh pah-ree-ehn-tehs/ah-mee-gohs)*
Thank you!	**¡Gracias!** *(Grah-see-ahs)*

TABLE 3–3
Pronunciation of Selected Words

TABLA 3–3
Pronunciación de palabras selectas

English	Spanish	Pronunciation
blood	**sangre**	*(sahn-greh)*
how many	**cuántos**	*(koo-ahn-tohs)*
last name	**apellido**	*(ah-peh-yee-doh)*
nausea	**náusea**	*(nah-oo-seh-ah)*
question	**pregunta**	*(preh-goon-tah)*
thank you	**gracias**	*(grah-see-ahs)*
week	**semana**	*(seh-mah-nah)*
where	**dónde**	*(dohn-deh)*
you know	**sabe**	*(sah-beh)*
you need	**necesita**	*(neh-seh-see-tah)*

Table 3–3 will help you with pronunciation of selected words.
La Tabla 3–3 le ayudará con la pronunciación de palabras selectas.
The nurse approaches Mrs. Vargas.
La enfermera se acerca a la señora Vargas.

Hello, Mrs. Vargas. I need to take your temperature and blood pressure.
Hola, señora Vargas. Necesito tomarle la temperatura y la presión.
(Oh-lah, seh-nyoh-rah Bahr-gahs. Neh-seh-see-toh toh-mahr-leh lah tehm-peh-rah-too-rah ee lah preh-see-ohn)

I also need a urine sample.
También necesito una muestra de orina.
(Tahm-bee-ehn neh-seh-see-toh oo-nah moo-ehs-trah deh oh-ree-nah)

Don't get up!
¡No se levante!
(Noh seh leh-bahn-teh)

Supportive measures include ensuring privacy and accepting various reactions to fear and pain. Explain all procedures, even when you think the patient does not understand the language. Try to demonstrate the procedure you are about to perform and what you expect. Commonly used commands are found in Table 3–4.

Las medidas que dan apoyo incluyen el asegurar un área privada y aceptar varias reacciones al miedo y al dolor. Explique todos los proce-

dimientos, aún cuando usted piense que el paciente no entienda el lenguaje. Trate de demostrar el procedimiento que va a hacer y lo que se espera del paciente. Los mandatos que se usan comúnmente están en la Tabla 3–4.

I have the bedpan.	**Tengo el bacín/pato.** *(Tehn-goh ehl bah-seen/pah-toh)*
Bend your knees!	**¡Doble las piernas!** *(Doh-bleh lahs pee-ehr-nahs)*
Pull up your hips!	**¡Levante la cadera!** *(Leh-bahn-teh lah kah-deh-rah)*
Do you have pain?	**¿Tiene dolor?** *(Tee-eh-neh doh-lohr)*
Where?	**¿Dónde?** *(Dohn-deh)*
Here is the toilet paper.	**Aquí está el papel de baño/higiénico.** *(Ah-kee ehs-tah ehl pah-pehl deh bah-nyoh/ee-hee-eh-nee-koh)*
Lower your legs.	**Baje las piernas.** *(Bah-heh lahs pee-ehr-nahs)*

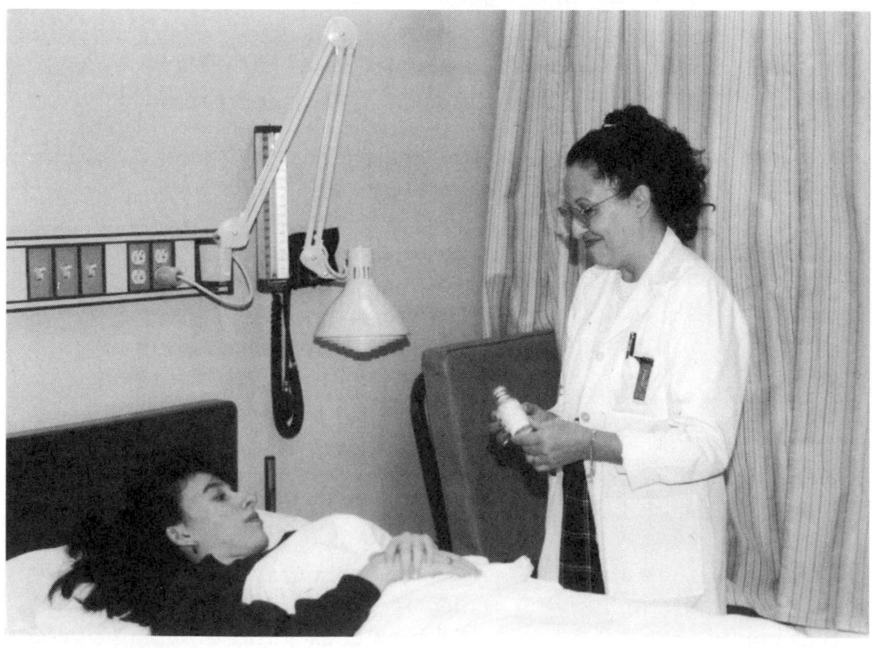

Figure 3–3 The nurse explains the directions on the bottle to the patient and asks a variety of questions.

TABLE 3–4
Common Commands

TABLA 3–4
Mandatos comunes

English	Spanish	Pronunciation
Bend!	**¡Doble!**	*(Doh-bleh)*
Call!	**¡Llame!**	*(Yah-meh)*
Choose!	**¡Escoja!**	*(Ehs-koh-hah)*
Get!	**¡Consiga!**	*(Kohn-see-gah)*
Get out!	**¡Fuera!**	*(Foo-eh-rah)*
Get up!	**¡Levántese!**	*(Leh-bahn-teh-seh)*
Lower!	**¡Baje!**	*(Bah-heh)*
Pull!	**¡Jale!**	*(Hah-leh)*
Tell me!	**¡Dígame!**	*(Dee-gah-meh)*
Wake up!	**¡Despierte!**	*(Dehs-pee-ehr-teh)*

Rest.
Descanse.
(Des-kahn-seh)

Later on, they will take X-rays.
Más tarde, le van a tomar rayos X.
(Mahs tahr-deh leh bahn ah toh-mahr rah-yohs eh-kiss)

Then they will take blood samples.
Luego le van a tomar muestras de sangre.
(Loo-eh-goh leh bahn ah toh-mahr moo-ehs-trahs deh sahn-greh)

Here is the bell.
Aquí está la campana.
(Ah-kee ehs-tah lah kahm-pah-nah)

Call if you need help.
Llame si necesita ayuda.
(Yah-meh see neh-seh-see-tah ah-yoo-dah)

In the waiting area, Mr. Vargas speaks to the receptionist.
En la sala de espera, el señor Vargas habla con la recepcionista.
See Table 3–5 for pronunciation of selected words.
Vea la Tabla 3–5 para la pronunciación de palabras selectas.

I am going to ask you some questions.
Voy a hacerle unas preguntas.
(Boy ah ah-sehr-leh oo-nahs preh-goon-tahs)

What is your address?
¿Cuál es su dirección?
(Koo-ahl ehs soo dee-rehk-see-ohn)

The name of the street . . .
El nombre de la calle...
(Ehl nohm-breh deh lah kah-yeh)

Telephone number?
¿Número de teléfono?
(Noo-meh-roh deh teh-leh-foh-noh)

TABLE 3–5 Pronunciation of Selected Words | **TABLA 3–5 Pronunciación de palabras selectas**

English	Spanish	Pronunciation
address	**dirección**	*(dee-rehk-see-ohn)*
health	**salud**	*(sah-lood)*
here	**aquí**	*(ah-kee)*
insurance	**seguro**	*(seh-goo-roh)*
number	**número**	*(noo-meh-roh)*
work	**trabajo**	*(trah-bah-hoh)*
you sign	**firme**	*(feer-meh)*

Number of: **Número de:**
(Noo-meh-roh deh)

Health insurance? **¿Seguro de salud?**
Seh-goo-roh deh sah-lood)

Medicaid? **¿Medicaid?**
(Meh-dee-kehd)

Social Security? **¿Seguro Social?**
(Seh-goo-roh Soh-see-ahl)

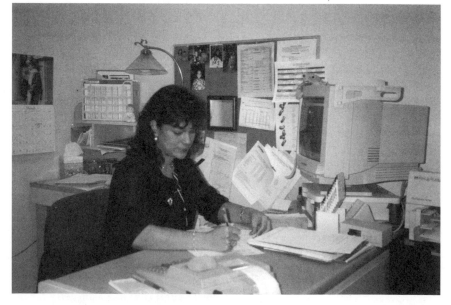

Figure 3–4 Patient information is carefully documented.

Where do you work? **¿Dónde trabaja?**
(Dohn-deh trah-bah-hah)

Work phone number? **¿Teléfono del trabajo?**
(Teh-leh-foh-noh dehl trah-bah-hoh)

Sign here, please. **Firme aquí, por favor.**
(Feer-meh ah-kee, pohr fah-bohr)

Thank you! **¡Gracias!**
(Grah-see-ahs)

Memorization of numbers is helpful when you are asking for addresses or phone numbers. Table 3–6.

Memorizar los números le ayuda cuando pida direcciones o números de teléfono. Tabla 3–6.

TABLE 3–6
Helpful Numbers

TABLA 3–6
Números útiles

Number	English	Spanish	Pronunciation
1	one	**uno**	*(oo-noh)*
2	two	**dos**	*(dohs)*
3	three	**tres**	*(trehs)*
4	four	**cuatro**	*(koo-ah-troh)*
5	five	**cinco**	*(seen-koh)*
6	six	**seis**	*(seh-ees)*
7	seven	**siete**	*(see-eh-teh)*
8	eight	**ocho**	*(oh-choh)*
9	nine	**nueve**	*(noo-eh-beh)*
10	ten	**diez**	*(dee-ehs)*
15	fifteen	**quince**	*(keen-seh)*
20	twenty	**veinte**	*(beh-een-teh)*
30	thirty	**treinta**	*(treh-een-tah)*
40	forty	**cuarenta**	*(koo-ah-rehn-tah)*
50	fifty	**cincuenta**	*(seen-koo-ehn-tah)*
60	sixty	**sesenta**	*(seh-sehn-tah)*
70	seventy	**setenta**	*(seh-tehn-tah)*
80	eighty	**ochenta**	*(oh-chehn-tah)*
90	ninety	**noventa**	*(noh-behn-tah)*
100	one hundred	**cien**	*(see-ehn)*

Chapter Four | Capítulo cuatro

In the Hospital | En el hospital

When someone asks you for directions in Spanish, knowing key words is essential. Do not hesitate to use your hands or draw a map that the patient can use as a guide. He will appreciate it. Table 4–1 will help you with pronunciation of selected words.

Cuando alguien le pide direcciones en español, es esencial saber palabras clave. No vacile en usar las manos o dibujar un mapa que el paciente puede usar como guía. El lo apreciará. La Tabla 4–1 le ayudará con la pronunciación de palabras selectas.

Good morning! — **¡Buenos días!**
(Boo-eh-nohs dee-ahs)

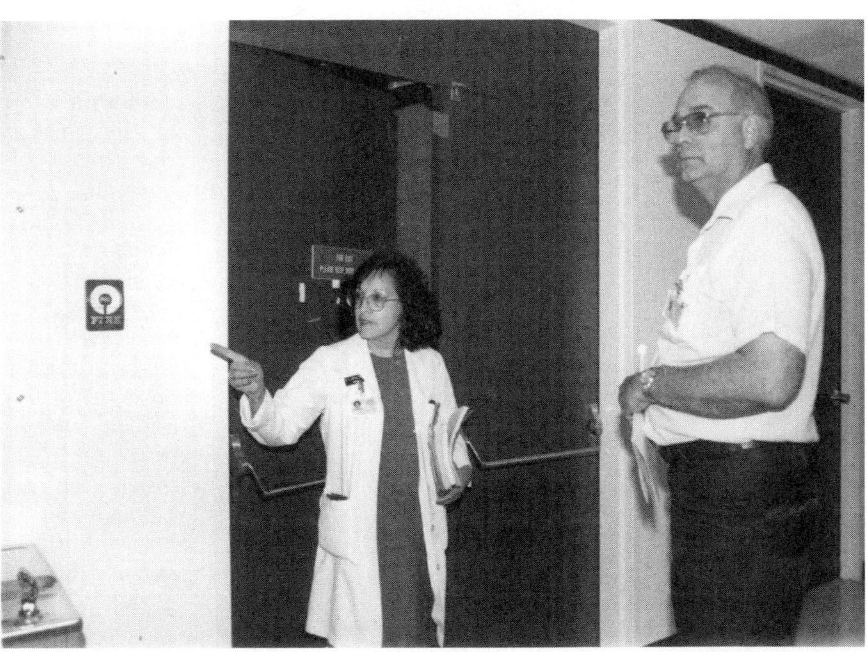

Figure 4–1 Knowing key words is essential when giving directions.

TABLE 4–1 Pronunciation of Selected Words | **TABLA 4–1 Pronunciación de palabras selectas**

English	Spanish	Pronunciation
administration	**administración**	*(ahd-mee-nee-strah-see-ohn)*
arrow	**flecha**	*(fleh-chah)*
building	**edificio**	*(eh-dee-fee-see-oh)*
cafeteria	**cafetería**	*(kah-feh-teh-ree-ah)*
clinic	**clínica**	*(klee-nee-kah)*
directions	**direcciones**	*(dee-rehk-see-ohn-ehs)*
elevator	**elevador**	*(eh-leh-bah-dohr)*
fire escape	**escape de fuego**	*(ehs-kah-peh deh foo-eh-goh)*
hesitate	**vacilar**	*(bah-see-lahr)*
laboratory	**laboratorio**	*(lah-boh-rah-toh-ree-oh)*
lobby	**vestíbulo**	*(behs-tee-boo-loh)*
stairs	**escalera**	*(ehs-kah-leh-rah)*
surgery	**cirugía**	*(see-roo-hee-ah)*
tower	**torre**	*(toh-reh)*

Is this ____ Hospital? — **¿Es este el Hospital ____?** *(Ehs ehs-teh ehl ohs-pee-tahl ____)*

I need to go to the surgery clinic. — **Necesito ir a la clínica de cirugía.** *(Neh-seh-see-toh eer ah lah klee-nee-kah deh see-roo-hee-ah)*

Can you give me directions? — **¿Me puede dar direcciones?** *(Meh poo-eh-deh dahr dee-rek-see-ohn-ehs)*

Yes, go to the end of the hall. — **Sí, vaya al final del pasillo.** *(See, bah-yah ahl feen-ahl dehl pah-see-yoh)*

Can you see the fire extinguisher? — **¿Ve el extinguidor de fuego?** *(Beh ehl ehx-teen-ghee-dohr deh foo-eh-goh)*

It's in the middle of the wall. — **Está en el medio de la pared.** *(Ehs-tah ehn ehl meh-dee-oh deh lah pah-rehd)*

When you get there, turn right. — **Cuando llegue ahí, dé vuelta a la derecha.** *(Koo-ahn-doh yeh-gheh ah-ee, deh boo-ehl-tah ah lah deh-reh-chah)*

You will pass the cafeteria.	**Va a pasar la cafetería.** *(Bah ah pah-sahr lah kah-feh-teh-ree-ah)*
Go to the glass doors.	**Vaya a las puertas de vidrio.** *(Bah-yah ah lahs poo-ehr-tahs deh bee-dree-oh)*
The clinic is in another building.	**La clínica está en otro edificio.** *(Lah klee-nee-kah ehs-tah ehn oh-troh eh-dee-fee-see-oh)*

You may wish to memorize single words that will help you with directions. Table 4–2 has key words.

Puede memorizar palabras que le ayudarán con las direcciones. La Tabla 4–2 tiene palabras clave.

You have to cross the street.	**Tiene que cruzar la calle.** *(Tee-eh-neh keh kroo-sahr lah kah-yeh)*
Walk two blocks.	**Camine dos cuadras.** *(Kah-mee-neh dohs koo-ah-drahs)*
Then, turn to the left.	**Luego dé vuelta a la izquierda.** *(Loo-eh-goh deh boo-ehl-tah ah lah ees-kee-ehr-dah)*
The building has beige brick.	**El edificio tiene ladrillo crema.** *(Ehl eh-dee-fee-see-oh tee-eh-neh lah-dree-yoh kreh-mah)*

TABLE 4–2
Key Words

TABLA 4–2
Palabras clave

English	Spanish	Pronunciation
above	**arriba**	*(ah-ree-bah)*
below	**abajo**	*(ah-bah-hoh)*
blocks	**cuadras**	*(koo-ah-drahs)*
corner	**esquina**	*(ehs-kee-nah)*
hallway	**pasillo**	*(pah-see-yoh)*
left	**izquierda**	*(ees-kee-ehr-dah)*
right	**derecha**	*(deh-reh-chah)*
sign	**letrero**	*(leh-treh-roh)*
straight	**derecho**	*(deh-reh-choh)*
wall	**pared**	*(pah-rehd)*

It is a six-story building.	**Es un edificio de seis pisos.** *(Ehs oon eh-dee-fee-see-oh deh seh-ees pee-sohs)*
Take the elevator to the sixth floor.	**Tome el elevador al sexto piso.** *(Toh-meh ehl eh-leh-bah-dohr ahl sehx-toh pee-soh)*
The elevators are slow.	**Los elevadores son lentos.** *(Lohs eh-leh-bah-doh-rehs sohn lehn-tohs)*
Exit to the right.	**Salga a la derecha.** *(Sahl-gah ah lah deh-reh-chah)*
You will see the sign on the wall.	**Verá el letrero en la pared.** *(Beh-rah ehl leh-treh-roh ehn lah pah-rehd)*
Follow the red arrows.	**Siga las flechas rojas.** *(See-gah lahs fleh-chahs roh-hahs)*

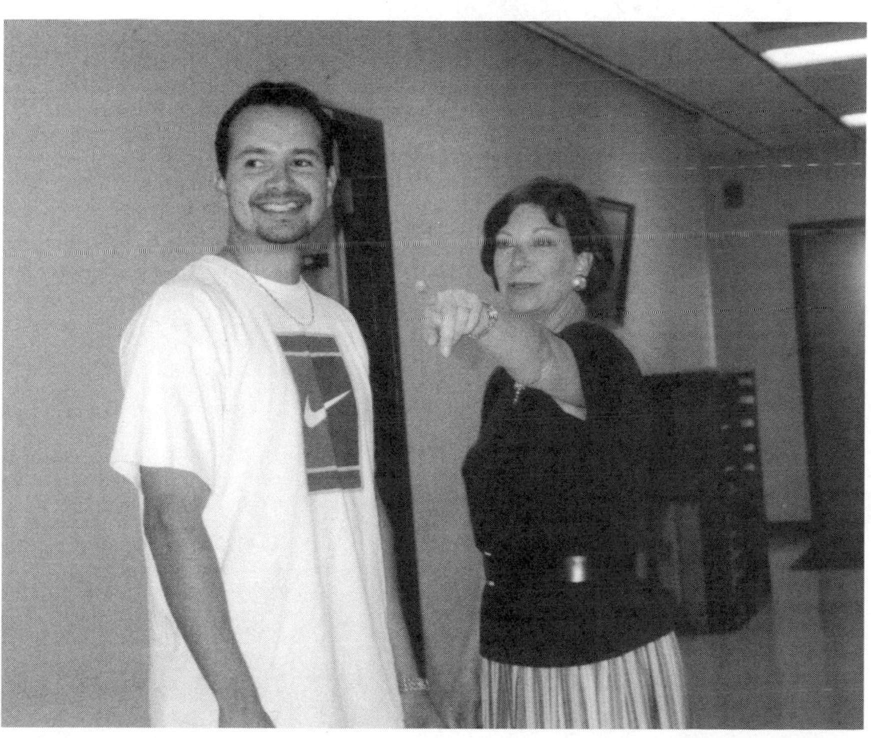

Figure 4–2 Use your hands or draw a map when giving directions to a non-English speaking patient.

There is a front desk.	**Hay un escritorio al frente.** *(Ah-ee oon ehs-kree-toh-ree-oh ahl frehn-teh)*
Ask the receptionist for a number.	**Pídale un número a la recepcionista.** *(Pee-dah-leh oon noo-meh-roh ah lah reh-sehp-see-ohn-ees-tah)*
Wait in the lobby.	**Espere en el vestíbulo.** *(Ehs-peh-reh ehn ehl behs-tee-boo-loh)*

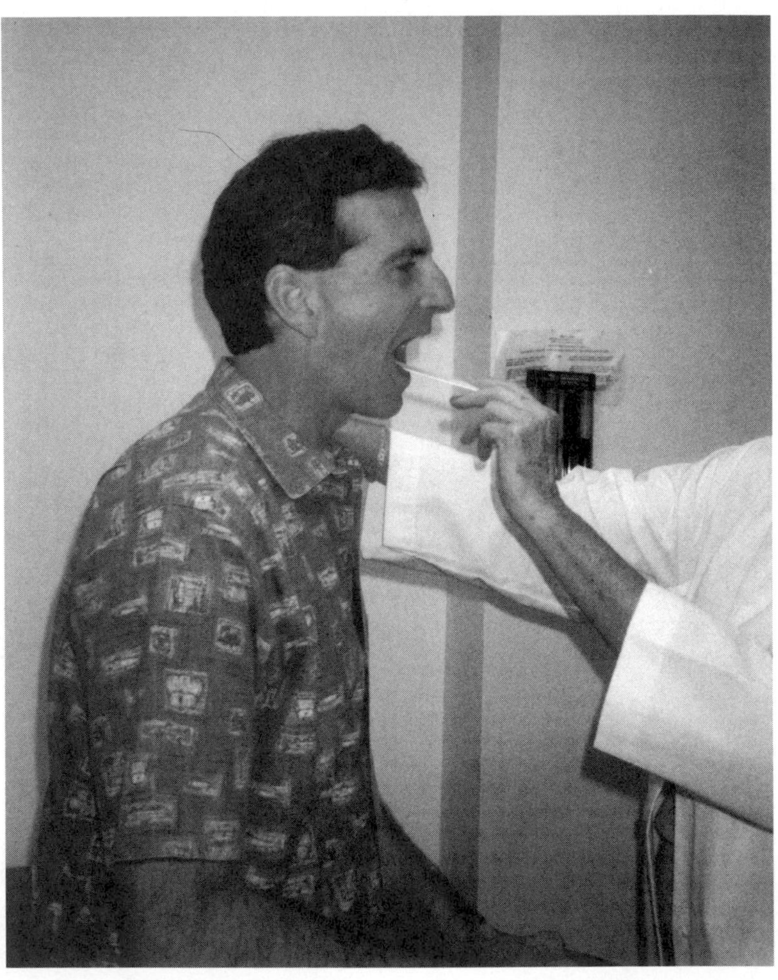

Figure 4–3 Memorizing a few verbs in Spanish will help you give the right commands even when you are unable to carry on a conversation.

You have to wait your turn.	**Tendrá que esperar su turno.** *(Tehn-drah keh ehs-peh-rahr soo tuhr-noh)*
Do you want to take the stairs?	**¿Quiere tomar la escalera?** *(Kee-eh-reh toh-mahr lah ehs-kah-leh-rah)*
They are around the corner.	**Están alrededor de la esquina.** *(Ehs-tahn ahl-reh-deh-dohr deh lah ehs-kee-nah)*
You can't miss them!	**¡Se dará cuenta!** *(Seh dah-rah coo-ehn-tah)*
The stairs will take you.	**La escalera lo llevará.** *(Lah ehs-kah-leh-rah loh yeh-bah-rah)*

Sometimes you will only remember a few words. No problem! Verbs usually come in handy because they are the essence of a sentence. You can help the patients if you recognize some useful verbs. Table 4–3.

Algunas veces sólo recordará pocas palabras. ¡No hay problema! Los verbos vienen a la mano porque son lo esencial de una oración. Puede ayudar a los pacientes si reconoce unos verbos útiles. Tabla 4–3.

You can cross at the walkway.	**Puede cruzar por el pasillo sobre la calle.** *(Poo-eh-deh kroo-sahr pohr ehl pah-see-yoh soh-breh lah kah-yeh)*

TABLE 4–3
Useful Verbs

TABLA 4–3
Verbos útiles

English	Spanish	Pronunciation
to ask	**preguntar**	*(preh-goon-tahr)*
to cross	**cruzar**	*(kroo-sahr)*
to follow	**seguir**	*(seh-geer)*
to give	**dar**	*(dahr)*
to hurt	**doler**	*(doh-lehr)*
to see	**ver**	*(behr)*
to take	**tomar**	*(toh-mahr)*
to tell	**decir**	*(deh-seer)*
to turn	**voltear/dar vuelta**	*(bohl-teh-ahr)/(dahr boo-ehl-tah)*
to wait	**esperar**	*(ehs-peh-rahr)*

I don't think so.	**No lo creo.** *(Noh loh kreh-oh)*
I am hurting a lot.	**Tengo mucho dolor.** *(Tehn-goh moo-choh doh-lohr)*
If it is far, could I drive?	**Si está lejos, ¿podría manejar?** *(See ehs-tah leh-hohs, poh-dree-ah mah-neh-hahr)*
Is there a policeman?	**¿Hay un policía?** *(Ah-ee oon poh-lee-see-ah)*
I need better directions.	**Necesito mejores direcciones.** *(Neh-seh-see-toh meh-hoh-rehs dee-rehk-see-ohn-ehs)*
I am afraid to get lost.	**Tengo miedo de perderme.** *(Tehn-goh mee-eh-doh deh pehr-dehr-meh)*
This is a large place.	**Este es un lugar grande.** *(Ehs-teh ehs oon loo-gahr grahn-deh)*
I will not find the street.	**No encontraré la calle.** *(Noh ehn-kohn-trah-reh lah kah-yeh)*
What is the name?	**¿Cuál es el nombre?** *(Koo-ahl ehs ehl nohm-breh)*
Can you write the name?	**¿Puede escribir el nombre?** *(Poo-eh-deh ehs-kree-beer ehl nohm-breh)*
I have a piece of paper.	**Tengo un pedazo de papel.** *(Tehn-goh oon peh-dah-soh deh pah-pehl)*
But I don't have a pencil.	**Pero no tengo lápiz.** *(Peh-roh noh tehn-goh lah-pees)*
I don't have a pen either.	**Tampoco tengo una pluma.** *(Tahm-poh-koh tehn-goh oo-nah ploo-mah)*

Since you are sensitive to the patient's needs, you decide that he is going to need more help than just writing the directions to the clinic. Reassurance sometimes does not help.

Como es sensitivo a las necesidades del paciente, decide que él necesita más ayuda que sólo escribir las direcciones a la clínica. El volverlo a asegurar a veces no ayuda.

Sit here and wait.	**Siéntese aquí y espere.** *(See-ehn-teh-seh ah-kee ee ehs-peh-reh)*

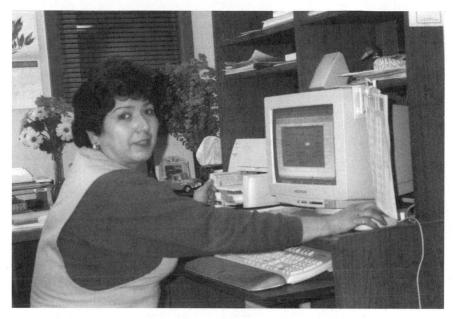

Figure 4–4 The secretary helps the patient by verifying his appointment.

I'll call for a wheelchair. **Pedire una silla de ruedas.** *(Peh-dee-reh oo-nah see-yah deh roo-eh-dahs)*

This is an employee. **Este es un empleado.** *(Ehs-teh ehs oon ehm-pleh-ah-doh)*

He will take you. **El lo llevará.** *(Ehl loh yeh-bah-rah)*

Sit down, please. **Siéntese, por favor.** *(See-ehn-teh-seh pohr fah-bohr)*

Place your feet here. **Ponga los pies aquí.** *(Pohn-gah lohs pee-ehs ah-kee)*

Over the stool. **Sobre el taburete.** *(Soh-breh ehl tah-boo-reh-teh)*

We have to go far. **Tenemos que ir lejos.** *(Teh-neh-mohs keh eer leh-hohs)*

Are you OK? **¿Está bien?** *(Ehs-tah bee-ehn)*

Let me know how you feel. **Dígame cómo se siente.** *(Dee-gah-meh koh-moh seh see-ehn-teh)*

I can stop.	**Puedo pararme.** *(Poo-eh-doh pah-rahr-meh)*
Where are you from?	**¿De dónde es usted?** *(Deh dohn-deh ehs oos-tehd)*
How did you get here?	**¿Cómo llegó aquí?** *(Koh-moh yeh-goh ah-kee)*
Is someone with you?	**¿Hay alguien con usted?** *(Ah-ee ahl-ghee-ehn kohn oos-tehd)*
Do you know how to return?	**¿Sabe cómo regresar?** *(Sah-beh koh-moh reh-greh-sahr)*

The patient has arrived at a different place. He is not familiar with his surroundings. There are many questions that he can ask. Table 4–4 has other questions that he may ask.

El paciente llegó a un lugar diferente. El no está familiarizado con su alrededor. Hay muchas preguntas que puede hacer. La Tabla 4–4 tiene otras preguntas que él puede hacer.

TABLE 4–4 Other Questions — **TABLA 4–4 Otras preguntas**

English	Spanish	Pronunciation
Is it far?	**¿Está lejos?**	*(Ehs-tah leh-hohs)*
How far?	**¿Qué tan lejos?**	*(Keh tahn leh-hohs)*
Do I have time?	**¿Tengo tiempo?**	*(Tehn-goh tee-ehm-poh)*
At what time do they close?	**¿A qué hora cierran?**	*(Ah keh oh-rah see-eh-rahn)*
What time is it?	**¿Qué hora es?**	*(Keh oh-rah ehs)*
Are there elevators?	**¿Hay elevadores?**	*(Ah-ee eh-leh-bah-doh-rehs)*
Are there ramps?	**¿Hay rampas?**	*(Ah-ee ram-pahs)*
Where is it?	**¿Dónde está?**	*(Dohn-deh ehs-tah)*
Is it the same color?	**¿Es del mismo color?**	*(Ehs dehl mees-moh koh-lohr)*
Should I drive?	**¿Debo de manejar?**	*(Deh-boh deh mah-neh-hahr)*
Is parking available?	**¿Hay estacionamiento?**	*(Ah-ee ehs-tah-see-ohn-ah-mee-ehn-toh)*
What is the name of the street?	**¿Cuál es el nombre de la calle?**	*(Koo-ahl ehs ehl nohm-breh deh lah kah-yeh)*
Can you go with me?	**¿Puede ir conmigo?**	*(Poo-eh-deh eer kohn-mee-goh)*

This is the clinic.
Esta es la clínica.
(Ehs-tah ehs lah klee-nee-kah)

Good morning, sir.
Buenos días, señor.
(Boo-eh-nohs dee-ahs, seh-nyohr)

I was told to come here.
Me dijeron que viniera aquí.
(Meh dee-heh-rohn keh bee-nee-eh-rah ah-kee)

I need to see Doctor White.
Necesito ver al doctor White.
(Neh-seh-see-toh behr ahl dohk-tohr White)

Have you been here before?
¿Ha estado aquí antes?
(Ah ehs-tah-doh ah-kee ahn-tehs)

If you have been here, I need your card.
Si ha estado aquí, necesito su tarjeta.
(See ah ehs-tah-doh ah-kee, neh-seh-see-toh soo tahr-heh-tah)

If you haven't, please fill out these papers.
Si no, por favor llene estos papeles.
(See noh, pohr fah-bohr yeh-neh ehs-tohs pah-peh-lehs)

I cannot read English . . . can you help me?
No puedo leer inglés... ¿puede ayudarme?
(Noh poo-eh-doh leh-ehr een-glehs... poo-eh-deh ah-yoo-dahr-meh)

Yes, please wait.
Sí, espere por favor.
(See, ehs-peh-reh pohr fah-bohr)

This is my first time here.
Esta es mi primera vez aquí.
(Ehs-tah ehs mee pree-meh-rah behs ah-kee)

In that case, tell me your whole name.
En ese caso, dígame su nombre completo.
(Ehn eh-seh kah-soh, dee-gah-meh soo nohm-breh kohm-pleh-toh)

What is your birthdate? year? month? day?
¿Cuál es la fecha de nacimiento? ¿año/mes/día?
(Koo-ahl ehs lah feh-chah deh nah-see-mee-ehn-toh) (ah-nyoh/mehs/dee-ah)

The computer says that you have an appointment.
La computadora dice que tiene cita.
(Lah kohm-poo-tah-doh-rah dee-seh keh tee-eh-neh see-tah)

You have to go to the floor directly.
Debe ir al piso directamente.
(Deh-beh eer ahl pee-soh dee-rehk-tah-mehn-teh)

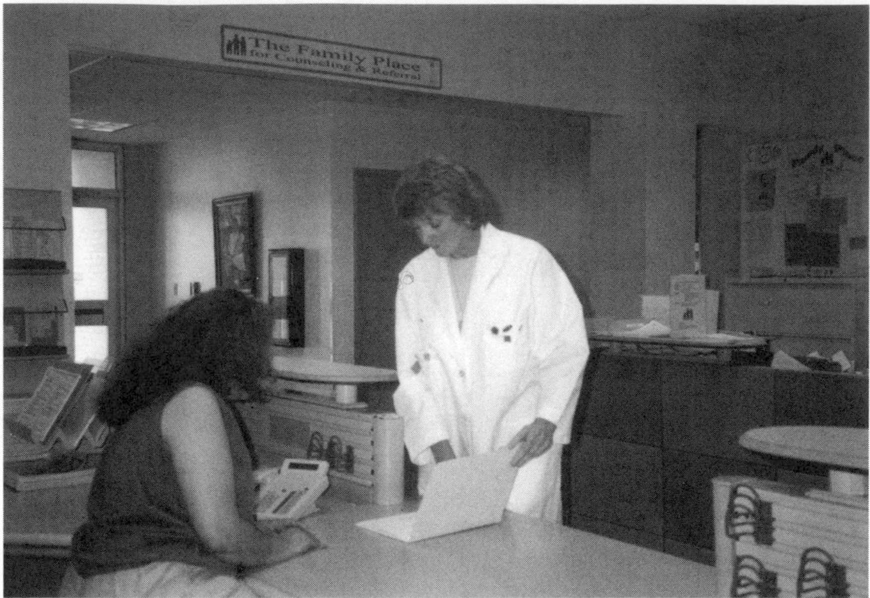

Figure 4–5 It is helpful to verify if the patient has an appointment before you give her any other directions.

The doctor will see you there.	**El doctor lo verá ahí.** *(Ehl dohk-tohr loh beh-rah ah-ee)*
The surgery floor is in the hospital towers.	**El piso de cirugía está en las torres del hospital.** *(Ehl pee-soh deh see-roo-hee-ah ehs-tah ehn lahs toh-rehs dehl ohs-pee-tahl)*
Ask for unit Six A.	**Pregunte por la unidad Seis A.** *(Preh-goon-teh pohr lah oo-nee-dahd Seh-ees Ah)*
From here, turn to the left, then turn right.	**De aquí, dé vuelta a la izquierda, luego voltee a la derecha.** *(Deh ah-kee, deh boo-ehl-tah ah lah ees-kee-ehr-dah, loo-eh-goh bohl-teh-eh ah lah deh-reh-chah)*
Follow the green line.	**Siga la línea verde.** *(See-gah lah lee-nee-ah behr-deh)*
The line is on the wall.	**La línea está en la pared.** *(Lah lee-nee-ah ehs-tah ehn lah pah-rehd)*

Watch for the arrow.	**Fíjese en la flecha.** *(Fee-heh-seh ehn lah fleh-chah)*
This will take you to the end of the hall.	**Esta lo llevará al final del pasillo.** *(Ehs-tah loh yeh-bah-rah ahl feen-ahl dehl pah-see-yoh)*
There, turn to the left.	**Ahí, voltee a la izquierda.** *(Ah-ee, bohl-teh-eh ah lah ees-kee-ehr-dah)*
The secretary will help.	**La secretaria lo ayudará.** *(Lah seh-kreh-tah-ree-ah loh ah-yoo-dah-rah)*
Good luck!	**¡Buena suerte!** *(Boo-eh-nah soo-ehr-teh)*

Chapter Five | Capítulo cinco

Admitting a Patient | Admitiendo al paciente

Many Hispanic patients take someone with them to the hospital. This person is able to translate for the patient. However, there's nothing like being able to greet the patient in his language and be able to elicit first-hand information. Do not be annoyed if the patient brings with him several members of his family. Hispanics tend to be supportive of each other and feel better when family is around. Be patient. Alert the patient that you will be asking many questions.

Muchos pacientes hispanos llevan a una persona con ellos al hospital. Esta persona sirve de intérprete; pero, no hay nada, como el poder saludar al paciente en su lengua y tomar información de primera. No se moleste si el paciente va acompañado por varios miembros de su familia. Los hispanos tienden a apoyarse uno al otro y se sienten mejor cuando hay familiares alrededor. Tenga paciencia. Avísele al paciente que va a hacerle muchas preguntas.

What can I help you with?	**¿En qué puedo ayudarlo?** *(Ehn keh poo-eh-doh ah-yoo-dahr-loh)*
Tell me why you are here.	**Dígame por qué está aquí.** *(Dee-gah-meh pohr keh ehs-tah ah-kee)*
What's happening?	**¿Qué le pasa?** *(Keh leh pah-sah)*
How did you get here?	**¿Cómo llegó aquí?** *(Koh-moh yeh-goh ah-kee)*
Did you come by car?	**¿Vino en carro?** *(Bee-noh ehn kah-roh)*
Did you arrive in a wheelchair?	**¿Llegó en silla de ruedas?** *(Yeh-goh ehn see-yah deh roo-eh-dahs)*
Did you walk?	**¿Caminó?** *(Kah-mee-noh)*

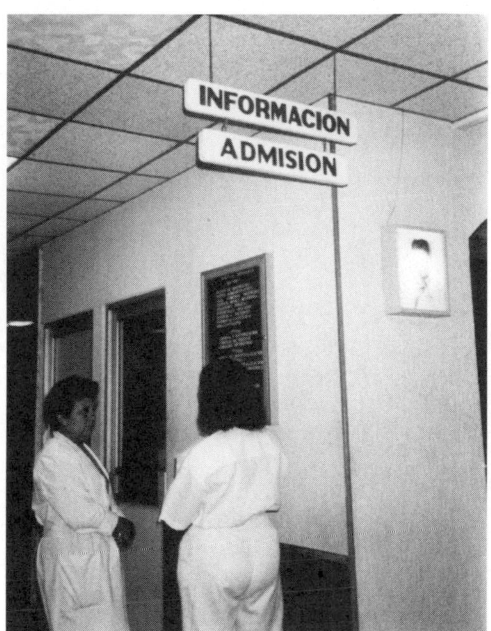

Figure 5–1 The admission office staff will ask for necessary information.

You have to give permission for treatment.	**Tiene que dar permiso para el tratamiento.** *(Tee-eh-neh keh dahr pehr-mee-soh pah-rah ehl trah-tah-mee-ehn-toh)*
Can you write?	**¿Puede escribir?** *(Poo-eh-deh ehs-kree-beer)*
Please sign here.	**Por favor, firme aquí.** *(Pohr fah-bohr, feer-meh ah-kee)*
What brought you to the hospital?	**¿Qué lo trajo al hospital?** *(Keh loh trah-hoh ahl ohs-pee-tahl)*
What problem do you have?	**¿Qué problema tiene?** *(Keh proh-bleh-mah tee-eh-neh)*
Do you have high blood pressure?	**¿Tiene la presión alta?** *(Tee-eh-neh lah preh-see-ohn ahl-tah)*
Are you dizzy?	**¿Tiene mareos?** *(Tee-eh-neh mah-reh-ohs)*
Do you get headaches?	**¿Tiene dolor de cabeza?** *(Tee-eh-neh doh-lohr deh kah-beh-sah)*

See Table 5–1 for similar medical terms.
Vea la Tabla 5–1 con términos médicos similares.

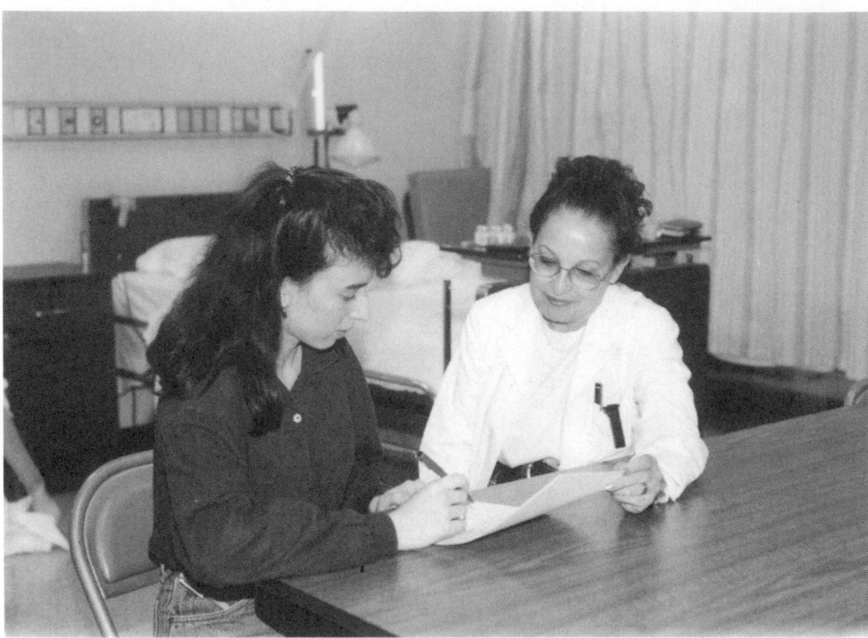

Figure 5–2 The patient is asked to sign permission for treatment.

TABLE 5–1
Similar Medical Terms

TABLA 5–1
Términos médicos similares

English	Spanish	Pronunciation
anemia	**anemia**	*(ah-neh-mee-ah)*
cardiac	**cardíaco**	*(kahr-dee-ah-koh)*
dehydrated	**deshidratado**	*(deh-see-drah-tah-doh)*
epilepsy	**epilepsia**	*(eh-pee-lehp-see-ah)*
inflammation	**inflamación**	*(een-flah-mah-see-ohn)*
neurotic	**neurótico**	*(neh-oo-roh-tee-koh)*
organ	**órgano**	*(ohr-gah-noh)*
pancreas	**páncreas**	*(pahn-kreh-ahs)*
rheumatic	**reumático**	*(reh-oo-mah-tee-koh)*
valve	**válvula**	*(bahl-boo-lah)*
vision	**visión**	*(bee-see-ohn)*
vomit	**vómito**	*(boh-mee-toh)*

I am going to ask many questions!	**¡Voy a hacerle muchas preguntas!** *(Boy ah ah-sehr-leh moo-chahs preh-goon-tahs)*
Do you speak English?	**¿Habla inglés?** *(Ah-blah een-glehs)*
Can you read?	**¿Puede leer?** *(Poo-eh-deh leh-ehr)*
Where do you work?	**¿Dónde trabaja?** *(Dohn-deh trah-bah-hah)*
What is your occupation?	**¿Qué clase de trabajo tiene?** *(Keh klah-seh deh trah-bah-hoh tee-eh-neh)*
How many years did you go to school?	**¿Cuántos años fue a la escuela?** *(Koo-ahn-tohs ah-nyohs foo-eh ah lah ehs-koo-eh-lah)*
What is your religion?	**¿Cuál es su religión?** *(Koo-ahl ehs soo reh-lee-hee-ohn)*
Who takes care of you at home?	**¿Quién lo cuida en casa?** *(Kee-ehn loh koo-ee-dah ehn kah-sah)*

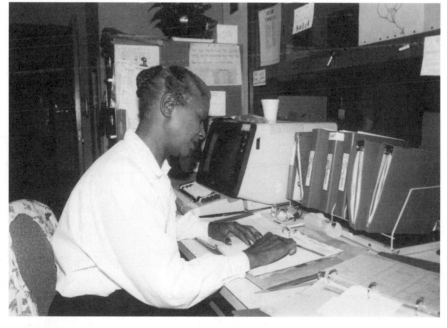

Figure 5–3 The floor/unit secretary may need to ask additional questions.

Table 5–2 will help you with pronunciation of commonly used words.
La Tabla 5–2 le ayudará con la pronunciación de palabras comunes.

Husband? Wife? Children?	**¿Esposo? ¿Esposa? ¿Hijos?** *(Ehs-poh-soh Ehs-poh-sah Ee-hohs)*
Do you have a family doctor?	**¿Tiene un doctor familiar?** *(Tee-eh-neh oon dohk-tohr fah-mee-lee-ahr)*
Do you have allergies?	**¿Tiene alergias?** *(Tee-eh-neh ah-lehr-hee-ahs)*
Are you allergic to foods?	**¿Es alérgico a comidas?** *(Ehs ah-lehr-hee-koh ah koh-mee-dahs)*
to drugs? to plants?	**¿a medicamentos? ¿a plantas?** *(ah meh-dee-kah-mehn-tohs ah plahn-tahs)*
Do you smoke?	**¿Fuma usted?** *(Foo-mah oos-tehd)*
How many cigarettes per day?	**¿Cuántos cigarrillos por día?** *(Koo-ahn-tohs see-gah-ree-yohs pohr dee-ah)*

TABLE 5–2
Pronunciation of Selected Words

TABLA 5–2
Pronunciación de palabras selectas

English	**Spanish**	**Pronunciation**
alcohol	**alcohol**	*(ahl-kohl)*
allergies	**alergias**	*(ah-lehr-hee-ahs)*
ask	**preguntar**	*(preh-goon-tahr)*
chest	**pecho**	*(peh-choh)*
help	**ayuda**	*(ah-yoo-dah)*
hospital	**hospital**	*(ohs-pee-tahl)*
last	**última**	*(ool-tee-mah)*
permission	**permiso**	*(pehr-mee-soh)*
read	**leer**	*(leh-ehr)*
reason	**razón**	*(rah-sohn)*
smoke	**fumar**	*(fooh-mahr)*
speak	**hablar**	*(ah-blahr)*
visit	**visita**	*(bee-see-tah)*
work	**trabajo**	*(trah-bah-hoh)*

Do you drink alcohol?	**¿Toma bebidas alcohólicas?** *(Toh-mah beh-bee-dahs ahl-koh-lee-kahs)*
What kind of drinks?	**¿Qué clase de bebidas?** *(Keh klah-seh deh beh-bee-dahs)*
How much do you drink per day?	**¿Cuánto alcohol toma por día?** *(Koo-ahn-toh ahl-kohl toh-mah pohr dee-ah)*
Do you use drugs/medicine?	**¿Usa drogas/medicamento?** *(Oo-sah droh-gahs/meh-dee-kah-mehn-toh)*
What drugs/medicine do you use?	**¿Qué drogas/medicamento usa?** *(Keh droh-gahs/meh-dee-kah-mehn-toh oo-sah)*
Have you had blood transfusions?	**¿Ha tenido transfusiones de sangre?** *(Ah teh-nee-doh trahns-foo-see-ohn-ehs deh sahn-greh)*
Reaction to transfusions?	**¿Reacción a transfusiones?** *(Reh-ahk-see-ohn ah tranhs-foo-see-ohn-ehs)*
What medicines do you take?	**¿Qué medicinas toma?** *(Keh meh-dee-see-nahs toh-mah)*
When was the last time that you took medicine?	**¿Cuándo fue la última vez que tomó medicina?** *(Koo-ahn-doh foo-eh lah ool-tee-mah behs keh toh-moh meh-dee-see-nah)*
Have you had surgeries?	**¿Ha tenido operaciones?** *(Ah teh-nee-doh oh-peh-rah-see-ohn-ehs)*
What kind of surgeries?	**¿Qué clase de operaciones?** *(Keh klah-seh deh oh-peh-rah-see-ohn-ehs)*
Have you had broken bones?	**¿Ha tenido huesos rotos/fracturados?** *(Ah teh-nee-doh oo-eh-sohs roh-tohs/frahk-too-rah-dohs)*
Car accidents?	**¿Accidentes de auto?** *(Ahk-see-dehn-tehs deh ah-oo-toh)*
Did you bring valuables?	**¿Trajo algo de valor?** *(Trah-hoh ahl-goh deh bah-lohr)*
glasses?	**¿anteojos/lentes?** *(ahn-teh-oh-hohs/lehn-tehs)*
jewelry? cash?	**¿joyas? ¿dinero?** *(hoh-yahs dee-neh-roh)*

artificial eye?	**¿ojo artificial?** *(oh-hoh ahr-tee-fee-see-ahl)*
hearing aid?	**¿aparato para oír?** *(ah-pah-rah-toh pah-rah oh-eer)*
dentures?	**¿dentadura postiza?** *(dehn-tah-doo-rah pohs-tee-sah)*
The hospital is not responsible.	**El hospital no se hace responsable.** *(Ehl ohs-pee-tahl noh seh ah-seh rehs-pohn-sah-bleh)*
Do you have special problems?	**¿Tiene problemas especiales?** *(Tee-eh-neh proh-bleh-mahs ehs-peh-see-ah-lehs)*
Do you take a special diet?	**¿Toma dieta especial?** *(Toh-mah dee-eh-tah ehs-peh-see-ahl)*
What foods do you like?	**¿Qué alimentos le gustan?** *(Keh ah-lee-mehn-tohs leh goos-tahn)*
What foods do you dislike?	**¿Qué alimentos le disgustan?** *(Keh ah-lee-mehn-tohs leh dees-goos-tahn)*

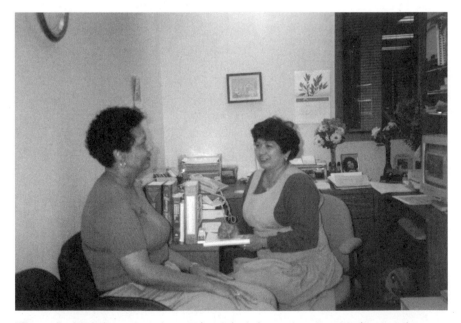

Figure 5–4 It is important to get the right information. Repeat the question when you are not sure that the patient understood what you were asking.

Do you need to see a dietitian? — **¿Necesita ver a la dietista?** *(Neh-seh-see-tah behr ah lah dee-eh-tees-tah)*

Table 5–3 gives a list of special diets.
La Tabla 5–3 le da una lista de dietas especiales.

Do you have — **¿Tiene** *(Tee-eh-neh)*

- tuberculosis? — **¿tuberculosis?** *(too-behr-koo-loh-sees)*
- chest pain? — **¿dolor en el pecho?** *(doh-lohr ehn ehl peh-choh)*
- diabetes? — **¿diabetes?** *(dee-ah-beh-tehs)*
- cancer? — **¿cáncer?** *(kahn-sehr)*

How many persons in your family? — **¿Cuántas personas forman su familia?** *(koo-ahn-tahs pehr-soh-nahs fohr-mahn soo fah-mee-lee-ah)*

Do you live by yourself? — **¿Vive solo?** *(Bee-beh soh-loh)*

How do you spend the day? — **¿Cómo pasa el día?** *(Koh-moh pah-sah ehl dee-ah)*

At what time do you get up? — **¿A qué hora se levanta?** *(Ah keh oh-rah seh leh-bahn-tah)*

At what time do you go to bed? — **¿A qué hora se acuesta?** *(Ah keh oh-rah seh ah-koo-ehs-tah)*

TABLE 5–3
Types of Diets

TABLA 5–3
Tipos de dietas

English	Spanish	Pronunciation
regular	**regular**	*(reh-goo-lahr)*
diabetic	**diabética**	*(dee-ah-beh-tee-kah)*
liquid	**líquida**	*(lee-kee-dah)*
low cholesterol	**poco colesterol**	*(poh-koh koh-lehs-teh-rohl)*
low fat	**poca grasa**	*(poh-kah grah-sah)*
low sodium	**baja en sal/poca sal**	*(bah-hah ehn sahl/poh-kah sahl)*
pureed	**puré**	*(poo-reh)*

How many hours do you sleep?	**¿Cuántas horas duerme?** *(Koo-ahn-tahs oh-rahs doo-ehr-meh)*
Do you sleep during the day?	**¿Duerme durante el día?** *(Doo-ehr-meh doo-rahn-teh ehl dee-ah)*
How long?	**¿Cuánto tiempo?** *(Koo-ahn-toh tee-ehm-poh)*
Who helps you at home?	**¿Quién le ayuda en casa?** *(Kee-ehn leh ah-yoo-dah ehn kah-sah)*
Can you do house chores?	**¿Puede hacer quehaceres?** *(Poo-eh-deh ah-sehr keh-ah-seh-rehs)*
Do you get tired easily?	**¿Se cansa con facilidad?** *(Seh kahn-sah kohn fah-see-lee-dahd)*
Do you need to see a social worker?	**¿Necesita ver a la trabajadora social?** *(Neh-seh-see-tah behr ah lah trah-bah-hah-doh-rah soh-see-ahl)*
Do you want to see a priest?	**¿Necesita ver al sacerdote?** *(Neh-seh-see-tah behr ahl sah-sehr-doh-teh)*

See Table 5–4 for more helpful words and phrases.
Vea la Tabla 5–4 con más palabras y frases útiles.

I will show you your room.	**Le mostraré su cuarto.** *(Leh mohs-trah-reh soo koo-ahr-toh)*
You cannot smoke here.	**No puede fumar aquí.** *(Noh poo-eh-deh foo-mahr ah-kee)*
This is the call bell.	**Este es el timbre.** *(Ehs-teh ehs ehl teem-breh)*

TABLE 5–4
Helpful Words and Phrases

TABLA 5–4
Palabras y frases útiles

English	Spanish	Pronunciation
chaplain	**capellán**	*(kah-peh-yahn)*
hospital policy	**reglas del hospital**	*(reh-glahs dehl ohs-pee-tahl)*
instructions	**instrucciones**	*(eens-trook-see-ohn-ehs)*
no smoking	**no se permite fumar**	*(noh seh pehr-mee-teh foo-mahr)*
priest	**sacerdote/cura**	*(sah-sehr-doh-teh/koo-rah)*
routine	**la rutina**	*(lah roo-tee-nah)*
visiting hours	**horas de visita**	*(oh-rahs deh bee-see-tah)*

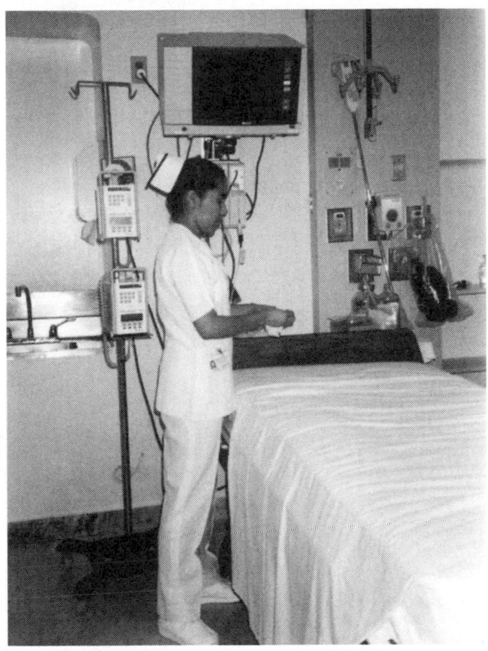

Figure 5–5 Hospital rooms are not always comfortable and they are sometimes frightening.

The meals are served	**Los alimentos se sirven** *(Lohs ah-lee-mehn-tohs seh seer-behn)*
at seven A.M.	**a las siete de la mañana.** *(ah lahs see-eh-teh deh lah mah-nyah-nah)*
at eleven thirty.	**a las once y media.** *(ah lahs ohn-seh ee meh-dee-ah)*
at five P.M.	**a las cinco de la tarde.** *(ah lahs seen-koh deh lah tahr-deh)*
Phone for local calls.	**Teléfono para llamadas locales.** *(Teh-leh-foh-noh pah-rah yah-mah-dahs loh-kah-lehs)*
This is the radio.	**Este es el radio.** *(Ehs-teh ehs ehl rah-dee-oh)*
The television has four channels.	**El televisor tiene cuatro canales.** *(Ehl teh-leh-bee-sohr tee-eh-neh koo-ah-troh kah-nah-lehs)*

There is an educational channel.	**Hay un canal educativo.** *(Ah-ee oon kah-nahl eh-doo-kah-tee-boh)*
These buttons move the bed up/down.	**Estos botones mueven la cama arriba/abajo.** *(Ehs-tohs boh-toh-nehs moo-eh-behn lah kah-mah ah-ree-bah/ah-bah-hoh)*
You can raise the head.	**Puede levantar la cabeza.** **(Poo-eh-deh leh-bahn-tahr lah kah-beh-sah)**
You can raise the feet.	**Puede levantar los pies.** *(Poo-eh-deh leh-bahn-tahr lohs pee-ehs)*
The rails lower down.	**El barandal se baja.** *(Ehl bah-rahn-dahl seh bah-hah)*
Visits are from two to eight P.M.	**Las visitas son de las dos a las ocho de la noche.** *(Lahs bee-see-tahs sohn deh lahs dohs ah lahs oh-choh deh lah noh-cheh)*
Wear this bracelet all the time.	**Use esta pulsera todo el tiempo.** *(Oo-seh ehs-tah pool-seh-rah toh-doh ehl tee-ehm-poh)*
Your towels are in the bathroom.	**Sus toallas están en el baño.** *(Soos too-ah-yahs ehs-tahn ehn ehl bah-nyoh)*
There is an emergency light.	**Hay una luz para emergencias.** *(Ah-ee oo-nah loos pah-rah eh-mehr-hehn-see-ahs)*
Pull the cord in the bathroom.	**Jale el cordón en el baño.** *(Hah-leh ehl kohr-dohn ehn ehl bah-nyoh)*
The bell will sound.	**La campana sonará.** *(Lah kahm-pah-nah soh-nah-rah)*
Your family will bring you clothes.	**Su familia le traerá ropa.** *(Soo fah-mee-lee-ah leh trah-eh-rah roh-pah)*
Change into this gown.	**Póngase esta bata.** *(Pohn-gah-seh ehs-tah bah-tah)*
Rest now.	**Descanse ahora.** *(Dehs-kahn-seh ah-oh-rah)*
Do you have questions?	**¿Tiene dudas?** *(Tee-eh-neh doo-dahs)*
I will return to ask you more questions.	**Regresaré para hacerle más preguntas.** *(Reh-greh-sah-reh pah-rah ah-sehr-leh mahs preh-goon-tahs)*

Table 5–5 will help you review common questions.
La Tabla 5–5 le ayudará a repasar preguntas comunes.

TABLE 5–5 Common Questions | **TABLA 5–5 Preguntas comunes**

English	Spanish	Pronunciation
Can you . . . ?	**¿Puede usted... ?**	***(Poo-eh-deh oos-tehd)***
Do you have . . . ?	**¿Tiene... ?**	***(Tee-eh-neh)***
Have you had . . . ?	**¿Ha tenido... ?**	***(Ah teh-nee-doh)***
How did you?	**¿Cómo hizo?**	***(Koh-moh ee-soh)***
How many?	**¿Cuántos?**	***(Koo-ahn-tohs)***
What is . . . ?	**¿Qué es... ?**	***(Keh ehs)***
What kind?	**¿Qué clase?**	***(Keh klah-seh)***
What's the matter?	**¿Qué pasa?**	***(Keh pah-sah)***

Chapter Six | **Capítulo seis**

The Clerical Staff

Las secretarias

The clerical staff is very important. They are the ones that first greet the patient. Their ability to be pleasant and courteous and to give the appropriate information will speed up the process of admitting the patient to the hospital or referring him to another department.

Las secretarias son muy importantes. Ellas son las primeras personas que saludan al paciente. La habilidad de ser amables y atentas y de dar información apropiada asegura que el proceso de admitir al paciente al hospital o de mandarlo a otro departamento sea mas rápido.

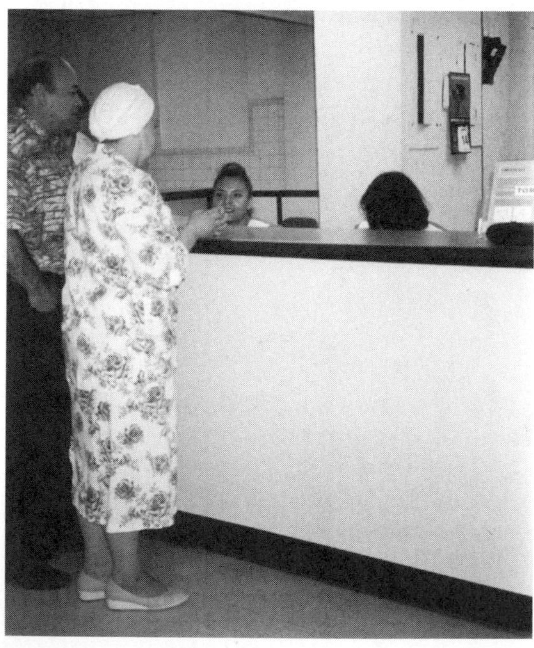

Figure 6–1 Gathering appropriate information helps the patient.

Good afternoon!	**¡Buenas tardes!** *(Boo-eh-nahs tahr-dehs)*
Are you the patient?	**¿Es usted el/la paciente?** *(Ehs oos-tehd ehl/lah pah-see-ehn-teh)*
Do you speak English?	**¿Habla usted inglés?** *(Ah-blah oos-tehd een-glehs)*
Is he/she with you?	**¿El/Ella viene con usted?** *(Ehl/Eh-yah bee-eh-neh kohn oos-tehd)*
Does he/she speak English?	**¿El/Ella habla inglés?** *(Ehl/Eh-yah ah-blah een-glehs)*
How may I help you?	**¿En qué puedo servirle?** *(Ehn keh poo-eh-doh sehr-beer-leh)*
What happened to you?	**¿Qué le pasó?** *(Keh leh pah-soh)*
Please sit down.	**Por favor, siéntese.** *(Pohr fah-bohr, see-ehn-teh-seh)*
I need to ask you some questions.	**Necesito hacerle unas preguntas.** *(Neh-seh-see-toh ah-sehr-leh oo-nahs preh-goon-tahs)*
I have to enter the information in the computer.	**Tengo que poner la información en la computadora.** *(Tehn-goh keh poh-nehr lah een-fohr-mah-see-ohn ehn lah kohm-poo-tah-doh-rah)*
What is your name?	**¿Cómo se llama usted?** *(Koh-moh seh yah-mah oos-tehd)*
What is your last name?	**¿Cómo se apellida?** *(Koh-moh seh ah-peh-gee-dah)*
Have you been in this hospital?	**¿Ha estado en este hospital?** *(Ah ehs-tah-doh ehn ehs-teh ohs-pee-tahl)*
Have you been to the emergency room?	**¿Ha estado en el cuarto de emergencia/urgencias?** *(Ah ehs-tah-doh ehn ehl koo-ahr-toh deh eh-mehr-hehn-see-ah/oor-hehn-see-ahs)*
When was the last time you were here?	**¿Cuándo fué la última vez que estuvo aquí?** *(Koo-ahn-doh foo-eh lah ool-tee-mah behs keh ehs-too-boh ah-kee)*
Is this your first time in the hospital?	**¿Es su primera vez en el hospital?** *(Ehs soo pree-meh-rah behs ehn ehl ohs-pee-tahl)*

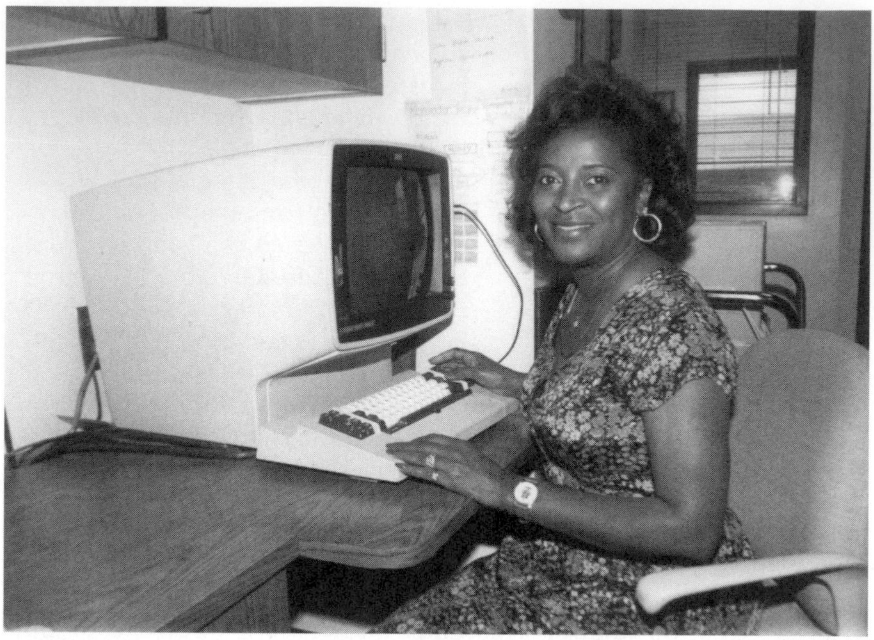

Figure 6–2 Most information is entered in the computer.

Do you have a hospital card?	**¿Tiene usted tarjeta de hospital?** *(Tee-eh-neh oos-tehd tahr-heh-tah deh ohs-pee-tahl)*
What is your social security number?	**¿Cuál es su número de Seguro Social?** *(Koo-ahl ehs soo noo-meh-roh deh Seh-goo-roh Soh-see-ahl)*
Please repeat slowly.	**Por favor, repita despacio.** *(Pohr fah-bohr, reh-pee-tah dehs-pah-see-oh)*
Date of birth?	**¿Fecha de nacimiento?** *(Feh-chah deh nah-see-mee-ehn-toh)*
When (in what year) were you born?	**¿En qué año nació?** *(Ehn keh ah-nyoh nah-see-oh)*
How old are you?	**¿Cuántos años tiene?** *(Koo-ahn-tohs ah-nyohs tee-eh-neh)*
Do you have health insurance?	**¿Tiene seguro de salud?** *(Tee-eh-neh seh-goo-roh deh sah-lood)*

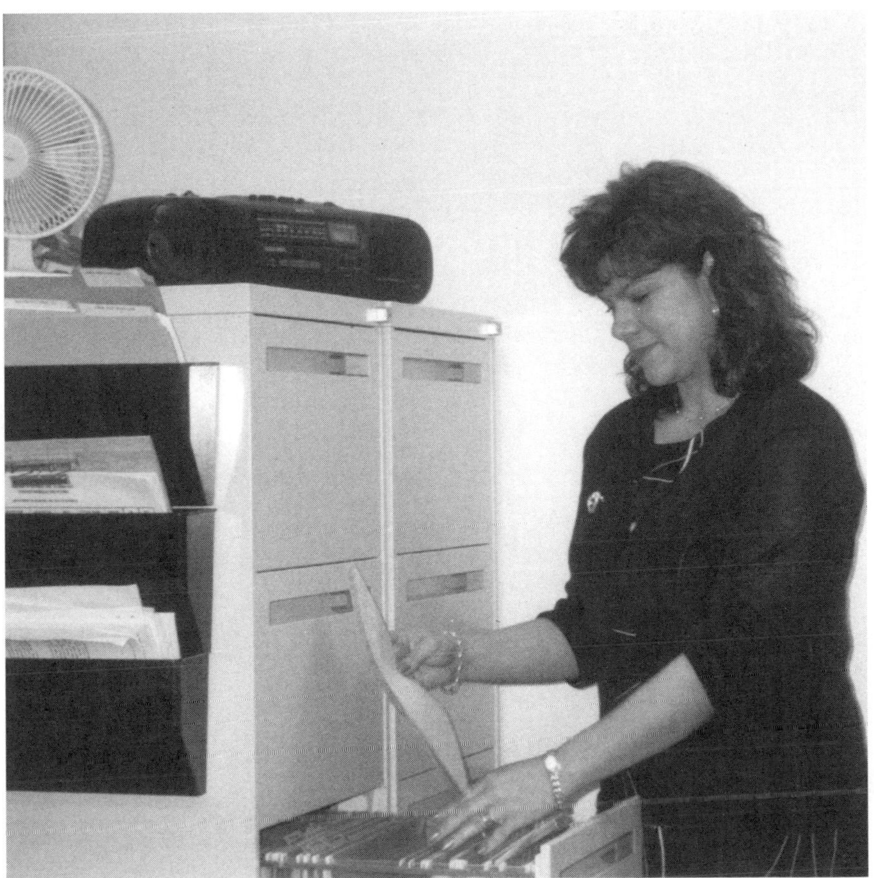

Figure 6–3 All the patient's information must be completed.

What is the name of the insurance?	**¿Cuál es el nombre del seguro?** *(Koo-ahl ehs ehl nohm-breh dehl seh-goo-roh)*
Will it pay for the hospital?	**¿Paga por la hospitalización?** *(Pah-gah pohr lah ohs-pee-tah-lee-sah-see-ohn)*
Who is going to pay the hospital?	**¿Quién va a pagar el hospital?** *(Kee-ehn bah ah pah-gahr ehl ohs-pee-tahl)*
Do you have Medicare?	**¿Tiene Medicare?** *(Tee-eh-neh Meh-dee-kehr)*

Do you have your Medicare card?	**¿Tiene su tarjeta de Medicare?** *(Tee-eh-neh soo tahr-heh-tah deh Meh-dee-kehr)*
Do you have a driver's license?	**¿Tiene licencia para manejar?** *(Tee-eh-neh lee-sehn-see-ah pah-rah mah-neh-hahr)*
What is your address?	**¿Cuál es su dirección?** *(Koo-ahl ehs soo dee-rehk-see-ohn)*
Where do you live?	**¿Dónde vive usted?** *(Dohn-deh bee-beh oos-tehd)*
What is the street name?	**¿Cuál es el nombre de la calle?** *(Koo-ahl ehs ehl nohm-breh deh lah kah-yeh)*
Is that an apartment?	**¿Es apartamento?** *(Ehs ah-pahr-tah-mehn-toh)*
Is it a house?	**¿Es una casa?** *(Ehs oo-nah kah-sah)*
What is the zip code?	**¿Cuál es el código postal?** *(Koo-ahl ehs ehl koh-dee-goh pohs-tahl)*
What is your phone number?	**¿Cuál es su número de teléfono?** *(Koo-ahl ehs soo noo-meh-roh deh teh-leh-foh-noh)*
Do you work?	**¿Trabaja usted?** *(Trah-bah-hah oos-tehd)*
Where do you work?	**¿Dónde trabaja usted?** *(Dohn-deh trah-bah-hah oos-tehd)*
What is the address?	**¿Cuál es la dirección?** *(Koo-ahl ehs lah dee-rehk-see-ohn)*
Is it here in town?	**¿Está en esta ciudad?** *(Ehs-tah ehn ehs-tah see-oo-dahd)*
What work do you do?	**¿Qué trabajo hace usted?** *(Keh trah-bah-hoh ah-seh oos-tehd)*
Where were you born?	**¿Dónde nació usted?** *(Dohn-deh nah-see-oh oos-tehd)*
Are you single?	**¿Es usted soltero (*m.*)/soltera (*f.*)?** *(Ehs oos-tehd sohl-teh-roh/sohl-teh-rah)*
Are you married?	**¿Es usted casado/casada?** *(Ehs oos-tehd kah-sah-doh/kah-sah-dah)*
Are you divorced?	**¿Es usted divorciado/divorciada?** *(Ehs oos-tehd dee-bohr-see-ah-doh/dee-bohr-see-ah-dah)*

Are you a widow/widower?	**¿Es usted viuda/viudó?** *(Ehs oos-tehd bee-oo-dah/bee-oo-doh)*
Common-law wife/husband?	**¿Unión libre?** *(Oo-nee-ohn lee-breh)*
What is your religion?	**¿Cuál es su religión?** *(Koo-ahl ehs soo reh-lee-heh-ohn)*
Who can we call in case of an emergency?	**¿A quién le llamamos en caso de emergencia?** *(Ah kee-ehn leh yah-mah-mohs ehn kah-soh deh eh-mehr-hehn-see-ah)*
Do you have a family doctor?	**¿Tiene usted doctor familiar?** *(Tee-eh-neh oos-tehd dohk-tohr fah-mee-lee-ahr)*
Do you want to see our doctor?	**¿Quiere ver a nuestro doctor?** *(Kee-eh-reh behr ah noo-ehs-troh dohk-tohr)*
Do you prefer to call your doctor?	**¿Prefiere llamar a su doctor?** *(Preh-fee-eh-reh yah-mahr ah soo dohk-tohr)*
You must pay a deposit.	**Debe pagar un depósito.** *(Deh-beh pah-gahr oon deh-poh-see-toh)*
You don't have to pay cash/in full.	**No tiene que pagar en efectivo/al contado.** *(Noh tee-eh-neh keh pah-gahr ehn eh-fehk-tee-boh/ahl kohn-tah-doh)*
You can pay on terms.	**Puede pagar a plazos.** *(Poo-eh-deh pah-gahr ah plah-sohs)*
You need to sign this form.	**Debe firmar esta forma.** *(Deh-beh feer-mahr ehs-tah fohr-mah)*
You are giving us permission to treat you here.	**Nos da permiso de tratarlo aquí.** *(Nohs dah pehr-mee-soh deh trah-tahr-loh ah-kee)*
Please sign here.	**Por favor, firme aquí.** *(Pohr fah-bohr, feer-meh ah-kee)*
Can you write?	**¿Puede escribir?** *(Poo-eh-deh ehs-kree-beer)*
You can write an "X".	**Puede escribir una "X".** *(Poo-eh-deh ehs-kree-beer oo-nah eh-kees)*
How long have you been sick?	**¿Desde cuándo está enfermo/enferma?** *(Dehs-deh koo-ahn-doh ehs-tah ehn-fehr-moh/ehn-fehr-mah)*

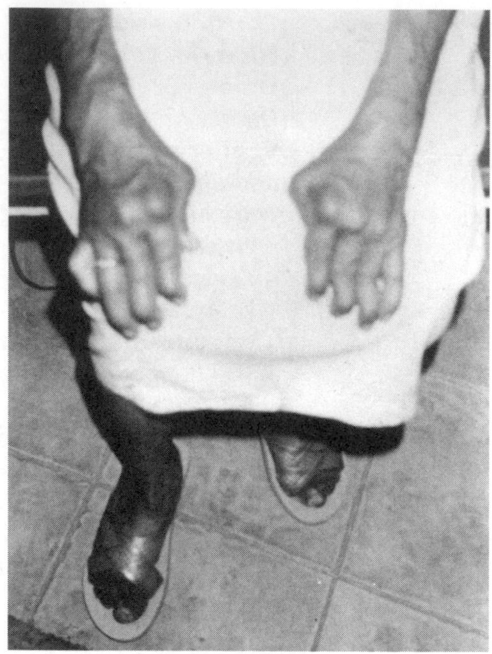

Figure 6–4 Sometimes, because of debilitating illness, a person cannot sign but is able to place a mark on the line.

Days? Months?	**¿Días? ¿Meses?** *(Dee-ahs Meh-sehs)*
Why are you here?	**¿Por qué está aquí?** *(Pohr keh ehs-tah ah-kee)*
What is the worst problem?	**¿Cuál es su peor problema?** *(Koo-ahl ehs soo peh-ohr proh-bleh-mah)*
What is hurting you?	**¿Qué le duele?** *(Keh leh doo-eh-leh)*
Start at the beginning.	**Comience desde el principio.** *(Koh-mee-ehn-seh dehs-deh ehl preen-see-pee-oh)*
When did this happen?	**¿Cuándo le pasó esto?** *(Koo-ahn-doh leh pah-soh ehs-toh)*
Do you have relatives/ friends?	**¿Tiene parientes/amigos?** *(Tee-eh-neh pah-ree-ehn-tehs/ah-mee-gohs)*

Where are they?	**¿Dónde están?** *(Dohn-deh ehs-tahn)*
What is your brother's/ sister's name?	**¿Cómo se llama su hermano/hermana?** *(Koh-moh seh yah-mah soo ehr-mah-noh/ehr-mah-nah)*
What is your husband's/ wife's name?	**¿Cómo se llama su esposo/esposa?** *(Koh-moh seh yah-mah soo ehs-poh-soh/ehs-poh-sah)*
Thank you for the information.	**Gracias por la información.** *(Grah-see-ahs pohr lah een-fohr-mah-see-ohn)*
Please sit down in the waiting room.	**Por favor, siéntese en la sala de espera.** *(Pohr fah-bohr, see-ehn-teh-seh ehn lah sah-lah deh ehs-peh-rah)*
There are a lot of patients.	**Hay muchos pacientes.** *(Ah-ee moo-chohs pah-see-ehn-tehs)*
You will have to wait.	**Tendrá que esperar usted.** *(Tehn-drah keh ehs-peh-rahr oos-tehd)*
Wait 30 minutes.	**Espere treinta minutos.** *(Ehs-peh-reh treh-een-tah mee-noo-tohs)*
You may be here about four hours.	**Estará aquí cerca de cuatro horas.** *(Ehs-tah-rah ah-kee sehr-kah deh koo-ah-troh oh-rahs)*
A nurse will see you.	**Una enfermera la atenderá.** *(Ooh-nah ehn-fehr-meh-rah lah ah-tehn-deh-rah)*
Do you need to call a taxi?	**¿Necesita llamar un taxi/carro de sitio?** *(Neh-seh-see-tah yah-mahr oon tahx-ee/kah-roh deh see-tee-oh)*
Do you want to go home?	**¿Quiere ir a su casa?** *(Kee-eh-reh eer ah soo kah-sah)*
You need to be admitted.	**Necesita internarse.** *(Neh-seh-see-tah een-tehr-nahr-seh)*
Please wait a few minutes.	**Por favor, espere unos minutos.** *(Poh fah-bohr, ehs-peh-reh oo-nohs mee-noo-tohs)*
I will call transportation.	**Llamaré al transporte.** *(Yah-mah-reh ahl trahns-pohr-teh)*

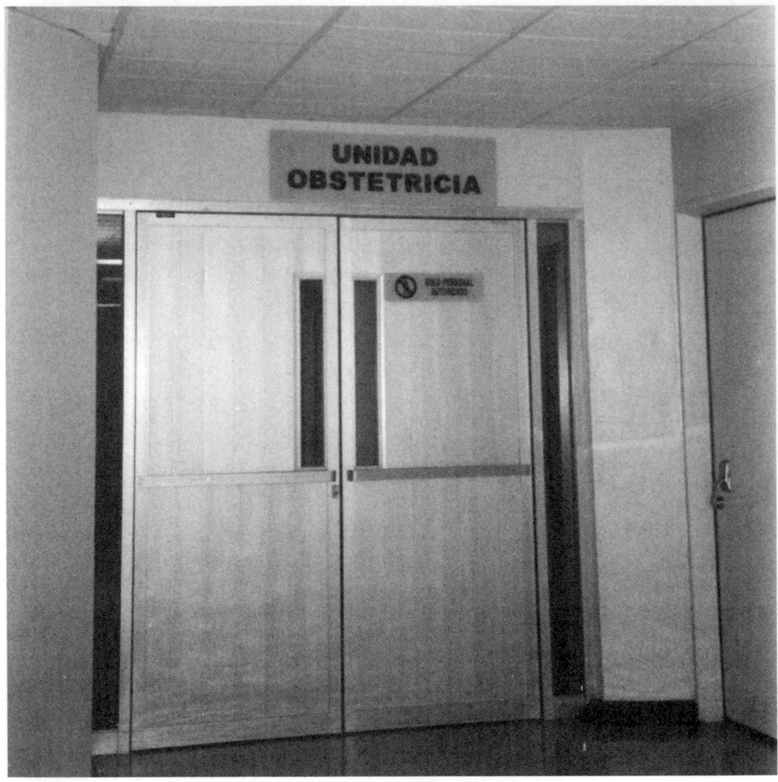

Figure 6–5 The name of the hospital unit is usually found by the door.

Someone will take you to your room.
Alguien lo llevará a su cuarto.
(Ahl-ghee-ehn loh yeh-bah-rah ah soo koo-ahr-toh)

You will be all right!
¡Va a estar bien!
(Bah ah ehs-tahr bee-ehn)

Don't worry!
¡No se preocupe!
(Noh seh preh-oh-koo-peh)

Unit 2

Unidad 2

Chapter Seven | Capítulo siete

A Visit to the Family Doctor
Una visita al médico familiar

Gonzalo Rivera, a 23-year-old male, visits a family doctor for the first time. He is afraid to go into the office. He has questions about his health habits.

Gonzalo Rivera, un hombre de veintitrés años, acude por primera vez al médico familiar. Siente miedo al entrar al consultorio porque tiene dudas sobre los hábitos de su salud.

—Doctor, I think I am infected with AIDS.

—Doctor, pienso que estoy infectado de SIDA.
(Dohk-tohr, pee-ehn-so keh ehs-toh-ee een-fek-tah-doh deh see-dah)

The doctor starts explaining about the disease.

El doctor le da una explicación sobre la enfermedad.

Fear about AIDS comes from ignorance about the true nature of the disease and those who have the virus. The means of transmission are through sexual contact, contact with contaminated blood products and body fluids, or from infected mother to fetus.

El miedo al SIDA proviene de la ignorancia sobre la naturaleza de la enfermedad y los efectos del virus. Los medios de transmisión son: contacto o relaciones sexuales, contacto con productos de la sangre, fluidos del cuerpo contaminados y madres con la enfermedad que infectan al feto.

The doctor asks the patient:

El doctor le pregunta al paciente:
(Ehl dohk-tohr leh preh-goon-tah ahl pah-see-ehn-teh)

Have you been exposed to any infectious diseases?

¿Ha estado expuesto a enfermedades infecciosas?
(Ah ehs-tah-doh ex-poo-ehs-toh ah ehn-fehr-meh-dah-dehs een-fek-see-oh-sahs)

Do you have any infectious disease now?	**¿Tiene alguna enfermedad infecciosa ahora?** *(Tee-eh-neh ahl-goo-nah ehn-fehr-meh-dahd een-fehk-see-oh-sah ah-oh-rah)*
Do you have sexual relations?	**¿Tiene relaciones sexuales?** *(Tee-eh-neh reh-lah-see-oh-nehs sex-oo-ah-lehs)*
With how many people?	**¿Con cuántas personas?** *(Kohn koo-ahn-tahs pehr-soh-nahs)*
Do you participate in homosexual relations?	**¿Participa en relaciones homosexuales?** *(Pahr-tee-see-pah ehn reh-lah-see-ohn-ehs oh-moh-sex-oo-ahl-ehs)*
Do you engage in protective sex?	**¿Practica el sexo seguro?** *(Prahk-tee-kah ehl sehx-oh seh-goo-roh)*

The doctor explains that AIDS was first reported in 1981. Persons with Acquired Immune Deficiency Syndrome develop a defect in their immune system. They are vulnerable to serious infections (referred to as opportunistic infections) that ordinarily pose little threat to an intact immune sys-

TABLE 7–1
Selected Words

TABLA 7–1
Palabras selectas

English	Spanish	Pronunciation
acquired	**adquirida**	*(ahd-kee-ree-dah)*
antibodies	**anticuerpos**	*(ahn-tee-koo-ehr-pohs)*
develop	**desarrollar**	*(deh-sah-roh-yahr)*
fear	**miedo**	*(mee-eh-doh)*
ignorance	**ignorancia**	*(eeg-noh-rahn-see-ah)*
immunodeficiency	**inmunodeficiencia**	*(een-moo-noh-deh-fee-see-ehn-see-ah)*
nature	**naturaleza**	*(nah-too-rah-leh-sah)*
pneumonia	**pulmonía/neumonía**	*(neh-oo-moh-nee-ah/pool-moh-nee-ah)*
opportunistic	**oportunista**	*(oh-pohr-too-nees-tah)*
panic	**pánico**	*(pah-nee-koh)*
precaution	**precaución**	*(preh-kah-oo-see-ohn)*
preliminary	**preliminar**	*(preh-lee-mee-nahr)*
sneeze	**estornudo**	*(ehs-tohr-noo-doh)*
syndrome	**síndrome**	*(seen-droh-meh)*
transfusion	**transfusión**	*(trahns-foo-see-ohn)*

tem. Common problems among AIDS patients are: *pneumocystis carinii* pneumonia; a type of tumor, Kaposi's sarcoma; problems with the central nervous system that may cause forgetfulness, personality changes, or impaired motor skills. In addition, diarrhea and weight loss are common.

El doctor le explica que el SIDA se reportó por primera vez en 1981. Las personas con este síndrome tienen un defecto en su sistema inmunitario. Ellos son vulnerables a las infecciones serias (llamadas infecciones oportunistas) que amenazan al sistema inmunológico. Los pacientes con SIDA tienen problemas como: neumonía producida por el *pneumocystis carinii*; una especie de tumor llamado Sarcoma de Kaposi; alteraciones en el sistema nervioso central que pueden causar el olvido de las cosas, cambios en la personalidad, daños en las habilidades motoras. Adicionalmente, diarreas frecuentes y pérdida de peso son comunes.

The patient asks:	**El paciente pregunta:** *(Ehl pah-see-ehn-teh preh-goon-tah)*
—What causes AIDS?	**—¿Qué causa el SIDA?** *(Keh kah-oo-sah ehl see-dah)*
A virus known as HIV . . .	**El virus causal del SIDA se conoce como VIH...** *(Ehl bee-roos kah-oo-sahl dehl see-dah seh koh-noh-seh koh-moh beh-ee-ah-cheh [VIH])*
—Who is at risk of getting AIDS?	**—¿Quién está en riesgo de contraer el SIDA?** *(Kee-ehn ehs-tah ehn ree-ehs-goh deh kohn-trah-ehr ehl see-dah)*
Sexually active homosexual and bisexual males or females;	**Homosexuales activos y hombres o mujeres bisexuales;** *(Oh-moh-sehx-oo-ah-lehs ahk-tee-bohs ee ohm-brehs oh moo-heh-rehs bee-sehx-oo-ah-lehs)*
intravenous drug abusers;	**los que abusan de las drogas intravenosas;** *(Lohs keh ah-boo-sah deh lahs droh-gahs een-trah-beh-noh-sahs)*
hemophiliacs and recipients of blood/blood components.	**hemofílicos, donadores de sangre o transfusión con sangre contaminada;** *(eh-moh-fee-lee-kohs, doh-nah-doh-rehs deh sahn-greh oh trahns-foo-see-ohn kohn sahn-greh kohn-tah-mee-nah-dah)*

fetus of infected mothers.

fetos de madres contaminadas.
(feh-tohs deh mah-drehs kohn-tah-mee-nah-dahs)

—If you become infected with HIV, what is the risk of getting AIDS?

—Si ha sido infectado con VIH, ¿cuál es el riesgo de contraer el SIDA?
(See ah see-doh een-fehk-tah-doh kohn VIH, koo-ahl ehs ehl ree-ehs-goh deh kohn-trah-ehr ehl see-dah)

About 31% of infected individuals will develop AIDS within six to seven years.

Cerca del 31 por ciento de individuos infectados desarrollan SIDA dentro de seis a siete años.
(Sehr-kah dehl treh-een-tah ee oon pohr see-ehn-toh deh een-dee-bee-doo-ohs een-fehk-tah-dohs deh-sah-roh-yahn see-dah dehn-troh deh seh-ees ah see-eh-teh ah-nyohs)

Studies show that many infected persons remain in good health.

Los estudios muestran que muchas personas infectadas quedan con buena salud.
(Lohs ehs-too-dee-ohs moo-ehs-trahn keh moo-chahs pehr-soh-nahs een-fehk-tah-dahs keh-dahn kohn boo-eh-nah sah-lood)

Infected persons can transmit the virus.

Las personas infectadas pueden transmitir el virus.
(Lahs pehr-soh-nahs een-fehk-tah-dahs poo-eh-dehn trahns-mee-teer ehl bee-roos)

—Can casual contact cause AIDS?

—¿Los contactos eventuales pueden causar SIDA?
(Lohs kohn-tahk-tohs eh-behn-too-ah-lehs poo-eh-dehn kah-oo-sahr see-dah)

HIV is not transmissible by casual contact, nor . . .

El VIH no es transmitido en forma casual, ni por...
(Ehl VIH noh ehs trahns-mee-tee-doh ehn fohr-mah kah-soo-ahl, nee pohr:

living in same house as infected persons;

vivir en la misma casa con personas infectadas;
(bee-beer ehn lah mees-mah kah-sah kohn pehr-soh-nahs een-fehk-tah-dahs)

eating food handled by persons with AIDS; | **comer comida preparada por personas infectadas con SIDA;** *(koh-mehr koh-mee-dah preh-pah-rah-dah pohr pehr-soh-nahs een-fehk-tah-dahs kohn see-dah)*

coughing, sneezing, kissing, or swimming with infected persons. | **tos, estornudo, besar, o nadar con personas infectadas.** *(tohs, ehs-tohr-noo-doh, beh-sahr oh nah-dahr kohn pehr-soh-nahs een-fehk-tah-dahs)*

—Is there a laboratory test for AIDS? | **—¿Hay pruebas de laboratorio para detectar el SIDA?** *(Ah-ee proo-eh-bahs deh lah-boh-rah-toh-ree-oh pah-rah deh-tehk-tahr ehl see-dah)*

No, but there is a test for antibodies. | **No, pero hay prueba de anticuerpos.** *(Noh, peh-roh ah-ee prooh-eh-bah deh ahn-tee-koo-ehr-pohs)*

—What are the symptoms? | **—¿Cuáles son los síntomas?** *(Koo-ah-lehs sohn lohs seen-toh-mahs)*

Most have no symptoms. | **La mayoría no tiene síntomas.** *(Lah mah-yoh-ree-ah noh tee-eh-neh seen-toh-mahs)*

Some develop: tiredness, fever, loss of appetite, weight loss, diarrhea, night sweats. | **Algunos desarrollan: cansancio, fiebre, falta de apetito, pérdida de peso, diarrea, sudor nocturno.** *(Ahl-goo-nohs deh-sah-roh-yahn kahn-sahn-see-oh, fee-eh-breh, fahl-tah deh ah-peh-tee-toh, pehr-dee-dah deh peh-soh, dee-ah-reh-ah, soo-dohr nohk-toor-noh)*

—How is AIDS diagnosed? | **—¿Cómo se diagnostica el SIDA?** *(Koh-moh seh dee-ahg-nohs-tee-kah ehl see-dah)*

Diagnosis is based on evaluation of indicators: immune system function and T-cell count, presence of opportunistic diseases, unexplained dementia, and detection of HIV antibodies. | **El diagnóstico se basa en la evaluación de indicadores: la función del sistema inmunológico y la cuenta de células T, presencia de enfermedades oportunistas, demencia inexplicada y el descubrimiento de anticuerpos VIH.**

(Ehl dee-ahg-nohs-tee-koh seh bah-sah ehn la eh-bah-loo-ah-see-ohn deh een-dee-kah-doh-rehs: lah foon-see-ohn dehl sees-teh-mah een-moo-noh-loh-hee-koh ee lah koo-ehn-tah deh seh-loo-lahs Teh, preh-sehn-see-ah deh ehn-fehr-meh-dah-dehs oh-pohr-too-nees-tahs, deh-mehn-see-ah een-ehx-plee-kah-dah ee ehl dehs-koo-bree-mee-ehn-toh deh ahn-tee-koo-ehr-pohs VIH)

—What are some of the diseases affecting persons with AIDS?

—¿Cuáles son las enfermedades que aparecen en personas infectadas con SIDA?

(Koo-ah-lehs sohn lahs ehn-fehr-meh-dah-dehs keh ah-pah-reh-sehn ehn pehr-soh-nahs een-fehk-tah-dahs kohn see-dah)

About 85% of AIDS patients have had one or both:

Cerca del 85 por ciento de pacientes con SIDA han tenido una o ambas:

(Sehr-kah dehl oh-chehn-tah ee seen-koh pohr see-ehn-toh deh pah-see-ehn-tehs kohn see-dah ahn teh-nee-doh oo-nah oh ahm-bahs:)

Pneumocystis carinii pneumonia (PCP), and/or

Neumonía por *pneumocystis carinii* (PCP), y/o

(neh-oo-moh-nee-ah pohr neh-oo-moh-sees-tees kah-ree-nee ee/oh)

Kaposi's sarcoma.

Sarcoma de Kaposi.

(Sahr-koh-mah deh kah-poh-see)

—How serious is AIDS?

—¿Qué tan serio es el SIDA?

(Keh tahn seh-ree-oh ehs ehl see-dah)

AIDS has a high fatality rate approaching 100%.

El SIDA tiene una tasa cercana al 100 por ciento de mortalidad.

(Ehl see-dah tee-eh-neh oo-nah tah-sah sehr-kah-nah ahl see-ehn pohr see-ehn-toh deh mohr-tah-lee-dahd)

The majority of patients have a life span of about 18–24 months.

La mayoría de los pacientes tienen una sobrevivencia aproximada de dieciocho a veinticuatro meses.

(Lah mah-yoh-ree-ah deh lohs pah-see-ehn-tehs tee-eh-nehn oo-nah soh-breh-bee-behn-see-ah ah-prohx-ee-mah-dah deh dee-ehs-ee-oh-choh ah veh-een-tee-koo-ah-troh meh-sehs)

—Is there a danger from donated blood?

—¿Qué peligro hay por sangre donada?

(Keh peh-lee-groh ah-ee pohr sahn-greh doh-nah-dah)

The risk of contracting HIV is not high. Blood banks and other centers use sterile equipment and disposable needles.

El riesgo de contraer VIH no es alto. Los bancos de sangre y otros centros usan equipos estériles y agujas desechables.

(Ehl ree-ehs-goh deh kohn-trah-ehr VIH noh ehs ahl-toh. Lohs bahn-kohs deh sahn-greh ee oh-trohs sehn-trohs oo-sahn eh-kee-pohs ehs-teh-ree-lehs ee ah-goo-hahs deh-seh-chah-blehs)

—What can be done to prevent AIDS?

—¿Qué se puede hacer para prevenir el SIDA?

(Keh seh poo-eh-deh ah-sehr pah-rah preh-beh-neer ehl see-dah)

The U.S. Public Health Service recommends:

El Departamento de Salud Pública de los Estados Unidos recomienda:

(Ehl Deh-pahr-tah-mehn-toh deh Sah-lood Poo-blee-kah deh lohs Ehs-tah-dohs Oo-nee-dohs reh-koh-mee-ehn-dah)

1. Know sexual background/habits of partners.

   Conozca los hábitos sexuales de su pareja.

   (Koh-nohs-kah lohs ah-bee-tohs sex-oo-ah-lehs deh soo pah-reh-hah)

2. Use a condom or prophylactic.

   Use un condón o profiláctico.

   (Oo-seh oon kohn-dohn oh proh-fee-lahk-tee-koh)

3. If your partner is in a high risk group, cease sexual relations.

   Si su compañera está en el grupo de alto riesgo, suspenda las relaciones sexuales.

   (See soo kohm-pah-nyeh-rah ehs-tah ehn ehl groo-poh deh ahl-toh ree-ehs-goh, soos-pehn-dah lahs reh-lah-see-ohn-ehs sehx-oo-ahl-ehs)

4. Eliminate multiple sexual partners.

4. Elimine múltiples compañeros sexuales.

(Eh-lee-mee-neh mool-tee-plehs kohm-pha-nyeh-rohs sehx-oo-ah-lehs)

5. Don't use intravenous drugs with contaminated needles; don't share needles or syringes.

5. No use drogas intravenosas con agujas contaminadas; no comparta agujas o jeringas.

(Noh oos-eh droh-gahs een-trah-veh-noh-sahs kohn ah-goo-hahs kohn-tah-mee-nah-dahs; noh kohm-pahr-tah ah-goo-hahs oh hehr-een-gahs)

Chapter Eight | Capítulo ocho

A Visit to the Pediatrician | Una visita a la pediatra

It is important that children visit the pediatrician from infancy in order to evaluate their growth and development and to administer the prescribed immunizations. Mrs. Mora decides to take her two children to the pediatrician. The infant is one month old and the other child is six years old.

Es importante que desde los primeros meses de vida, los niños visiten a la pediatra para valorar su desarrollo, crecimiento y vacunación. La señora Mora decide llevar a sus hijos a la consulta: un niño de un mes y el otro de seis años.

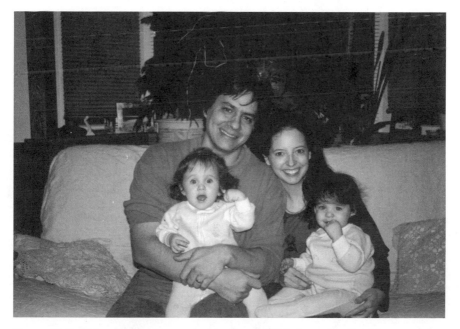

Figure 8–1 All family members must be assessed during a family visit.

Hello, Mrs. Mora.	**Hola, señora Mora.** *(Oh-lah, seh-nyoh-rah Moh-rah)*
How are you?	**¿Cómo está?** *(Koh-moh ehs-tah)*
I am the doctor.	**Yo soy la doctora.** *(Yoh soh-eeh lah dohk-toh-rah)*

A variety of greetings and common expressions will help you to get acquainted with the patients. Table 8–1.

Una variedad de saludos y expresiones comunes le ayudarán a darse a conocer con los pacientes. Tabla 8–1.

I am here to examine the baby.	**Estoy aquí para examinar al bebé.** *(Ehs-toh-ee ah-kee pah-rah ehx-ah-mee-nahr ahl beh-beh)*
I will start by taking vital signs.	**Voy a empezar por tomar los signos vitales.** *(Boy ah ehm-peh-sahr pohr toh-mahr lohs seeg-nohs bee-tah-lehs)*
When was he/she born?	**¿Cuándo nació?** *(koo-ahn-doh nah-see-oh)*
Where?	**¿Dónde?** *(Dohn-deh)*
Was the delivery normal?	**¿Fue normal el parto?** *(Foo-eh nohr-mahl ehl pahr-toh)*

TABLE 8–1
Greetings and Common Expressions

TABLA 8–1
Saludos y expresiones comunes

English	Spanish	Pronunciation
Good morning!	¡Buenos días!	*(Boo-eh-nohs dee-ahs)*
Good evening! (Good night!)	¡Buenas noches!	*(Boo-eh-nahs noh-chehs)*
Pardon me!	¡Perdóneme!	*(Pehr-doh-neh-meh)*
Excuse me!	¡Excúseme!	*(Ehx-koo-seh-meh)*
Good afternoon!	¡Buenas tardes!	*(Boo-eh-nahs tahr-dehs)*
Thank you!	¡Gracias!	*(Grah-see-ahs)*
Please!	¡Por favor!	*(Pohr fah-bohr)*
Good!	¡Bueno!	*(Boo-eh-noh)*
Go on!	¡Síga!	*(See-gah)*

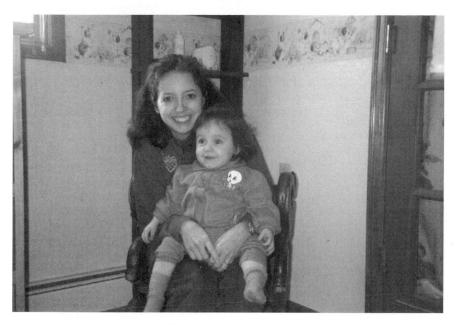

Figure 8–2 During a home visit the health care worker has an opportunity to talk to the mother about her baby.

Note that questions in Spanish use the interrogation symbol at the beginning and at the end of the question. It is helpful to memorize some common pronouns used in questions. Table 8–2.

Note que las preguntas en español usan el símbolo interrogativo al principio y al final de la pregunta. Es conveniente memorizar algunos pronombres comunes que se usan en las preguntas. Tabla 8–2.

Was he premature? — **¿Fue prematuro?** *(Foo-eh preh-mah-too-roh)*

Has the child been ill? — **¿Ha estado enfermo el niño?** *(Ah ehs-tah-doh ehn-fehr-moh ehl nee-nyoh)*

Is he/she . . . — **¿Está...** *(Ehs-tah...)*

- eating well? — **comiendo bien?** *(koh-mee-ehn-doh bee-ehn)*
- sleeping well? — **durmiendo bien?** *(door-mee-ehn-doh bee-ehn)*
- breast-feeding? — **tomando pecho?** *(toh-mahn-doh peh-choh)*
- taking formula? — **tomando fórmula?** *(toh-mahn-doh fohr-moo-lah)*

TABLE 8–2 **Common Interrogative Expressions**	**TABLA 8–2** **Expresiones interrogativas comunes**	
English	**Spanish**	**Pronunciation**
Who? (one person)	¿Quién?	*(Kee-ehn)*
Who? (several people)	¿Quiénes?	*(Kee-ehn-ehs)*
What?	¿Qué?	*(Keh)*
Which?	¿Cuál?	*(Koo-ahl)*
Which (ones)?	¿Cuáles?	*(Koo-ah-lehs)*
How?	¿Cómo?	*(Koh-moh)*
How many?	¿Cuántos? (*m.*)	*(Koo-ahn-tohs)*
	¿Cuántas? (*f.*)	*(Koo-ahn-tahs)*
How much?	¿Cuánto? (*m.*)	*(Koo-ahn-toh)*
	¿Cuánta? (*f.*)	*(Koo-ahn-tah)*
When?	¿Cuándo?	*(Koo-ahn-doh)*
Where?	¿Dónde?	*(Dohn-deh)*
Why?	¿Por qué?	*(Pohr keh)*
For what?	¿Para qué?	*(Pah-rah keh)*

What formula does he take? **¿Qué fórmula toma?** *(Keh fohr-moo-lah toh-mah)*

How many ounces does he take? **¿Cuántas onzas toma?** *(Koo-ahn-tahs ohn-sahs toh-mah)*

How often do you feed the baby? **¿Qué tan a menudo alimenta al bebé?** *(Keh tahn ah meh-noo-doh ah-lee-mehn-tah ahl beh-beh)*

Do you feed every three hours? **¿Le da de comer cada tres horas?** *(Leh dah deh koh-mehr kah-dah trehs oh-rahs)*

This is a new formula. **Esta es una fórmula nueva.** *(Ehs-tah ehs oo-nah fohr-moo-lah noo-eh-bah)*

Table 8–3 helps you with the pronunciation of selected words.

La Tabla 8–3 le asiste con la pronunciación de palabras selectas.

Does he/she have: fever/diarrhea/colic? **¿Tiene: fiebre/diarrea/cólico?** *(Tee-eh-neh: fee-eh-breh/dee-ah-rreh-ah/koh-lee-koh)*

TABLE 8–3 Pronunciation of Selected Words

TABLA 8–3 Pronunciación de palabras selectas

English	Spanish	Pronunciation
colic	**cólico**	*(koh-lee-koh)*
cough	**tos**	*(tohs)*
diarrhea	**diarrea**	*(dee-ah-reh-ah)*
diaper	**pañal**	*(pah-nyahl)*
family	**familia**	*(fah-mee-lee-ah)*
fever	**fiebre**	*(fee-eh-breh)*
formula	**fórmula**	*(fohr-moo-lah)*
I am	**yo soy**	*(yoh soh-ee)*
medicine	**medicina**	*(meh-dee-see-nah)*
nurse	**enfermera**	*(ehn-fehr-meh-rah)*
sleep	**sueño**	*(soo-eh-nyoh)*

Does the baby sleep all night?
¿Duerme el bebé toda la noche?
(Doo-ehr-meh ehl beh-beh toh-dah lah noh-cheh)

How many times does he wake up?
¿Cuántas veces se despierta?
(Koo-ahn-tahs beh-sehs seh dehs-pee-ehr-tah)

Does he cry a lot?
¿Llora mucho?
(Yoh-rah moo-choh)

When was the last time he had a bowel movement?
¿Cuándo fue la última vez que evacuó/hizo del baño?
(Koo-ahn-doh foo-eh lah ool-tee-mah behs keh eh-bah-koo-oh/ee-soh dehl bah-nyoh)

Is he urinating well?
¿Orina bien?
(Oh-ree-nah bee-ehn)

Have you seen blood in the urine?
¿Ha visto sangre en la orina?
(Ah bees-toh sahn-greh ehn lah oh-ree-nah)

How many diapers have you changed since yesterday?
¿Cuántos pañales le ha cambiado desde ayer?
(Koo-ahn-tohs pah-nyah-lehs leh ah kahm-bee-ah-doh dehs-deh ah-yehr)

When did you notice the skin rash?
¿Cuándo se dió cuenta de la piel rosada?
(Koo-ahn-doh seh dee-oh koo-ehn-tah deh lah pee-ehl roh-sah-dah)

How many times has he vomited?	**¿Cuántas veces ha vomitado?** *(Koo-ahn-tahs beh-sehs ah boh-mee-tah-doh)*
Is it a lot?	**¿Es mucho?** *(Ehs moo-choh)*
Does the vomit have blood?	**¿Tiene sangre el vómito?** *(Tee-eh-neh sahn-greh ehl boh-mee-toh)*
What color?	**¿De qué color?** *(Deh keh koh-lohr)*
Does it have undigested food?	**¿Tiene restos de comida?** *(Tee-eh-neh rehs-tohs deh koh-mee-dah)*
Does it smell bad?	**¿Huele mal?** *(Oo-eh-leh mahl)*
Is he coughing?	**¿Está tosiendo?** *(Ehs-tah toh-see-ehn-doh)*

Write on an index card some of the common verbs from Table 8–4. They will come in handy in the clinical setting.

Escriba en una tarjeta algunos verbos comunes de la Tabla 8–4. Serán convenientes en el área clínica.

TABLE 8–4
Useful Verbs

TABLA 8–4
Verbos útiles

English	Spanish	Pronunciation
boil	**hervir**	*(ehr-beer)*
change	**cambiar**	*(kahm-bee-ahr)*
cough	**toser**	*(toh-sehr)*
cry	**llorar**	*(yoh-rahr)*
dress	**vestir**	*(behs-teer)*
drink	**beber/tomar**	*(beh-behr/toh-mahr)*
eat	**comer**	*(koh-mehr)*
feel	**sentir**	*(sehn-teer)*
give	**dar**	*(dahr)*
leave	**dejar**	*(deh-hahr)*
make	**hacer**	*(ah-sehr)*
play	**jugar**	*(hoo-gahr)*
see	**ver**	*(behr)*
take	**tomar/llevar**	*(toh-mahr/yeh-bahr)*

Does he cough only at night?	**¿Tose sólo de noche?** *(Toh-seh soh-loh deh noh-cheh)*
Is it a dry cough?	**¿Es tos seca?** *(Ehs tohs seh-kah)*
Moist cough?	**¿Tos húmeda?** *(Tohs oo-meh-dah)*
Does the cough produce vomit?	**¿La tos le produce vómito?** *(Lah tohs leh proh-doo-seh boh-mee-toh)*
Dress the baby with few clothes.	**Vista al bebé con poca ropa.** *(Bees-tah ahl beh-beh kohn poh-kah roh-pah)*
Leave the area uncovered.	**Deje el área descubierta.** *(Deh-heh ehl ah-reh-ah dehs-koo-bee-ehr-tah)*
Do not put on plastic pants.	**No le ponga calzones de plástico.** *(Noh leh pohn-gah kahl-sohn-ehs deh plahs-tee-koh)*
Take the temperature rectally.	**Tome la temperatura por el recto.** *(Toh-meh lah tehm-peh-rah-too-rah pohr ehl rehk-toh)*
Normal rectal temperature should be 100.4 degrees Fahrenheit.	**La temperatura normal en el recto es de 100.4 grados Fahrenheit.** *(Lah tehm-peh-rah-too-rah nohr-mahl ehn ehl rehk-toh ehs deh see-ehn poon-toh koo-ah-troh grah-dohs Fah-rehn-heh-eet)*
Give him/her the medicine every four hours.	**Déle la medicina cada cuatro horas.** *(Deh-leh lah meh-dee-see-nah kah-dah koo-ah-troh oh-rahs)*
Boil the water he drinks.	**Hierva el agua que toma.** *(Ee-ehr-bah ehl ah-goo-ah keh toh-mah)*
Sterilize the bottles.	**Esterilice las botellas/los biberones.** *(Ehs-teh-ree-lee-seh lahs boh-teh-yahs/lohs bee-beh-roh-nehs)*
You can feed him/her solid foods.	**Puede darle alimentos sólidos.** *(Poo-eh-deh dahr-leh ah-lee-mehn-tohs soh-lee-dohs)*
Wash well all fruits and vegetables.	**Lave bien frutas y verduras.** *(Lah-beh bee-ehn froo-tahs ee behr-doo-rahs)*

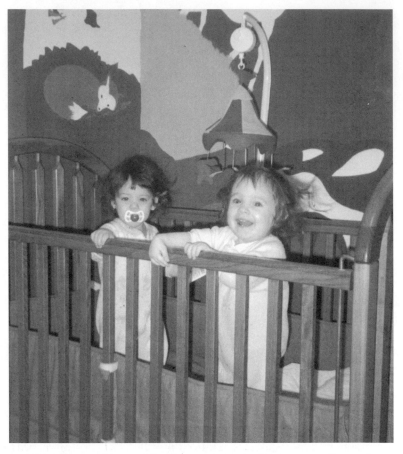

Figure 8–3 A home visit provides you an opportunity to assess the environment and see if there are other needs that you must address.

Wash hands before eating.	**Lave las manos antes de comer.** *(Lah-beh lahs mah-nohs ahn-tehs deh koh-mehr)*
Don't let him put dirt in his mouth.	**No deje que se meta tierra en la boca.** *(Noh deh-heh keh seh meh-tah tee-eh-rah ehn lah boh-kah)*
Make the baby burp.	**Haga que el bebé eructe/repita.** *(Ah-gah keh ehl beh-beh eh-rook-teh/reh-pee-tah)*

Keep the baby awake.	**Mantenga al bebé despierto.** *(Mahn-tehn-gah ahl beh-beh dehs-pee-ehr-toh)*
Don't let the baby sleep more than three hours during the day.	**No deje que el bebé duerma más de tres horas durante el día.** *(Noh deh-heh keh ehl beh-beh doo-ehr-mah mahs deh trehs oh-rahs doo-rahn-teh ehl dee-ah)*
Watch if he sleeps quietly.	**Vigile si su sueño es tranquilo.** *(Bee-hee-leh see soo soo-eh-nyoh ehs trahn-kee-loh)*
Watch if he has abnormal movements.	**Vigile si presenta movimientos anormales.** *(Bee-hee-leh see preh-sehn-tah moh-bee-mee-ehn-tohs ah-nohr-mah-lehs)*
Give him/her the medicine with a dropper.	**Déle la medicina con gotero.** *(Deh-leh lah meh-dee-see-nah kohn goh-teh-roh)*

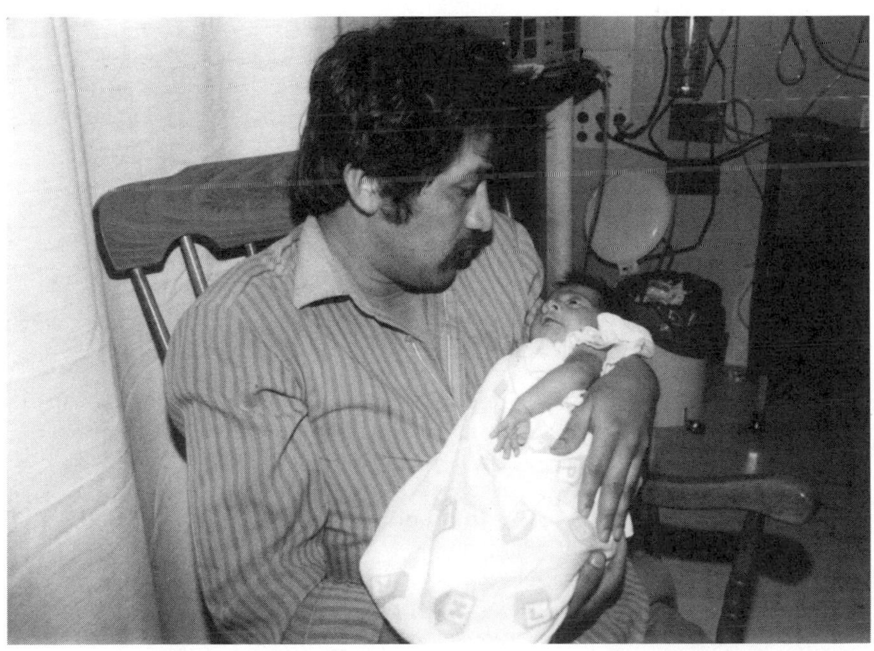

Figure 8–4 Observe the father's interaction with his child. Note how they get along.

It is a good idea to talk to the parents when you examine the baby or older children. Ask direct questions of older children and call them by their names. Also, observe if the parents and the child get along. Table 8–5 has common questions.

Es buena idea hablar con los padres cuando examine al bebé o a niños mayores. Hágales preguntas directamente a los niños mayores y llámeles por su nombre. También observe si los padres y el niño se llevan bien. La Tabla 8-5 tiene preguntas comunes.

I want to examine the older child.	**Quiero examinar al niño mayor.** *(Kee-eh-roh ehx-ah-mee-nahr ahl nee-nyoh mah-yohr)*
The one who is 6 years old.	**El que tiene seis años.** *(Ehl keh tee-eh-neh seh-ees ah-nyohs)*
Does he go to school?	**¿Va a la escuela?** *(Bah ah lah ehs-koo-eh-lah)*
Does he sleep well?	**¿Duerme bien?** *(Doo-ehr-meh bee-ehn)*
Does he wet the bed?	**¿Moja la cama?** *(Moh-hah lah kah-mah)*
Does he play outdoors?	**¿Juega afuera de la casa?** *(Joo-eh-gah ah-foo-eh-rah deh lah kah-sah)*
Does he have any friends?	**¿Tiene amigos?** *(Tee-eh-neh ah-mee-gohs)*

TABLE 8–5
Simple Questions

TABLA 8–5
Preguntas sencillas

English	Spanish	Pronunciation
Do you understand?	**¿Entiende?**	*(Ehn-tee-ehn-deh)*
What is this?	**¿Qué es esto?**	*(Keh ehs ehs-toh)*
Why not?	**¿Por qué no?**	*(Pohr keh noh)*
What's going on?	**¿Qué pasa?**	*(Keh pah-sah)*
Since when?	**¿Desde cuándo?**	*(Dehs-deh koo-ahn-doh)*
For what?	**¿Para qué?**	*(Pah-rah keh)*
Never?	**¿Nunca?**	*(Noon-kah)*
Are you hungry?	**¿Tiene hambre?**	*(Tee-eh-neh ahm-breh)*
Are you thirsty?	**¿Tiene sed?**	*(Tee-eh-neh sehd)*
Is that enough?	**¿Es suficiente?**	*(Ehs soo-fee-see-ehn-teh)*
Is that too much?	**¿Es mucho?**	*(Ehs moo-choh)*
Can you feel this?	**¿Siente esto?**	*(See-ehn-teh ehs-toh)*

Do any of your children have:	**¿Algunos de sus niños tienen:** *(Ahl-goo-nohs deh soos nee-nyohs tee-eh-nehn)*
asthma?	**asma?** *(ahs-mah)*
cold/flu?	**resfriado/gripa?** *(rehs-free-ah-doh/gree-pah)*
chickenpox?	**varicela?** *(bah-ree-seh-lah)*
diphtheria?	**difteria?** *(deef-teh-ree-ah)*
measles?	**sarampión?** *(sah-rahm-pee-ohn)*
mumps?	**paperas?** *(pah-peh-rahs)*
pneumonia?	**pulmonía?** *(pool-moh-nee-ah)*
convulsions?	**convulsiones?** *(kohn-bool-see-ohn-ehs)*
nausea and vomiting?	**náusea y vómitos?** *(nah-oo-seh-ah ee boh-mee-tohs)*
hearing defects?	**defectos del oído?** *(deh-fehk-tohs dehl oh-ee-doh)*
delayed speech?	**tardío del lenguaje?** *(tahr-dee-oh dehl lehn-goo-ah heh)*
visual defects?	**defectos de la vista?** *(deh-fehk-tohs deh lah bees-tah)*
bad coordination?	**mala coordinación?** *(mah-lah kohr-dee-nah-see-ohn)*
Is he hyperactive?	**¿Es inquieto/latoso?** *(Ehs een-kee-eh-toh/lah-toh-soh)*
Does the school have complaints about him?	**¿Tiene quejas de la escuela?** *(Tee-eh-neh keh-hahs deh lah ehs-koo-eh-lah)*

In general, when speaking to a child, the familiar you (tu) is used.
Generalmente se usa la forma familiar de usted cuando habla con un niño.

What is your name?	**¿Cómo te llamas?** *(Koh-moh teh yah-mahs)*
My name is . . .	**Mi nombre es... /Me llamo...** *(Mee nohm-breh ehs/Meh yah-moh)*

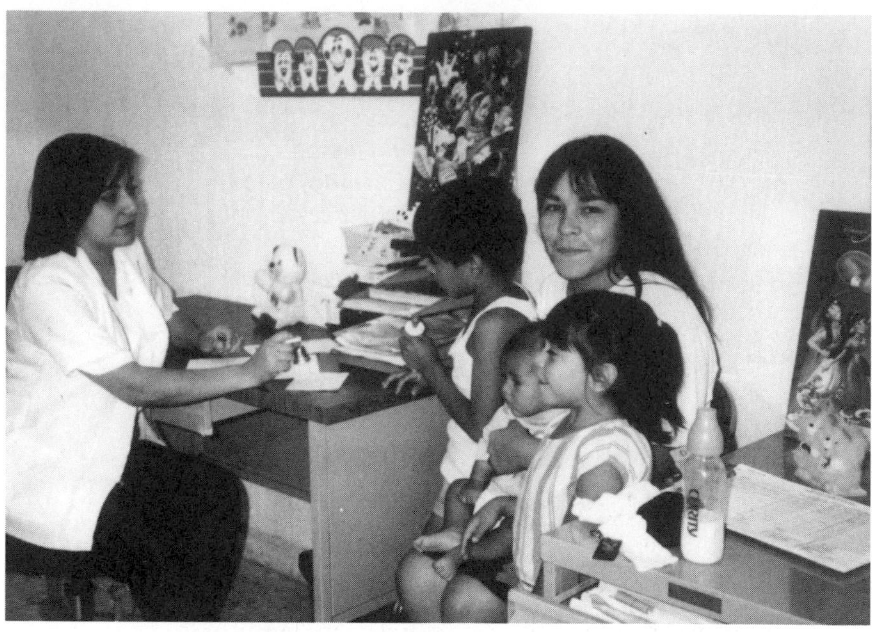

Figure 8–5 The nurse must ask questions about the growth and development of each child.

I would like to talk to you!	**¡Me gustaría hablar contigo!** *(Meh goos-tah-ree-ah ah-blahr kohn-tee-goh)*
Do you have time?	**¿Tienes tiempo?** *(Tee-eh-nehs tee-ehm-poh)*
Are you in a hurry?	**¿Estás de prisa?** *(Ehs-tahs deh pree-sah)*
Do you like going to school?	**¿Te gusta ir a la escuela?** *(Teh goos-tah eer ah lah ehs-koo-eh-lah)*
What grade are you in?	**¿En qué año estás?** *(Ehn keh ah-nyoh ehs-tahs)*
What subject do you like best?	**¿Qué materia te gusta más?** *(Keh mah-teh-ree-ah teh goos-tah mahs)*
What kind of grades do you make?	**¿Qué calificaciones sacas?** *(Keh kah-lee-fee-kah-see-ohn-ehs sah-kahs)*
Do you play sports?	**¿Juegas deportes?** *(Joo-eh-gahs deh-pohr-tehs)*

Which kind?	**¿Qué clase?** *(Keh klah-seh)*
How many friends do you have?	**¿Cuántos amigos tienes?** *(Koo-ahn-tohs ah-mee-gohs tee-eh-nehs)*
Do you need help with school work?	**¿Necesitas ayuda con la tarea?** *(Neh-seh-see-tahs ah-yoo-dah kohn lah tah-reh-ah)*
Who helps you?	**¿Quién te ayuda?** *(Kee-ehn teh ah-yoo-dah)*
Do you have vision problems?	**¿Tienes problemas con la visión?** *(Tee-eh-nehs proh-bleh-mahs kohn lah bee-see-ohn?)*
Do you wear glasses?	**¿Usas anteojos/lentes?** *(Oo-sahs ahn-teh-oh-hohs/lehn-tehs)*
Can you see the blackboard well?	**¿Puedes ver bien el pizarrón?** *(Poo-eh-dehs behr bee-ehn ehl pee-sah-rohn)*
Do you miss school a lot?	**¿Faltas mucho a la escuela?** *(Fahl-tahs moo-choh ah lah ehs-koo-eh-lah)*
Do you get distracted easily?	**¿Te distraes fácilmente?** *(Teh dees-trah-ehs fah-seel-mehn-teh)*
Who takes you to school?	**¿Quién te lleva a la escuela?** *(Kee-ehn teh yeh-bah ah lah ehs-koo-eh-lah)*
Do you walk to school?	**¿Caminas a la escuela?** *(Kah-mee-nahs ah lah ehs-koo-eh-lah)*
Do you eat breakfast/lunch?	**¿Tomas desayuno/almuerzo?** *(Toh-mahs deh-sah-yoo-noh/ahl-moo-ehr-soh)*
Do you have problems with your teeth?	**¿Tienes problemas con los dientes?** *(Tee-eh-nehs proh-bleh-mahs kohn lohs dee-ehn-tehs)*
At what time do you go to sleep?	**¿A qué hora te acuestas a dormir?** *(Ah keh oh-rah teh ah-koo-ehs-tahs ah dohr-meer)*
How many hours do you sleep?	**¿Cuántas horas duermes?** *(Koo-ahn-tahs oh-rahs doo-ehr-mehs)*
Do you wake up at night?	**¿Te despiertas en la noche?** *(Teh dehs-pee-ehr-tahs ehn lah noh-che)*
What house chores do you do?	**¿Qué quehaceres haces?** *(Keh keh-ah-seh-rehs ah-sehs)*
How do you feel?	**¿Cómo te sientes?** *(Koh-moh teh see-ehn-tehs)*

Have you been sick?	**¿Has estado enfermo/enferma?** *(Ahs ehs-tah-doh ehn-fehr-moh/ enferma)*
Is there anything that worries you?	**¿Hay algo que te preocupa?** *(Ah-ee ahl-goh keh teh preh-oh-koo-pah)*
Who do you talk to?	**¿Con quién hablas?** *(Kohn kee-ehn ah-blahs)*
Do you have questions?	**¿Tienes preguntas?** *(Tee-eh-nehs preh-goon-tahs)*
Thank you for talking to me!	**¡Gracias por hablar conmigo!** *(Grah-see-ahs pohr ah-blahr kohn-mee-goh)*
I will talk to your mother again.	**Hablaré con tu mamá otra vez.** *(Ah-blah-reh kohn too mah-mah oh-trah behs)*
Good-bye!	**¡Hasta luego!** *(Ahs-tah loo-eh-goh)*

Chapter Nine | Capítulo nueve

A Visit to the Cardiologist | Una visita al cardiólogo

Mrs. Ortiz is at the cardiologist's office. She was sent by her family doctor who found heart problems and hypertension.

La señora Ortiz está en el consultorio del cardiólogo. La envió su médico familiar porque encontró una alteración en su corazón y en su presión arterial.

Good morning, Mrs. Ortiz!	**¡Buenos días, señora Ortiz!** *(Boo-eh-nohs dee-ahs, seh-nyo-rah ohr-tees)*
—Good morning, doctor.	**—¡Buenos días, doctor!** *(Boo-eh-nohs dee-ahs, dohk-tohr)*
How old are you?	**¿Cuántos años tiene?** *(Koo-ahn-tohs ah-nyohs tee-eh-neh)*
—Forty-five years (old).	**—Cuarenta y cinco años.** *(Koo-ah-rehn-tah ee seen-koh ah-nyohs)*
Do you smoke?	**¿Fuma usted?** *(Foo-mah oo-stehd)*
—Yes.	**—Sí.** *(See)*
How many cigarettes per day?	**¿Cuántos cigarrillos al día?** *(Koo-ahn-tohs see-gah-ree-yohs ahl dee-ah)*
—Fifteen per day.	**—Quince al día.** *(Keen-seh ahl dee-ah)*
Do you have high blood pressure?	**¿Tiene la presión alta?** *(Tee-eh-neh lah preh-see-ohn ahl-tah)*
Do you have chest pain?	**¿Tiene dolor en el pecho?** *(Tee-eh-neh doh-lohr ehn ehl peh-choh)*
—Occasionally.	**—Ocasionalmente.** *(Oh-kah-see-ohn-ahl-mehn-teh)*

Palpitations?

¿Palpitaciones?
(Pahl-pee-tah-see-ohn-ehs)

—Once in a while.

—De vez en cuando.
(Deh behs ehn koo-ahn-doh)

Have you had pain in the left arm?

¿Ha sentido dolor en el brazo izquierdo?
(Ah sehn-tee-doh doh-lohr ehn ehl brah-soh ees-kee-ehr-doh)

—Yes, last week.

—Sí, la semana pasada.
(See, lah seh-mah-nah pah-sah-dah)

How long did it last?

¿Cuánto duró?
(Koo-ahn-toh doo-roh)

—Only five minutes.

—Sólo cinco minutos.
(Soh-loh seen-koh mee-noo-tohs)

When you have pain, do you get nauseated?

Cuando tiene dolor, ¿le da náuseas?
(Koo-ahn-doh tee-eh-neh doh-lohr, leh dah nah-oo-seh-ahs)

—No.

—No.
(Noh)

Do you have relatives with cardiac problems?

¿Tiene familiares con problemas cardíacos?
(Tee-eh-neh fah-mee-lee-ah-rehs kohn proh-bleh-mahs kahr-dee-ah-kohs)

—Yes, my dad.

—Sí, mi papá.
(See, mee pah-pah)

What happened to him?

¿Qué le pasó?
(Keh leh pah-soh)

—He had high cholesterol, and he had surgery.

—Tenía colesterol alto y le hicieron cirugía.
(Teh-nee-ah koh-lehs-teh-rohl ahl-toh ee leh ee-see-eh-rohn see-roo-hee-ah)

Have you had rheumatic fever?

¿Ha tenido fiebre reumática?
(Ah teh-nee-doh fee-eh-breh reh-oo-mah-tee-kah)

—No.

—No.
(Noh)

Have you had headaches?

¿Ha tenido dolor de cabeza?
(Ah teh-nee-doh doh-lohr deh kah-beh-sah)

—Often, two times per week.

—Seguido, dos veces por semana.
(Seh-gee-doh, dohs beh-sehs pohr seh-mah-nah)

Have you passed out?	**¿Se ha desmayado?** *(Seh ah dehs-mah-yah-doh)*
—No, never.	**—No, nunca.** *(Noh, noon-kah)*
Do you have dizzy spells?	**¿Tiene mareos?** *(Tee-eh-neh mah-reh-ohs)*
Swelling of the ankles?	**¿Hinchazón en los tobillos?** *(Een-chah-sohn ehn lohs toh-bee-yohs)*
—Yes, in the afternoon.	**—Sí, por la tarde.** *(See, pohr lah tahr-deh)*
Are you diabetic?	**¿Es diabética?** *(Ehs dee-ah-beh-tee-kah)*
—I am pre-diabetic. I control it with diet.	**—Soy prediabética. Me controlo con dieta.** *(Soh-ee preh-dee-ah-beh-tee-kah. Meh kohn-troh-loh kohn dee-eh-tah)*
Do you drink alcohol?	**¿Toma bebidas alcohólicas?** *(Toh-mah beh-bee-dahs ahl-koh-lee-kahs)*
—Only at parties.	**—Sólo en las fiestas.** *(Soh-loh ehn lahs fee-ehs-tahs)*

The cardiologist examines Mrs. Ortiz. He finds a blood pressure of 160/100, a splitting of the second heart sound, and jugular pulsation.

El cardiólogo examina a la señora Ortiz. Le encuentra presión de 160/100, un desdoblamiento del segundo ruido cardíaco y leve injurgitación de la yugular.

TABLE 9–1
Useful Words

TABLA 9–1
Palabras útiles

English	Spanish	Pronunciation
diabetes	**diabetes**	*(dee-ah-beh-tehs)*
electrocardiogram	**electrocardiograma**	*(eh-lehk-troh-kahr-dee-oh-grah-mah)*
general chemistry	**química sanguínea**	*(kee-mee-kah sahn-gee-neh-ah)*
jugular vein	**vena yugular**	*(beh-nah yoo-goo-lahr)*
pacemaker	**marcapasos**	*(mahr-kah-pah-sohs)*
palpitations	**palpitaciones**	*(pahl-pee-tah-see-oh-nehs)*
paralysis	**parálisis**	*(pah-rah-lee-sees)*
prescription	**receta**	*(reh-seh-tah)*
rheumatic fever	**fiebre reumática**	*(fee-eh-breh reh-oo-mah-tee-kah)*
swollen ankles	**tobillos hinchados**	*(toh-bee-yohs een-chah-dohs)*

TABLE 9–2
Useful Words

TABLA 9–2
Palabras útiles

English	**Spanish**	**Pronunciation**
aneurysm	**aneurisma**	*(ah-neh-oo-rees-mah)*
angina	**angina**	*(ahn-hee-nah)*
aorta	**aorta**	*(ah-ohr-tah)*
arteriosclerosis	**arterioesclerosis**	*(ahr-teh-ree-oh-ehs-kleh-roh-sees)*
chest pain	**dolor de pecho**	*(doh-lohr deh peh-choh)*
complete blood count	**biometría hemática**	*(bee-oh-meh-tree-ah eh-mah-tee-kah)*
dizzy spell	**desmayo/mareo**	*(dehs-mah-yoh/mah-reh-oh)*
headache	**dolor de cabeza**	*(doh-lohr deh kah-beh-sah)*
thrombus	**coágulo**	*(koh-ah-goo-loh)*

Mrs. Ortiz, you need to go to the hospital.

Señora Ortiz, necesita ir al hospital.
(Seh-nyoh-rah Ohr-tees, neh-seh-see-tah eer ahl ohs-pee-tahl)

I am going to order:
a complete blood count, general chemistry, urine, antiestreptolysin, throat culture, electrocardiogram, and chest X-ray.

Voy a ordenar:
química sanguínea completa, química general, orina, anti-estreptolicinas, exudado faríngeo, electrocardiograma radiografía de tórax.
(Boy ah ohr-deh-nahr: Kee-mee-kah sahn-gee-nee-ah kohm-pleh-tah, kee-mee-kah geh-neh-rahl, oh-ree-nah, ahn-tee-ehs-trehp-toh-lee-see-nahs, ehx-oo-dah-doh fah-reen-heh-oh, eh-lehk-troh-kahr-dee-oh-grah-mah ee rah-dee-oh-grah-fee-ah deh toh-rahx)

Mrs. Ortiz, take this pill every 8 hours for 10 days.

Señora Ortiz, tome esta pastilla cada ocho horas por diez días.
(Seh-nyoh-rah Ohr-tees, toh-meh ehs-tah pahs-tee-yah kah-dah oh-choh oh-rahs pohr dee-ehs dee-ahs)

I will let you know about the exams.

Le avisaré sobre los exámenes.
(Leh ah-bee-sah-reh soh-breh lohs ehx-ah-meh-nehs)

Chapter Ten | Capítulo diez

A Visit to the Endocrinologist

Una visita al endocrinólogo

The family doctor finds that his patient is a diabetic because of his symptoms and the results of the laboratory exams. He sends him to an endocrinologist who explains the following.

El médico familiar detecta que su paciente es diabético por sus síntomas y los resultados de laboratorio. Lo envía al endocrinólogo quien le explica lo siguiente.

Diabetes mellitus is characterized by the body's inability to utilize glucose.

La diabetes mellitus se caracteriza por la incapacidad del cuerpo para utilizar glucosa.

(Lah dee-ah-beh-tehs meh-lee-toos seh kah-rahk-teh-ree-sah pohr lah een-kah-pah-see-dahd dehl koo ehr-poh pah-rah oo-tee-lee-sahr gloo-koh-sah)

Diminished amounts of insulin to meet requirements is called non-insulin-dependent DM.

A la disminución de insulina requerida se le llama diabetes no-insulino-dependiente.

(Ah lah dees-mee-noo-see-ohn deh een-soo-lee-nah reh-keh-ree-dah seh leh yah-mah dee-ah-beh-tehs noh-een-soo-lee-noh-deh-pehn-dee-ehn-teh)

It is also an imbalance between the availability and the requirements of insulin.

Es también un desequilibrio entre la disponibilidad y los requerimientos de insulina.

(Ehs tahm-bee-ehn oon deh-seh-kee-lee-bree-oh ehn-treh la dees-poh-nee-bee-lee-dahd ee lohs reh-keh-ree-mee-ehn-tohs deh een-soo-lee-nah)

Absence of insulin in the body is called insulin-dependent DM.	**A la ausencia de insulina se le llama diabetes insulino-dependiente.** *(Ah lah ah-oo-sehn-see-ah deh een-soo-lee-nah seh leh yah-mah dee-ah-beh-tehs een-soo-lee-noh-deh-pehn-dee-ehn-teh)*

The endocrinologist continues to talk to the patient.
El endocrinólogo continúa hablando con el paciente.

I see from your history that weight has always been a problem.	**Veo en su historia que su peso siempre ha sido un problema.** *(Beh-oh ehn soo ees-toh-ree-ah keh soo peh-soh see-ehm-preh ah see-doh oon proh-bleh-mah)*
Is that right?	**¿Es cierto?** *(Ehs see-ehr-toh)*
—It has been.	**—Ha sido.** *(Ah see-doh)*
I see your sister and grandfather had diabetes.	**Veo que su hermana y abuelo tenían diabetes.** *(Beh-oh keh soo ehr-mah-nah ee ah-boo-eh-loh teh-nee-ahn dee-ah-beh-tehs)*
—My grandfather died from complications of an amputation because of DM.	**—Mi abuelo murió por complicaciones de una amputación debida a DM.** *(Mee ah-boo-eh-loh moo-ree-oh pohr kohm-plee-kah-see-oh-nehs deh oo-nah ahm-poo-tah-see-ohn deh-bee-dah ah DM)*
—My sister is now being treated.	**—Mi hermana está en tratamiento.** *(Mee ehr-mah-nah ehs-tah ehn trah-tah-mee-ehn-toh)*
How old are you?	**¿Cuántos años tiene?** *(Koo-ahn-tohs ah-nyohs tee-eh-neh)*
—I am 44 years old.	**—Tengo 44 años.** *(Tehn-goh koo-ah-rehn-tah ee koo-ah-troh ah-nyohs)*
Are you a smoker?	**¿Es fumador?** *(Ehs foo-mah-dohr)*
—Yes.	**—Sí.** *(See)*

How many packs a day?	**¿Cuántas cajetillas al día?** *(Koo-ahn-tahs kah-heh-tee-yahs ahl dee-ah)*
—One and a half.	**—Una y media.** *(Oo-nah ee meh-dee-ah)*
I want to do some testing.	**Quiero hacer una prueba.** *(Kee-eh-roh ah-sehr oon-ah proo-eh-bah)*
Have you had a fasting glucose level done?	**¿Le han hecho examen de glucosa en ayunas?** *(Leh ahn eh-choh ehx-ah-mehn deh gloo-koh-sah ehn ah-yoo-nahs)*
—No, I don't think so.	**—No, no lo creo.** *(Noh, noh loh kreh-oh)*
Tomorrow, at 7:00 A.M., go to the lab and have your blood drawn.	**Mañana a las siete vaya al laboratorio para tomar una muestra de sangre.** *(Mah-nyah-nah ah lahs see-eh-teh bah-yah ahl lah-boh-rah-toh-ree-oh pah-rah toh-mahr oo-nah moo-ehs-trah deh sahn-greh)*
—I can do that.	**—Puedo hacerlo.** *(Poo-eh-doh ah-sehr-loh)*
Be sure not eat or drink anything after 9:00 P.M.	**No tome nada después de las nueve de la noche.** *(Noh toh-meh nah-dah dehs-poo-ehs deh lahs noo-eh-beh deh lah noh-cheh)*

TABLE 10–1
Selected Words

TABLA 10–1
Palabras selectas

English	Spanish	Pronunciation
absence	**ausencia**	*(ah-oo-sehn-see-ah)*
available	**disponible**	*(dees-poh-nee-bleh)*
dependent	**dependiente**	*(deh-pehn-dee-ehn-teh)*
disorder	**desorden**	*(deh-sohr-dehn)*
hypoglycemia	**hipoglicemia**	*(ee-poh-glee-seh-mee-ah)*
ketoacidosis	**cetoacidosis**	*(seh-toh-ah-see-doh-sees)*
pathophysiology	**fisiopatología**	*(fee-see-oh-pah-toh-loh-gee-ah)*
requirements	**requerimiento**	*(reh-keh-ree-mee-ehn-toh)*
risk	**riesgo**	*(ree-ehs-goh)*
utilize	**utilizar**	*(oo-tee-lee-sahr)*

—Sure.	**—Seguro.** *(Seh-goo-roh)*
After the bloodwork, you may have your breakfast.	**Después de tomar la muestra, puede desayunar.** *(Dehs-poo-ehs deh toh-mahr lah moo-ehs-trah, poo-eh-deh deh-sah-yoo-nahr)*
—Great.	**—Bien.** *(Bee-ehn)*
Also, make an appointment for Wednesday.	**También, pida cita para el miércoles.** *(Tahm-bee-ehn, pee-dah see-tah pah-rah ehl mee-ehr-koh-lehs)*
—I will do that.	**—Lo haré.** *(Loh ah-reh)*
Please do the following:	**Por favor, haga lo siguiente:** *(Pohr fah-bohr ah-gah loh see-gee-ehn-teh)*
Take the medicines daily.	**Tome las medicinas diariamente.** *(Toh-meh lahs meh-dee-see-nahs dee-ah-ree-ah-mehn-teh)*
Eat a 1,500 calorie diet.	**Lleve la dieta de 1,500 calorías.** *(Yeh-beh lah dee-eh-tah deh meel-kee-nee-ehn-tahs kah-loh-ree-ahs)*
Keep a general hygiene: bath, nail cutting, sleep.	**Medidas de higiene general: baño, recorte de uñas, dormir.** *(Meh-dee-dahs deh ee-hee-eh-neh heh-neh-rahl: bah-nyo, reh-kohr-teh deh oo-nyahs, dohr-meer)*

TABLE 10–2
Selected Words

TABLA 10–2
Palabras selectas

English	Spanish	Pronunciation
glycosuria	**glucosuria**	*(gloo-koh-soo-ree-ah)*
lipoatrophy	**lipotrofia**	*(lee-poh-troh-fee-ah)*
nephropathy	**nefropatía**	*(neh-froh-pah-tee-ah)*
neuropathy	**neuropatía**	*(neh-oo-roh-pah-tee-ah)*
polydipsia	**polidipsia**	*(poh-lee-deep-see-ah)*
polyphagia	**polifagia**	*(poh-lee-fah-hee-ah)*
polyuria	**poliuria**	*(poh-lee-oo-ree-ah)*
retinopathy	**retinopatía**	*(reh-tee-noh-pah-tee-ah)*

Use comfortable clothes and shoes.	**Use ropa y zapatos cómodos.** *(Oo-seh roh-pah ee sah-pah-tohs koh-moh-dohs)*
Avoid scratching or cutting your skin.	**Evite rasguños o heridas en la piel.** *(Eh-bee-teh rahs-goo-nyohs oh eh-ree-dahs ehn lah pee-ehl)*
Exercise.	**Haga ejercicio.** *(Ah-gah eh-hehr-see-see-oh)*
Go to the dentist every six months.	**Vaya al dentista cada seis meses.** *(Bah-yah ahl dehn-tees-tah kah-dah seh-ees meh-sehs)*
Go to the ophthalmologist every year.	**Vaya al oftalmólogo cada año.** *(Bah-yah ahl ohf-tahl-moh-loh-goh kah-dah ah-nyoh)*

Chapter Eleven | Capítulo once

A Visit to the OB-GYN

Una visita al gineco-obstetra

Mrs. García visits the obstetrician when she finds out that she is pregnant. The doctor orders blood and urine exams to see the patient's health status. After examining her, he tells her the tentative date of delivery. He also gives her an appointment so she can learn about breast exams.

La señora García visita al gineco-obstetra cuando se entera de que está embarazada. El doctor le ordena los exámenes de sangre y orina para saber el estado de salud de la paciente. Después de examinarla le dice cuál será la fecha del parto. También le da una cita para que acuda a una plática sobre el cáncer de los senos.

Mrs. García is a 32-year-old woman who delivered a baby and the doctor is visiting her in her room. He tells her that she will be discharged tomorrow. He also tells her that she must follow directions carefully so that everything turns out all right.

La señora García, de 32 años, fue atendida en su parto y el doctor la visita en su cuarto. Le comunica que mañana le dará de alta. También le dice que debe seguir cuidadosamente las recomendaciones que se le den para que todo salga bien.

Mrs. García, tomorrow you will be discharged from the hospital.

Señora García, mañana sale usted del hospital.

(Seh-nyoh-rah Gahr-see-ah, mah-nyah-nah sah-leh oos-tehd dehl ohs-pee-tahl)

I will give you instructions for you and the baby.

Le daré instrucciones para usted y su bebé.

(Leh dah-reh eens-trook-see-ohn-ehs pah-rah oos-tehd ee soo beh-beh)

You will have to rest at least seven days.

Tendrá que guardar reposo al menos siete días.

(Tehn-drah keh goo-ahr-dahr reh-poh-soh ahl meh-nohs see-eh-teh dee-ahs)

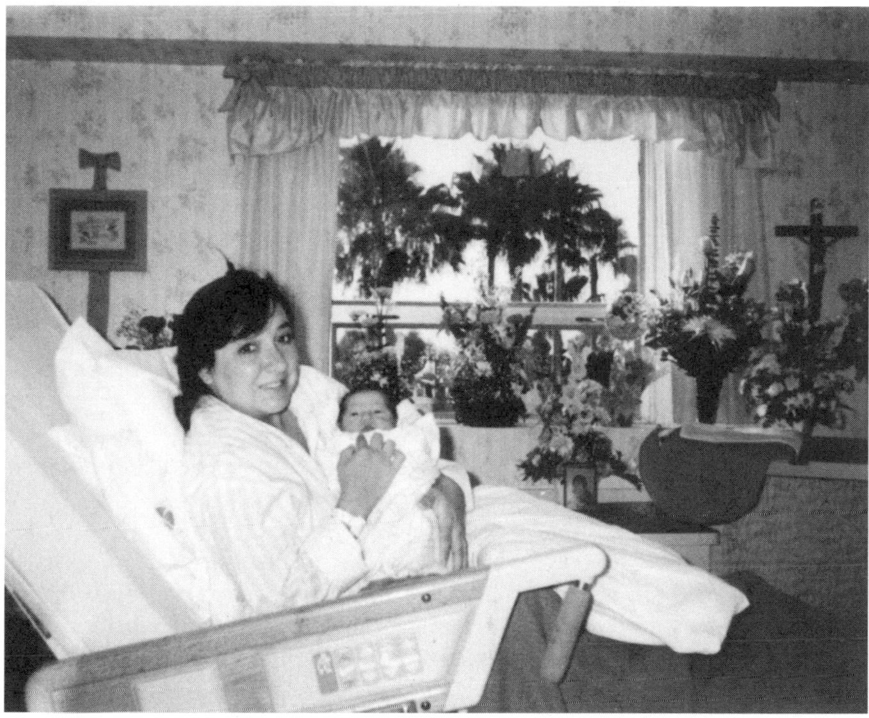

Figure 11–1 Discharge planning should start shortly after admission. Once the baby is born there are too many other issues to deal with.

TABLE 11–1 Discharge Recommendations

TABLA 11–1 Recomendaciones al dar de alta

English	Spanish	Pronunciation
birth control	**control de fertilidad**	*(kohn-trohl deh fehr-tee-lee-dahd)*
bleeding	**sangrado**	*(sahn-grah-doh)*
fats	**grasas**	*(grah-sahs)*
go	**acuda**	*(ah-koo-dah)*
hot sauces	**picante**	*(pee-kahn-teh)*
keep	**guardar**	*(goo-ahr-dahr)*
recommendations	**recomendaciones**	*(reh-koh-mehn-dah-see-ohn-ehs)*
rest	**reposo**	*(reh-poh-soh)*
will have	**tendrá**	*(tehn-drah)*
wound	**herida**	*(eh-ree-dah)*

Your diet should be low in fats and hot sauces.	**Su dieta debe ser baja en grasas y picantes.** *(Soo dee-eh-tah deh-beh sehr bah-hah ehn grah-sahs ee pee-kahn-tehs)*
Try to have a bowel movement every day.	**Procure hacer del baño diariamente.** *(Proh-koo-reh ah-sehr dehl bah-nyoh dee-ah-ree-ah-mehn-teh)*
Don't get constipated.	**No se deje estreñir.** *(Noh seh deh-heh ehs-treh-nyeer)*
Drink a lot of water and juices.	**Tome mucha agua y jugos.** *(Toh-meh moo-chah ah-goo-ah ee hoo-gohs)*
Watch that your wound doesn't get infected.	**Vigile que su herida no se infecte.** *(Bee-hee-leh keh soo eh-ree-dah noh seh een-fehk-teh)*
Watch your bleeding.	**Vigile su sangrado.** *(Bee-hee-leh soo sahn-grah-doh)*
If it is a lot, or there is fever, go to the hospital right away.	**Si es abundante, o aparece fiebre, acuda inmediatamente al hospital.** *(See ehs ah-boon-dahn-teh, oh ah-pah-reh-seh fee-eh-breh, ah-koo-dah een-meh-dee-ah-tah-mehn-teh ahl ohs-pee-tahl)*
Take a bath every day.	**Báñese todos los días.** *(Bah-nyeh-seh toh-dohs lohs dee-ahs)*
Clean your breasts thoroughly.	**Lave muy bien sus senos/pechos.** *(Lah-beh moo-eeh bee-ehn soohs seh-nohs/peh-chohs)*
Sleep at least six hours daily.	**Duerma por lo menos seis horas diarias.** *(Doo-ehr-mah pohr loh meh-nohs seh-ees oh-rahs dee-ah-ree-ahs)*
As soon as you can, go to your doctor for the birth control plan that you wish to use.	**En cuanto pueda, acuda a su doctor para el control de fertilidad que desee.** *(Ehn koo-ahn-toh poo-eh-dah, ah-koo-dah ah soo dok-tohr pah-rah ehl kohn-trohl deh fehr-tee-lee-dahd keh deh-seh-eh)*
About your baby. . .	**En cuanto a su bebé...** *(Ehn koo-ahn-toh ah soo beh-beh)*

Bathe him every day.	**Báñelo diariamente.** *(Bah-nyeh-loh dee-ah-ree-ah-mehn-teh)*
Watch his navel.	**Vigile su ombligo.** *(Bee-hee-leh soo ohm-blee-goh)*
Clean your nipples before you breastfeed.	**Lave sus pezones antes de dar pecho.** *(Lah-beh soos peh-soh-nehs ahn-tehs deh dahr peh-choh)*
Breast feed or give a bottle every three hours.	**Dé pecho o biberón cada tres horas.** *(Deh-leh peh-choh oh bee-beh-rohn kah-dah trehs oh-rahs)*
Help him to burp.	**Póngalo a repetir/eructar.** *(Pohn-gah-loh ah reh-peh-teer/eh-rook-tahr)*
Pat his back gently.	**Dé palmaditas en la espalda.** *(Deh pahl-mah-dee-tahs ehn lah ehs-pahl-dah)*
Watch his urine and his bowel movements.	**Vigile su orina y sus evacuaciones.** *(Bee-hee-leh sooh oh-ree-nah ee soos eh-bah-koo-ah-see-oh-nehs)*
Watch that his nose is clear.	**Vigile que su naríz esté libre.** *(Bee-hee-leh keh soo nah-rees ehs-teh lee-breh)*
Dress him with loose clothes.	**Póngale ropa cómoda.** *(Pohn-gah-leh roh-pah koh-moh-dah)*
Take him for vaccinations at two months.	**Llévelo a vacunar a los dos meses.** *(Yeh-beh-loh ah bah-koo-nahr ah lohs dohs meh-sehs)*
Watch his growth and development.	**Vigile su crecimiento y desarrollo.** *(Bee-hee-leh soo kreh-see-mee-ehn-toh ee deh-sah-roh-yoh)*
If you see anything wrong, take him to the doctor.	**Si nota algo malo, llévelo a su doctor.** *(See noh-tah ahl-goh mah-loh, yeh-beh-loh ah soo dohk-torh)*

TABLE 11–2 **Useful Words**	**TABLA 11–2** **Palabras útiles**	
English	**Spanish**	**Pronunciation**
burp	**repetir/eructar**	*(reh-peh-teer)/(eh-rook-tahr)*
development	**desarrollo**	*(deh-sah-roh-yoh)*
growth	**crecimiento**	*(kreh-see-mee-ehn-toh)*
I will see you	**la veré**	*(lah beh-reh)*
loose clothes	**ropa cómoda**	*(roh-pah koh-moh-dah)*
navel	**ombligo**	*(ohm-blee-goh)*
placing it	**colocándolo**	*(koh-loh-kahn-doh-loh)*
successful	**con éxito**	*(kohn ehx-ee-toh)*
vaccinations	**vacunas**	*(bah-koo-nahs)*

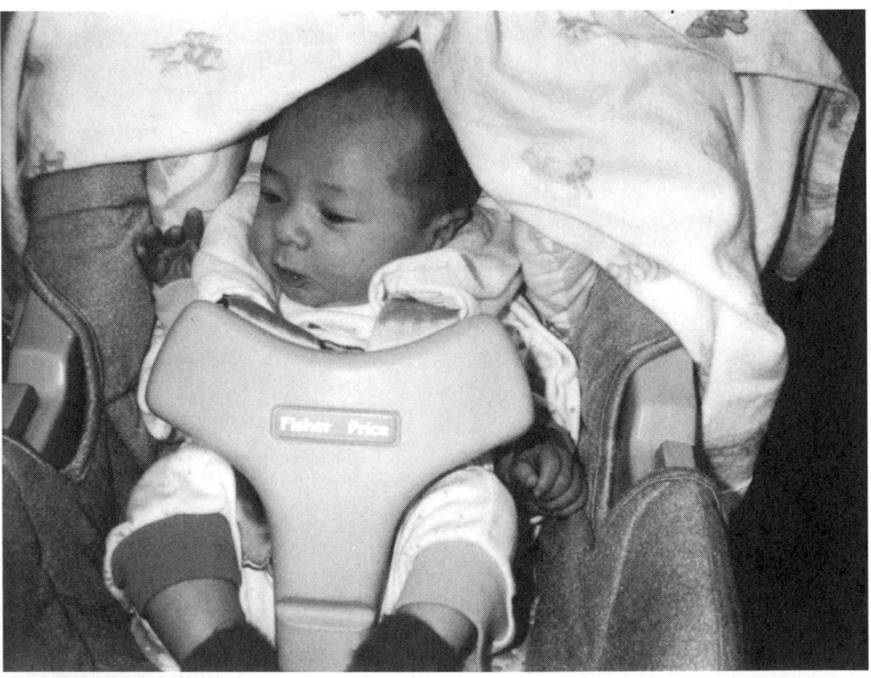

Figure 11–2 It is important to give mom written recommendations for the baby when she leaves the hospital.

If you follow these recommendations, everything will be all right.	**Si usted sigue estos consejos, todo saldrá con éxito.** *(See oos-tehd see-geh ehs-tohs kohn-seh-hohs, toh-doh sahl-drah kohn ehx-ee-toh)*
I will see you, Mrs. García.	**Hasta luego, señora García.** *(Ahs-tah loo-eh-goh, seh-nyoh-rah Gahr-see-ah)*
I will see you tomorrow.	**La veré mañana.** *(Lah beh-reh mah-nyah-nah)*

Mrs. García attends a talk that her doctor recommended. The talk is on the subject of cancer.

La señora García acude a la plática que le recomendó el doctor. La plática es sobre el cáncer.

More than 200 diseases have been identified as cancer. They are classified as such because they share common characteristics, progress in similar manner, and are treated similarly. The American Cancer Society defines cancer as a large group of diseases characterized by uncontrolled growth and spread of abnormal cells.

Más de 200 enfermedades se han identificado como cáncer. Se clasifican según sus características comunes, su progresión de manera semejante y su tratamiento similar. La Sociedad Americana de Cáncer define al cáncer como un grupo grande de enfermedades caracterizadas por un crecimiento anormal de las células.

TABLE 11–3 Selected Words — **TABLA 11–3 Palabras selectas**

English	Spanish	Pronunciation
characteristics	**características**	*(kahr-ahk-teh-rees-tee-kahs)*
classification	**clasificación**	*(klah-see-fee-kah-see-ohn)*
classified	**clasificado**	*(klah-see-fee-kah-doh)*
classify	**clasifique**	*(klah-see-fee-keh)*
detect	**descubra**	*(dehs-koo-brah)*
detection	**detección**	*(deh-tehk-see-ohn)*
diagnostic	**diagnóstico**	*(dee-ahg-nohs-tee-koh)*
identified	**identificado**	*(ee-dehn-tee-fee-kah-doh)*
illness	**enfermedad**	*(ehn-fehr-meh-dahd)*
terminal	**terminal**	*(tehr-mee-nahl)*

TABLE 11–4
Selected Words

TABLA 11–4
Palabras selectas

English	Spanish	Pronunciation
abnormal	**anormal**	*(ah-nohr-mahl)*
benign	**benigno**	*(beh-neeg-noh)*
cancer	**cáncer**	*(kahn-sehr)*
change	**cambio**	*(kahm-bee-oh)*
chemotherapy	**quimioterapia**	*(kee-mee-oh-tehr-ah-pee-ah)*
common	**común**	*(koh-moon)*
early	**temprano**	*(tehm-prah-no)*
growth	**crecimiento**	*(kreh-see-mee-ehn-toh)*
progression	**progresión**	*(proh-greh-see-ohn)*
similar	**similar**	*(see-mee-lahr)*

Pay attention to the following signs so you can detect cancer early.

Preste atención a las siguientes señas para que detecte el cáncer oportunamente.
(Prehs-teh ah-tehn-see-ohn ah lahs see-gee-ehn-tehs seh-nyahs pah-rah keh deh-tehk-teh ehl kahn-sehr oh-pohr-too-nah-mehn-teh)

1. Change in bowel or bladder habits.
   1. Cambio en el hábito de la orina o el excremento.
   (Kahm-bee-oh ehn ehl ah-bee-toh deh lah oh-ree-nah oh ehl ehx-kreh-mehn-toh)
2. A sore that does not heal.
   2. Un grano que no se cura.
   (Oon grah-noh keh noh seh koo-rah)
3. Unusual bleeding or discharge.
   3. Sangrado o flujo profuso.
   (Sahn-grah-doh oh floo-hoh proh-foo-soh)
4. Lump in breast or elsewhere.
   4. Bolita en el pecho o en otra parte.
   (Boh-lee-tah ehn ehl peh-choh oh ehn oh-trah pahr-teh)
5. Indigestion or difficulty swallowing.
   5. Indigestión o dificultad al tragar.
   (Een-dee-hehs-tee-ohn oh dee-fee-kool-tahd ahl trah-gahr)

6. Change in wart or mole.	**6. Cambio en verruga o lunar.** *(Kahm-bee-oh ehn loo-nahr oh beh-ruh-gah)*
7. Nagging cough or horseness.	**7. Tos persistente o afónico.** *(Tohs pehr-sees-tehn-teh oh ah-foh-nee-koh)*
Other recommendations for Mrs. García include:	**Otras recomendaciones para la señora García incluyen:** *(Oh-trahs reh-koh-mehn-dah-see-oh-nehs pah-rah lah sehn-yohr-ah Gahr-see-ah een-kloo-yehn)*
Perform monthly breast self exam.	**Haga un autoexamen del pecho cada mes.** *(Ah-gah-seh oon ah-oo-toh-ehx-ah-mehn dehl peh-choh kah-dah mehs)*
Have a yearly Pap smear.	**Haga una prueba de papanicolau cada año.** *(Ah-gah oo-nah proo-eh-bah deh pah-pah-nee-koh-lah-oo kah-dah ah-nyoh)*
For men: watch urinary problems, evaluate yearly the size of the prostrate.	**En hombres: vigile los problemas de la orina, haga el examen de la próstata cada año.** *(Ehn ohm-brehs: bee-hee-leh lohs proh-bleh-mahs deh lah oh-ree-nah, ah-gah ehl ehx-ah-mehn deh lah prohs-tah-tah kah-dah ah-nyoh)*

TABLE 11–5
Selected Words

TABLA 11–5
Palabras selectas

English	Spanish	Pronunciation
endoscopy	**endoscopia**	*(ehn-dohs-koh-pee-ah)*
surgeon	**cirujano**	*(see-roo-hah-noh)*
surgery	**cirugía**	*(see-roo-hee-ah)*
terms	**términos**	*(tehr-mee-nohs)*
tests	**pruebas**	*(proo-eh-bahs)*
tissue	**tejido**	*(teh-hee-doh)*
treatment	**tratamiento**	*(trah-tah-mee-ehn-toh)*
tumor	**tumor**	*(too-mohr)*
warning	**advertencia**	*(ahd-behr-tehn-see-ah)*

TABLE 11–6
Selected Words

TABLA 11–6
Palabras selectas

English	Spanish	Pronunciation
emergencies	**emergencias**	*(eh-mehr-hehn-see-ahs)*
examinations	**exámenes**	*(ehx-ah-meh-nehs)*
factors	**factores**	*(fahk-toh-rehs)*
imaging	**imagen**	*(ee-mah-hehn)*
laboratory	**laboratorio**	*(lah-boh-rah-toh-ree-oh)*
magnetic	**magnético**	*(mahg-neh-tee-koh)*
malignant	**maligno**	*(mah-leeg-noh)*
modifiers	**modificadores**	*(moh-dee-fee-kah-doh-rehs)*
oncology	**oncología**	*(ohn-koh-loh-hee-ah)*
prevention	**prevención**	*(preh-behn-see-ohn)*
radiologic	**radiológico**	*(rah-dee-oh-loh-hee-koh)*
radiotherapy	**radioterapia**	*(rah-dee-oh-teh-rah-pee-ah)*
recovery	**recuperación**	*(reh-koo-peh-rah-see-ohn)*
rehabilitation	**rehabilitación**	*(reh-ah-bee-lee-tah-see-ohn)*
resonance	**resonancia**	*(reh-sohn-ahn-see-ah)*
risk	**riesgo**	*(ree-ehs-goh)*
signs	**señales**	*(seh-nyah-lehs)*
sites	**sitios**	*(see-tee-ohs)*
studies	**estudios**	*(ehs-too-dee-ohs)*

Some forms of cancer are curable. Methods employed to detect cancer include physical exams, magnetic resonance imaging (MRI), or blood samples. Once the cancer is detected, treatment such as chemotherapy or radiotherapy is initiated. Many factors influence the recovery period. For some people, rehabilitation is difficult.

Algunas formas de cáncer son curables. Los métodos que se emplean para detectar el cáncer incluyen exámenes físicos, la imagen de resonancia magnética y muestras de sangre. Una vez que se detecta el cáncer, tratamiento tal como la quimioterapia o radioterapia se inicia. Muchos factores influencian el periodo de recuperación. Para algunas personas la rehabilitación es difícil.

Chapter Twelve — Capítulo doce

Amputations — Amputaciones

There are approximately 420,000 amputees in the United States with an annual increase of about 5%. The majority of these amputations are lower extremity amputations. Amputations can be performed through the joint or the bone itself. The term for an amputation through the joint is called disarticulation. General sites of the amputation are described by the joint nearest to the location of the amputation (i.e., lower shin or calf amputation is called below-the-knee amputation).

Hay aproximadamente 420,000 (cuatrocientos veinte mil) amputados en los Estados Unidos con un crecimiento anual de aproximadamente 5 por ciento. La mayoría de estas amputaciones son más frecuentes en extremidades inferiores. Se pueden ejecutar amputaciones por las articulaciones o el hueso mismo. El término de una amputación por la articulación se llama desarticulación. Los sitios generales de la amputación son descritos por la articulación cercana a la amputación (por ejemplo, la operación abajo de la rodilla es llamada amputación de la pantorrilla).

Dialogue:	**Diálogo:** *(Dee-ah-loh-goh)*
—Good morning, doctor!	**—¡Buenos días, doctor!** *(Boo-eh-nohs dee-ahs, dohk-tohr)*
—I have looked at the information we discussed yesterday.	**—He revisado la información que discutimos ayer.** *(Heh reh-bee-sah-doh lah een-fohr-mah-see-ohn keh dees-koo-tee-mohs ah-yehr)*
Good morning, Ms. Martinez.	**Buenos días, señorita Martínez.** *(Boo-eh-nohs dee-ahs, seh-nyoh-ree-tah Mahr-tee-nehs)*
We will start with diagnostic studies to assess how severe your problem might be.	**Empezaremos con estudios para evaluar la gravedad de su problema.**

(Ehm-peh-sah-reh-mohs kohn ehs-too-dee-ohs pah-rah eh-bah-loo-ahr lah grah-beh-dahd deh soo pro-bleh-mah)

We will begin with the use of angiography.

Comenzaremos con el estudio de angiografía.

(Koh-mehn-sah-reh-mohs kohn ehl ehs-too-dee-oh deh ahn-gee-oh-grah-fee-ah)

—What is that?

—¿Qué es eso?

(Keh ehs eh-soh)

It is a procedure used to see how open the veins are throughout the leg.

Es un procedimiento para valorar las venas de su pierna.

(Ehs oon proh-seh-dee-mee-ehn-toh pah-rah bah-loh-rahr lahs beh-nahs deh soo pee-ehr-nah)

—How is it done?

—¿Cómo se hace?

(Koh-moh seh ah-seh)

We inject a radioactive dye into the blood vessels and view the flow of blood through the vessels.

Se inyecta un medio de contraste en los vasos sanguíneos y se valora el flujo de la sangre por las venas.

(Seh een-yehk-tah oon meh-dee-oh deh kohn-trahs-teh ehn lohs bah-sohs sahn-ghee-neh-ohs ee seh bah-lor-ah ehl floo-ho deh lah sahn-greh pohr lahs beh-nahs)

—Can I be poisoned by the radiation?

¿Puedo ser dañada por la radiación?

(Poo-eh-doh sehr dah-nyah-dah pohr lah rah-dee-ah-see-ohn)

No. We control the amount of radiation you receive. We know which limits to trace throughout your system.

No. Controlamos la cantidad de radiación que recibe. Sabemos qué límites hay que seguir por todo el sistema.

(Noh. Kohn-troh-lah-mohs lah kahn-tee-dahd deh rah-dee-ah-see-ohn keh reh-see-beh. Sah-beh-mohs keh lee-mee-tehs ah-ee keh seh-gheer pohr toh-doh ehl sees-teh-mah)

I need for you to sign this permission slip so that the procedure might be done.

Necesito que firme usted el permiso, para realizar este estudio.

(Neh-seh-see-toh keh feer-meh oos-tehd ehl pehr-mee-soh, pah-rah reh-ah-lee-sahr ehs-teh ehs-too-dee-oh)

TABLE 12–1
Selected Words

TABLA 12–1
Palabras selectas

English	Spanish	Pronunciation
amputation	**amputación**	*(ahm-poo-tah-see-ohn)*
amputee	**amputado**	*(ahm-poo-tah-doh)*
care	**cuidado**	*(koo-ee-dah-doh)*
clinical	**clínico**	*(klee-nee-koh)*
complication	**complicación**	*(cohm-plee-kah-see-ohn)*
diagnostic	**diagnóstico**	*(dee-ahg-nohs-tee-koh)*
elderly	**anciano**	*(ahn-see-ah-noh)*
emergency	**emergencia**	*(eh-mehr-hen-see-ah)*
incidence	**incidencia**	*(een-see-dehn-see-ah)*
indications	**indicaciones**	*(een-dee-kah-see-oh-nehs)*
interventions	**intervenciones**	*(een-tehr-behn-see-ohn-ehs)*
management	**manejo**	*(mah-neh-hoh)*
medical	**médico**	*(meh-dee-koh)*

Do you have any further questions?

¿Tiene más preguntas que hacer?
(Tee-eh-neh mahs preh-goon-tahs keh ah-sehr)

—Not right now, but I will discuss it with my family.

—No por ahora, pero lo discutiré con mi familia.
(Noh pohr ah-oh-rah, peh-roh loh dees-koo-tee-reh kohn mee fah-mee-lee-ah)

If they have further questions, Ms. Brown is your nurse and she will be able to answer them. If you have additional questions, call me and I will return and answer them all.

Si tienen más preguntas que hacer, la señorita Brown es su enfermera y podrá contestarlas. Si tiene preguntas adicionales, llámeme y vendré para contestarlas.
(See tee-eh-nehn mahs preh-goon-tahs keh ah-sehr, lah seh-nyoh-ree-tah Brown ehs soo ehn-fehr-meh-rah ee poh-drah kohn-tehs-tahr-lahs. See tee-eh-neh preh-goon-tahs ah-dee-see-oh-nah-lehs, yah-meh-meh ee behn-dreh pah-rah kohn-tehs-tahr-lahs)

—Thank you, doctor.

—Gracias, doctor.
(Grah-see-ahs dohk-tohr)

You are welcome.

De nada.
(Deh nah-dah)

TABLE 12–2 Selected Words | **TABLA 12–2 Palabras selectas**

English	Spanish	Pronunciation
nurse	**enfermera**	*(ehn-fehr-meh-rah)*
patient	**paciente**	*(pah-see-ehn-teh)*
phases	**fases**	*(fah-sehs)*
postoperative	**postoperatorio**	*(pohst-oh-peh-rah-toh-ree-oh)*
preoperative	**preoperatorio**	*(preh-oh-peh-rah-toh-ree-oh)*
procedures	**procedimientos**	*(proh-seh-dee-mee-ehn-tohs)*
replantation	**reimplantación**	*(reh-eehm-plahn-tah-see-ohn)*
surgery	**cirugía**	*(see-roo-hee-ah)*
surgical	**quirúrgico**	*(kee-roor-hee-koh)*
tests	**pruebas**	*(proo-eh-bahs)*
treatment	**tratamiento**	*(trah-tah-mee-ehn-toh)*
types	**tipos**	*(tee-pohs)*

Some of the issues that need to be discussed with the patient are listed below.

Algunos de los puntos que se necesitan discutir con el paciente están listados abajo.

Indications and incidence.	**Indicaciones e incidencias.** *(Een-dee-kah-see-oh-nehs eh een-see-dehn-see-ahs)*
Diagnostic tests and procedures.	**Pruebas de diagnóstico y procedimientos.** *(Proo-eh-bahs deh dee-ahg-nohs-tee-koh ee proh-seh-dee-mee-ehn-tohs)*
Medical and surgical treatment.	**Tratamiento médico y quirúrgico.** *(Trah-tah-mee-ehn-toh meh-dee-koh ee kee-roor-hee-koh)*
Complications.	**Complicaciones.** *(Kohm-plee-kah-see-oh-nehs)*
Nursing care of the patient.	**Cuidados del paciente.** *(Koo-ee-dah-dohs dehl pah-see-ehn-teh)*
Replantation.	**Reimplantación.** *(Reh-eem-plahn-tah-see-ohn)*
Indications.	**Indicaciones.** *(Een-dee-kah-see-oh-nehs)*

TABLE 12–3 Selected Words | **TABLA 12–3 Palabras selectas**

English	Spanish	Pronunciation
anatomic position	**posición anatómica**	*(poh-see-see-ohn ah-nah-toh-mee-kah)*
blood flow	**circulación sanguínea**	*(seer-koo-lah-see-ohn sahn-gee-neh-ah)*
blood stream	**arroyo de la sangre**	*(ah-roh-yoh deh lah sahn-greh)*
broken bone	**hueso* roto**	*(oo-eh-soh roh-toh)*
closed reduction	**reducción cerrada**	*(reh-dook-see-ohn seh-rah-dah)*
Colles' fracture	**fractura de Colles**	*(frahk-too-rah deh Koh-yehs)*
comminuted fractures	**fracturas conminutas**	*(frahk-too-rahs kohn-mee-noo-tahs)*
compound fractures	**fracturas compuestas**	*(frahk-too-rahs kohm-poo-ehs-tahs)*
diagnostic procedures	**procedimientos de diagnóstico**	*(proh-seh-dee-mee-ehn-tohs deh dee-ahg-nohs-tee-koh)*
diagnostic tests	**pruebas de diagnóstico**	*(proo-eh-bahs deh dee-ahg-nohs-tee-koh)*
hip fracture	**fractura de cadera**	*(frahk-too-rah deh kah-dehr-ah)*

*Note that the **h** is always silent.

Emergency care.

Cuidado de emergencia.
(Koo-ee-dah-doh deh eh-mehr-hehn-see-ah)

Nursing care of the patient having replantation surgery is very important to assure a successful outcome. Listed below are some key goals.

El cuidado de enfermería en el paciente que tiene cirugía de reimplantación es muy importante para asegurar la recuperación. Listadas abajo están algunas metas clave.

1. Identify clinical indications for amputations.

1. Identifique las indicaciones clínicas para amputaciones.
(Ee-dehn-tee-fee-keh lahs een-dee-kah-see-oh-nehs klee-nee-kahs pah-rah ahm-poo-tah-see-oh-nehs)

TABLE 12–4
Selected Words

TABLA 12–4
Palabras selectas

English	Spanish	Pronunciation
immature bone	**hueso* inmaduro**	*(oo-eh-soh een-mah-doo-roh)*
major complications	**complicaciones mayores**	*(kohm-plee-kah-see-oh-nes mah-yoh-rehs)*
mature bone	**hueso* maduro**	*(oo-eh-soh mah-doo-roh)*
medical treatment	**tratamiento médico**	*(trah-tah-mee-ehn-toh meh-dee-koh)*
open reduction	**reducción abierta**	*(reh-dook-see-ohn ah-bee-ehr-tah)*
patient walkers	**pacientes con andadera**	*(pah-see-ehn-tehs kohn ahn-dah-deh-rah)*
pelvic fracture	**fractura pélvica**	*(frahk-too-rah pehl-bee-kah)*
prolonged stress	**tensión prolongada**	*(tehn-see-ohn proh-lohn-gah-dah)*
pulmonary hypertension	**hipertensión pulmonar**	*(ee-pehr-tehn-see-ohn pool-moh-nahr)*
therapeutic measures	**medidas terapéuticas**	*(meh-dee-dahs teh-rah-peh-oo-tee-kahs)*
tissue damage	**daño del tejido**	*(dah-nyoh dehl teh-hee-doh)*
types of fractures	**tipos de fracturas**	*(tee-pohs deh frak-too-rahs)*

*Note that the **h** is always silent.

2. Describe different types of amputations.

2. Describa los diferentes tipos de amputaciones.
(Dehs-kree-bah lohs dee-feh-rehn-tehstee-pohs deh ahm-poo-tah-see-oh-nehs)

3. Discuss medical and surgical management of the amputated patient.

3. Discuta el manejo médico y quirúrgico del paciente amputado.
(Dees-koo-tah ehl mah-neh-hoh meh-dee-koh ee kee-roor-hee-koh dehl pah-see-ehn-teh ahm-poo-tah-doh)

4. Identify appropriate nursing interventions during the preoperative and postoperative phases of care.

4. Identifique las intervenciones y cuidados del paciente en el proceso preoperatorio y postoperatorio.

(Ee-dehn-tee-fee-keh lahs een-tehr-behn-see-oh-nehs ee koo-eeh-dah-dohs dehl pah-see-ehn-teh ehn ehl proh-seh-soh preh-oh-peh-rah-toh-ree-oh ee pohst-oh-peh-rah-toh-ree-oh)

5. Use the nursing process to develop a plan of care.

5. Use el proceso de enfermería para desarrollar un plan de cuidado.

(Oo-seh ehl proh-seh-soh deh ehn-fehr-meh-ree-ah pah-rah deh-sah-roh-yahr oon plahn deh koo-ee-dah-doh)

6. Try to ask about the surgery.

6. Procure pedir informes sobre la cirugía.

(Proh-koo-reh peh-deer een-fohr-mehs soh-breh lah see-roo-hee-ah)

7. Ask about rehabilitation.

7. Pregunte sobre la rehabilitación.

(Preh-goon-teh soh-breh lah reh-ah-bee-lee-tah-see-ohn)

8. Ask if you will use devices, prosthesis, or crutches.

8. Pregunte si va a usar aparatos, prótesis o muletas.

(Preh-goon-teh see bah ah oo-sahr ah-pah-rah-tohs, proh-teh-sees oh moo-leh-tahs)

9. Assess hemodynamic status.

9. Evalúe el estado hemodinámico.

(Eh-bah-loo-eh ehl ehs-tah-doh ee-moh-dee-nah-mee-koh)

10. Administer intravenous fluids and blood.

10. Administre sueros intravenosos y sangre.

(Ahd-mee-nees-treh soo-eh-rohs ee sahn-greh)

11. Assess circulatory status: color, capillary refill, coolness.

11. Evalúe el estado circulatorio: color, relleno capilar, piel fría.

(Eh-bah-loo-eh ehl ehs-tah-doh seer-koo-lah-toh-ree-oh: koh-lohr, reh-yeh-noh kah-pee-lahr, pee-ehl free-ah)

12. Elevate the limb to promote venous and lymphatic drainage.

12. Eleve el miembro para promover el desagüe venoso y linfático.

(Eh-leh-beh ehl mee-ehm-broh pah-rah proh-moh-behr ehl deh-sah goo-eh beh-noh-soh ee leen-fah-tee-koh)

TABLE 12–5
Selected Words

TABLA 12–5
Palabras selectas

English	Spanish	Pronunciation
alignment	**alineación**	*(ah-lee-neh-ah-see-ohn)*
angulation	**angulación**	*(ahn-goo-lah-see-ohn)*
assessment	**evalúo**	*(eh-bah-loo-oh)*
canes	**bastones**	*(bahs-toh-nehs)*
casts	**lanzamientos**	*(lahn-sah-mee-ehn-tohs)*
cells	**células**	*(seh-loo-lahs)*
complications	**complicaciones**	*(kohm-plee-kah-see-ohn-ehs)*
continuity	**continuidad**	*(kohn-tee-noo-ee-dahd)*
crutches	**muletas**	*(moo-leh-tahs)*
debris	**restos**	*(rehs-tohs)*
diagnosis	**diagnóstico**	*(dee-ahg-nohs-tee-koh)*
embolism	**embolia**	*(ehm-boh-lee-ah)*
etiology	**etiología**	*(eh-tee-oh-loh-hee-ah)*
evaluation	**evaluación**	*(eh-bah-loo-ah-see-ohn)*
external	**externo**	*(ehx-tehr-noh)*
fat	**gordura**	*(gohr-doo-rah)*
fixation	**fijación**	*(fee-hah-see-ohn)*
fractures	**fracturas**	*(frahk-too-rahs)*
fragments	**fragmentos**	*(frahg-mehn-tohs)*
goals	**metas**	*(meh-tahs)*

13. Observe blood pressure, pulse, and the level or urine.

13. Observe la presión de la sangre, el pulso y el nivel de la orina.
(Ohb-sehr-beh lah preh-see-ohn deh lah sahn-greh, ehl pool-soh ee ehl nee-behl deh lah oh-ree-nah)

14. Observe the patient's mental status.

14. Observe el estado mental del paciente.
(Ohb-sehr-beh ehl ehs-tah-doh mehn-tahl dehl pah-see-ehn-teh)

15. Allow time for ventilation of feelings.

15. Permita tiempo para ventilar sentimientos.
(Pehr-mee-tah tee-ehm-poh pah-rah behn-tee-lahr sehn-tee-mee-ehn-tohs)

16. Assure that family is informed of patient care.

16. Asegure que la familia esté informada sobre el cuidado del paciente.

(Ah-seh-goo-reh keh lah fah-mee-lee-ah ehs-teh een-fohr-mah-dah soh-breh ehl koo-ee-dah-doh dehl pah-see-ehn-teh)

17. Prepare discharge planning.

17. Prepare el plan para dar de alta. ***(Preh-pah-reh ehl plahn pah-rah dahr deh ahl-tah)***

Below, find definitions of procedures that will help you when explaining the surgical interventions or obtaining surgical permits prior to the surgery.

Abajo, encuentre definiciones sobre procedimientos que le ayudarán cuando explique las intervenciones quirúrgicas o al obtener permiso para la cirugía.

Amputation Removal of a limb, part of a limb, or an organ; may be done by surgical means or in an accident.

Amputación **Quitar un miembro, parte de un miembro o un órgano; se puede hacer por medios quirúrgicos o en un accidente.**

Amputee Individual who has undergone an amputation.

Amputado **Individuo que ha sufrido una amputación.**

Bone remodeling Process in which immature bone cells are gradually replaced by mature bone cells.

Remodelación del hueso **Proceso en el que se reemplazan gradualmente las células inmaduras del hueso por células maduras.**

Closed amputation Amputation in which a limb or part of a limb is removed and surgically closed.

Amputación cerrada **Amputación en la que un miembro o parte de un miembro se quita y se cierra.**

Closed or *simple fracture* Fracture in which the broken bone does not break through the skin.

Fractura simple **o** ***cerrada*** **Es la fractura en la que el hueso no rompe la piel.**

Closed reduction or *manipulation* Nonsurgical realignment of the bones to their previous anatomic position using traction, angulation, rotation, or a combination of these.

Manipulación o reducción cerrada **Es la alineación del hueso a su posición anatómica sin cirugía, usando previamente tracción, angulación, rotación o una combinación de éstos.**

Compartment syndrome Serious complication of a fracture caused by internal or external pressure to the affected area, resulting in decreased blood flow, pain, and tissue damage.

Síndrome del compartimiento **Complicación seria de una fractura causada por una presión interna o externa, que da como resultado disminución del flujo sanguíneo, dolor y daño en los tejidos.**

Complete fracture Fracture in which the break extends across the entire bone, dividing it into two separate pieces.

Fractura completa **Fractura en la que el espacio se extiende por el hueso, dividiéndolo en dos pedazos separados.**

Congenital amputation Deformity or absence of a limb or limbs that occurs during fetal development in the uterus.

Amputación congénita **Deformidad o ausencia de un miembro o miembros que ocurre durante desarrollo fetal en el útero.**

TABLE 12–6
Selected Words

TABLA 12–6
Palabras selectas

English	**Spanish**	**Pronunciation**
heal	**sano**	*(sah-noh)*
healing	**curación**	*(koo-rah-see-ohn)*
hip	**cadera**	*(kah-deh-rah)*
incision	**incisión**	*(een-see-see-ohn)*
infection	**infección**	*(een-fehk-see-ohn)*
internal	**interior**	*(een-teh-ree-ohr)*
interventions	**intervenciones**	*(een-tehr-behn-see-oh-nehs)*
lungs	**pulmones**	*(pool-moh-nehs)*
marrow	**médula**	*(meh-doo-lah)*
migrate	**emigrar**	*(eh-mee-grahr)*

Delayed union Fracture healing that does not occur in the normally expected time.

Retardo en la unión **La curación de la fractura que no ocurre en el tiempo normalmente esperado.**

Fat embolism Condition in which fat globules are released from the marrow of the broken bone into the blood stream, migrate to the lungs, and cause pulmonary hypertension.

Embolia de grasa **Condición en la que glóbulos grasosos se desprenden de la médula del hueso roto hacia la corriente sanguínea, emigrando hacia los pulmones, causando hipertensión pulmonar.**

Fixation Procedure done during the open reduction surgical procedure to attach the fragments of the broken bone together when reduction alone is not feasible.

Fijación **Procedimiento hecho durante la cirugía de reducción abierta para atar juntos los fragmentos del hueso roto cuando sólo la reducción no es factible.**

Fracture Break or disruption in the continuity of a bone.

Fractura **Descanso o ruptura en la continuidad de un hueso.**

Gangrene Necrosis or death of tissue, usually due to a deficient or absent blood supply; may result from inflammatory processes, injury, arteriosclerosis, frostbite, or diabetes mellitus.

Gangrena **Necrosis o muerte de tejido, normalmente debido a un suministro deficiente o ausente de sangre; puede resultar de procesos inflamatorios, lesiones, arterioesclerosis, congelamiento o diabetes mellitus.**

Guillotine amputation Type of amputation in which a limb or portion of a limb is severed from the body and the wound is left open; a type of open amputation.

Amputación de la guillotina **Tipo de amputación en el que un miembro o una porción de un miembro del cuerpo se desarticula y la herida queda abierta; es un tipo de amputación abierta.**

Incomplete fracture Fracture in which the bone breaks only partially across, leaving some portion of the bone intact.

Fractura incompleta **Fractura en la que el hueso se rompe sólo parcialmente dejando alguna porción del hueso intacta.**

Nonunion Failure of a fracture to heal.

Sin unión **Fracaso de una fractura para sanar.**

Open amputation Amputation that is left open; usually done in cases of infection or necrosis.

Amputación abierta **Amputación que se queda abierta; normalmente ocurre en casos de infección o necrosis.**

Open or *compound fracture* Fracture in which the fragments of the broken bone break through the skin.

Fractura abierta* o *compuesta **Fractura en la que los fragmentos del hueso roto salen por la piel.**

Open reduction Surgical procedure in which an incision is made at the fracture site, usually on patients with open (compound) or comminuted fractures, to cleanse the area of fragments and debris.

Reducción abierta **Procedimiento quirúrgico en el que se hace una incisión al sitio de la fractura, normalmente en pacientes con fracturas abiertas o conminutas (compuestas), para limpiar el área de fragmentos y restos.**

TABLE 12–7
Selected Words

TABLA 12–7
Palabras selectas

English	Spanish	Pronunciation
pain	**dolor**	*(doh-lohr)*
pelvis	**pelvis**	*(pehl-bees)*
realign	**realinear**	*(reh-ah-lee-nee-ahr)*
reduction	**reducción**	*(reh-dook-see-ohn)*
rotation	**rotación**	*(roh-tah-see-ohn)*
signs	**signos/señales**	*(seeg-nohs/seh-nyah-lehs)*
symptoms	**síntomas**	*(seen-toh-mahs)*
syndrome	**síndrome**	*(seen-droh-meh)*
traction	**tracción**	*(trak-see-ohn)*

Phantom limb Illusion, following an amputation of a limb, that the limb still exists; the sensation that pain exists in removed limb is called *phantom limb pain.*

Miembro fantasma **Ilusión, en la que el paciente piensa que el miembro todavía existe; la sensación de que duele y existe el miembro amputado se llama *miembro fantasma doloroso.***

Reduction Process of bringing the ends of the broken bone into proper alignment.

Reducción **Proceso de traer los extremos del hueso roto en alineación propia.**

Replantation Surgical reattachment of an organ to its original site; reimplantation.

Reimplantación **Reimplante quirúrgico de un órgano a su sitio original.**

Staged amputation Amputation that is done over the course of several surgeries; usually done to control the spread of infection or necrosis.

Amputación progresiva **Amputación que se vuelve hacer en el curso de varias cirugías, normalmente para controlar la propagación de la infección o necrosis.**

Stress fracture Fracture caused by either sudden force or prolonged stress.

Fractura de la tensión **Fractura causada por la fuerza súbita o prolongada.**

Stump The distal portion of an amputated limb.

Muñón **La porción distal donde se amputó el miembro.**

Chapter Thirteen | **Capítulo trece**

A Visit to the Surgeon

Una visita al cirujano

The surgeon is a doctor that has prepared for many years. He specializes in the treatment of diseases, injuries, and deformities.

El cirujano es un médico que se ha preparado varios años. Se especializa en el tratamiento de enfermedades, lesiones (heridas) y deformidades.

Mr. Garza arrives at doctor Ortega's office:

El señor Garza llega al consultorio del doctor Ortega:
(Ehl seh-nyohr Gahr-sah yeh-gah ahl kohn-sool-toh-ree-oh dehl dohk-tohr Ohr-teh-gah)

Hello, Mr. Garza. Tell me what is wrong.

Hola, señor Garza. Dígame qué le pasa.
(Oh-lah, seh-nyohr Gahr-sah. Dee-gah-meh keh leh pah-sah)

—Doctor, I have had pain for the last five hours.

—Doctor, desde hace cinco horas tengo dolor.
(Dohk-tohr, dehs-deh ah-seh seen-koh oh-rahs tehn-goh doh-lohr)

Tell me, where did the pain start?

Dígame, ¿dónde comenzó el dolor?
(Dee-gah-meh, dohn-deh koh-mehn-soh ehl doh-lohr)

—Here, below the sternum.

—Aquí, debajo del esternón.
(Ah-kee deh-bah-hoh dehl ehs-tehr-nohn)

Is the pain localized in the same place?

¿El dolor está fijo en el mismo lugar?
(Ehl doh-lohr ehs-tah fee-hoh ehn ehl mees-moh loo-gahr)

—No, it moved to the right side.

—No, se recorrió al lado derecho.
(Noh, seh reh-koh-ree-oh ahl lah-doh deh-reh-choh)

What other discomfort do you have?

¿Qué otra molestia tiene?
(Keh oh-trah moh-lehs-tee-ah tee-eh-neh)

—I have nausea, vomiting, fever, and general malaise.

—Tengo náuseas, vómito, fiebre y malestar general.
(Tehn-goh nah-oo-seh-ahs, boh-mee-toh, fee-eh-breh ee mahl-ehs-tahr heh-neh-rahl)

Lay down so I can examine you.

Acuéstese para explorarlo.
(Ah-koo-ehs-teh-seh pah-rah ehx-ploh-rahr-loh)

Tell me if it hurts more when I press or when I let go.

Dígame si le duele más al presionar o al retirar la mano.
(Dee-gah-meh see leh doo-eh-leh mahs ahl preh-see-oh-nahr oh ahl reh-tee-rahr lah mah-noh)

—When you let go.

—Al retirar la mano.
(Ahl reh-tee-rahr lah mah-noh)

He takes the temperature. It is 100 degrees.

Le toma la temperatura. Es de cien grados.
(Leh toh-mah lah tehm-peh-rah-too-rah. Ehs deh see-ehn grah-dohs)

Mr. Garza, you probably have appendicitis.

Señor Garza, probablemente tenga apendicitis.
(Seh-nyohr Gahr-sah, proh-bah-bleh-mehn-teh tehn-gah ah-pehn-dee-see-tees)

You must go to the hospital.

Debe ir al hospital.
(Deh-beh eer ahl ohs-pee-tahl)

At the hospital, Dr. Ortega orders blood and urine samples, and X-rays of the abdomen. The doctor checks the results, finds that the white blood cell (leukocytosis) count is high, and that the X-ray of the abdomen shows blurring of the psoas muscle.

Ya en el hospital el doctor Ortega solicita exámenes de sangre, de orina y radiografías del abdomen. El doctor revisa los resultados de los exámenes y encuentra que en la sangre hay un aumento en los glóbulos blancos (leucocitosis) y la radiografía del abdomen muestra borramiento de los psoas.

Mr. Garza is sent to the anesthesiologist who asks:

El señor Garza es enviado con el anestesista, quien pregunta:
(Ehl seh-nyohr Gahr-sah ehs ehn-bee-ah-doh kohn ehl ah-nehs-teh-sees-tah, kee-ehn preh-goon-tah)

Do you have allergies, asthma, high blood pressure, cardiac problems, diabetes?	**¿Tiene alergias, asma, alta presión, problemas cardíacos, diabetes?** *(Tee-eh-neh ah-lehr-hee-ahs, ahs-mah, ahl-tah preh-see-ohn, proh-bleh-mahs kahr-dee-ah-kohs, dee-ah-beh-tehs)*
Mr Garza responds: I am very healthy!	**El señor Garza responde: ¡Estoy muy sano!** *(Ehl seh-nyohr Gahr-sah rehs-pohn-deh: Ehs-toh-ee moo-ee sah-noh)*

He is sent back to the surgeon who tells him that he must have surgery as soon as possible. He explains to Mr. Garza what the surgery is about.

Se le regresa al cirujano, quien le dice que debe ser operado lo más pronto posible. Le explica en qué consiste la cirugía.

After a few hours, Mr. Garza is taken to his room where he recovers from surgery.

Después de unas horas, el señor Garza es llevado a su cuarto donde se recupera de la cirugía.

TABLE 13-1
Useful Words

TABLA 13-1
Palabras útiles

English	Spanish	Pronunciation
accept	**aceptar**	*(ah-sehp-tahr)*
analgesics	**analgésicos**	*(ahn-ahl-heh-see-kohs)*
antibiotics	**antibióticos**	*(ahn-tee-bee-oh-tee-kohs)*
appendicitis	**apendicitis**	*(ah-pehn-dee-see-tees)*
confirm	**confirmar**	*(kohn-feer-mahr)*
diagnosis	**diagnóstico**	*(dee-ahg-nohs-tee-koh)*
discomfort	**molestia**	*(moh-lehs-tee-ah)*
doctor's office	**oficina/consultorio**	*(oh-fee-see-nah/kohn-sool-toh-ree-oh)*
epigastrium	**epigastrio**	*(eh-pee-gahs-tree-oh)*
infections	**infecciones**	*(een-fehk-see-ohn-ehs)*
leukocytes	**leucocitos**	*(leh-oo-koh-see-tohs)*
order	**solicitar**	*(sohl-ee-see-tahr)*
organs	**órganos**	*(ohr-gah-nohs)*
problems	**problemas**	*(proh-bleh-mahs)*
sternum	**esternón**	*(ehs-tehr-nohn)*
surgeon	**cirujano**	*(see-roo-hah-noh)*
sutures	**suturas/puntos**	*(soo-too-rahs/poon-tohs)*
white cells	**glóbulos blancos**	*(gloh-boo-lohs blahn-kohs)*

How do you feel, Mr. Garza?	**¿Cómo se siente, señor Garza?** *(Koh-moh seh see-ehn-teh seh-nyohr Gahr-sah)*
—I am fine, doctor, thank you. I feel like new!	**—Muy bien, doctor, gracias. ¡Me siento como nuevo!** *(Moo-ee bee-ehn, dohk-tohr, grah-see-ahs. Meh see-ehn-toh koh-moh noo-eh-boh)*
Well, you are going home tomorrow, but you must return to my office in eight days so I can remove your sutures.	**Bueno, mañana se va a su casa, pero debe regresar a mi oficina en ocho días para retirar los puntos de sutura.** *(Boo-eh-noh, mah-nyah-nah seh ba hah soo kah-sah, peh-roh deh-beh reh-greh-sahr ah mee oh-fee-see-nah ehn oh-choh dee-ahs pah-rah reh-tee-rahr lohs poon-tohs deh soo-too-rah)*

TABLE 13-2 Useful Phrases / **TABLA 13-2 Frases útiles**

English	Spanish	Pronunciation
I have pain.	**Tengo dolor.**	*(Tehn-goh doh-lohr)*
The pain is on the side.	**El dolor está en el lado/costado.**	*(Ehl doh-lohr ehs-tah ehn ehl lah-doh/kohs-tah-doh)*
The pain is localized, sharp.	**El dolor está fijo, agudo.**	*(Ehl doh-lohr ehs-tah fee-hoh, ah-goo-doh)*
The pain is worse.	**El dolor es peor.**	*(Ehl doh-lohr ehs peh-ohr)*
I have nausea and fever.	**Tengo náusea y fiebre.**	*(Tehn-goh nah-oo-seh-ah ee fee-eh-breh)*
Do you have high blood pressure?	**¿Tiene alta presión?**	*(Tee-eh-neh ahl-tah preh-see-ohn)*
Do you have cardiac problems?	**¿Tiene problemas cardíacos?**	*(Tee-eh-neh proh-bleh-mahs kahr-dee-ah-kohs)*
Don't lift more than 5 pounds.	**No levante más de cinco libras.**	*(Noh leh-bahn-teh mahs deh seen-koh lee-brahs)*
Keep the area clean.	**Mantenga el área limpia.**	*(Mahn-tehn-gah ehl ah-reh-ah leem-pee-ah)*
Eat soft foods.	**Coma alimentos blandos.**	*(Koh-mah ah-lee-mehn-tohs blahn-dohs)*
You can go back to work in one week.	**Puede regresar al trabajo en una semana.**	*(Poo-eh-deh reh-greh-sahr ahl trah-bah-hoh ehn oo-nah seh-mah-nah)*

Take this antibiotic to prevent infections and this analgesic for pain.

Tome este antibiótico para evitar infecciones y este analgésico para el dolor.

(Toh-meh ehs-teh ahn-tee-bee-oh-tee-koh pah-rah eh-bee-tahr een-fehk-see-oh-nehs ee ehs-teh ah-nahl-heh-see-koh pah-rah ehl doh-lohr)

Do not lift more than ten pounds of weight.

No levante más de diez libras de peso.

(Noh leh-bahn-teh mahs deh dee-ehs lee-brahs deh peh-soh)

Eat soft foods.

Coma alimentos blandos.

(Koh-mah ah-lee-mehn-tohs blahn-dohs)

If you notice fever or any problems in the incision, go to my office immediately.

Si nota fiebre o problemas en la herida, vaya inmediatamente a mi oficina.

(See noh-tah fee-eh-breh oh proh-bleh-mahs ehn lah eh-ree-dah, bah-yah een-meh-dee-ah-tah-mehn-teh ah mee oh-fee-see-nah)

Chapter Fourteen — Capítulo catorce

A Visit to the Psychologist

Una visita al psicólogo

Acute and Chronic Psychological Problems

Problemas psicológicos agudos y crónicos

In our society, many stressors threaten a person's psychological well-being. Whether at home or at work, as an individual's responsibilities increase, so do his/her stress levels. The many roles that one is called to play on a daily basis provide an open field where stress can flourish.

En nuestra sociedad existen muchos factores estresantes que ame-

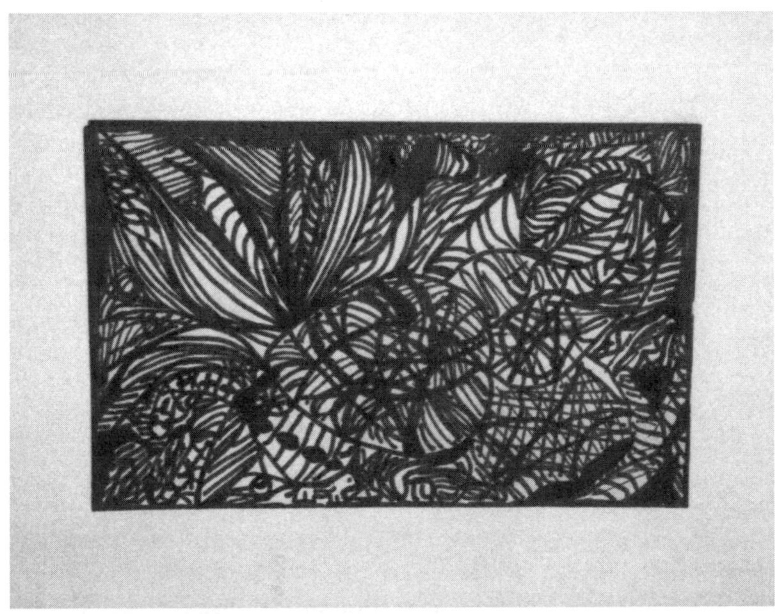

Figure 14–1 Drawing by Patricia Martinez.

nazan el bienestar psicológico de una persona. Ya sea en casa o en el trabajo, el aumento en las responsabilidades de un individuo incrementan el nivel del estrés. La variedad de roles que uno desempeña en la vida diaria proveen un campo libre donde puede florecer el estrés.

A careful assessment of contributing factors and a thorough psychosocial assessment should assist you in identifying the causes of the imbalance.

Una evaluación cuidadosa de factores y una asesoría psicosocial completa podrá asistirle en la identificación de las causas del problema.
(Oo-nah eh-bah-loo-ah-see-ohn koo-ee-dah-doh-sah deh fahk-toh-rehs ee oo-nah ah-seh-soh-ree-ah see-koh-soh-see-ahl kohm-pleh-tah poh-drah ahs-ees-teer-leh ehn lah ee-dehn-tee-fee-kah-see-ohn deh lahs kah-oo-sahs dehl proh-bleh-mah)

Very seldom do we visit a psychologist, since this implies that we have to talk about our problems, situations, feelings, and activities. This time, Juan and Roger decide to tell the psychologist about their problems.

Raras veces acudimos a consulta con un psicólogo, ya que implica platicarle nuestros problemas, situaciones, estados de ánimo y actividades. Esta vez Juan y Roger deciden contarle al psicólogo sus problemas.

Juan Peña recently changed jobs in order to increase his income. His wife delivered a baby girl one month ago. Two days ago, Juan developed abdominal pains and diarrhea. In addition, he feels short of breath intermittently.

Juan Peña cambió de trabajo recientemente para poder aumentar su salario. Su esposa dió a luz una bebita hace un mes. Hace dos días Juan desarrolló dolores de estómago y diarrea. Además, se siente falto de respiración constantemente.

Tell me, what brought you here?
—I feel overwhelmed, anxious.

Dígame, ¿qué lo trajo aquí?
(Dee-gah-meh, keh loh trah-hoh ah-kee)
—Me siento abatido, ansioso.
(Meh see-ehn-toh ah-bah-tee-doh, ahn-see-oh-soh)

What symptoms do you have?
—I have diarrhea and stomach pains.

¿Qué síntomas tiene?
(Keh seen-toh-mahs tee-eh-neh)
—Tengo diarrea y dolores de estómago.
(Tehn-goh dee-ah-reh-ah ee doh-loh-rehs deh ehs-toh-mah-goh)

TABLE 14–1
Selected Words

TABLA 14–1
Palabras selectas

English	Spanish	Pronunciation
abuse	**abuso**	*(ah-boo-soh)*
addictive	**adicto**	*(ah-deek-toh)*
analysis	**análisis**	*(ah-nah-lee-sees)*
anger	**enojo**	*(eh-noh-hoh)*
anxiety	**ansiedad**	*(ahn-see-eh-dahd)*
behavior	**conducta**	*(kohn-dook-tah)*
bereavement	**desamparo**	*(dehs-ahm-pah-roh)*
boredom	**fastidio**	*(fahs-tee-dee-oh)*
defense	**defensa**	*(deh-fehn-sah)*
dementia	**demencia**	*(deh-mehn-see-ah)*
dependence	**dependencia**	*(deh-pehn-dehn-see-ah)*
development	**desarrollo**	*(deh-sah-roh-yoh)*
diagnosis	**diagnóstico**	*(dee-ahg-nohs-tee-koh)*
difficulty	**dificultad**	*(dee-fee-kool-tahd)*
disorders	**desórdenes**	*(dehs-ohr-deh-nehs)*
evaluation	**evaluación**	*(eh-bah-loo-ah-see-ohn)*
findings	**hallazgos**	*(ah-yahs-gohs)*

Has anything changed in your life?
¿Ha cambiado algo en su vida?
(Ah kahm-bee-ah-doh ahl-goh ehn soo bee-dah)

—Well, I just changed jobs.
—Bueno, apenas cambié de trabajo.
(Boo-eh-noh, ah-peh-nahs kahm-bee-eh deh trah-bah-hoh)

Anything else?
¿Alguna otra cosa?
(Ahl-goo-nah oh-trah koh-sah)

—My wife just had a baby.
—Mi esposa tuvo un bebé.
(Mee ehs-poh-sah too-boh oon beh-beh)

Everybody experiences some anxiety.
Todo el mundo pasa por cierta ansiedad.
(Toh-doh ehl moon-doh pah-sah pohr see-ehr-tah ahn-see-eh-dahd)

Having continuous anxiety may cause serious problems.
El tener ansiedad continua puede llevar a problemas serios.
(Ehl teh-nehr ahn-see-eh-dahd kohn-tee-noo-ah poo-eh-deh yeh-bahr ah proh-bleh-mahs seh-ree-ohs)

—What kinds of problems?	**—¿Qué clase de problemas?** *(Keh klah-seh deh proh-bleh-mahs)*
Problems like ulcers, high blood pressure, and inability to enjoy life and the world.	**Problemas como úlceras, alta presión e incapacidad de gozar la vida y el mundo.** *(Proh-bleh-mahs koh-moh ool-seh-rahs, ahl-tah preh-see-ohn eh een-kah-pah-see-dahd deh goh-sahr lah bee-dah ee ehl moon-doh)*
Do you have trouble making friends at work?	**¿En su trabajo tiene dificultad para hacer amistades?** *(Ehn soo trah-bah-hoh tee-eh-neh dee-fee-kool-tahd pah-rah ah-sehr ah-mees-tah-dehs)*
How do you get along with your peers?	**¿Cómo se lleva usted con sus compañeros?** *(Koh-moh seh yeh-bah oos-tehd kohn soos kohm-pah-nyeh-rohs)*
Do you talk to your wife about your job?	**¿Trata de hablar con su esposa acerca de su trabajo?**

TABLE 14–2
Selected Words

TABLA 14–2
Palabras selectas

English	Spanish	Pronunciation
hope	**esperanza**	*(ehs-peh-rahn-sah)*
hostility	**hostilidad**	*(ohs-tee-lee-dahd)*
humanistic	**humanístico**	*(oo-mahn-ees-tee-koh)*
implementation	**implementación**	*(eem-pleh-mehn-tah-see-ohn)*
implications	**implicaciones**	*(eem-plee-kah-see-ohn-ehs)*
independence	**independencia**	*(een-deh-pehn-dehn-see-ah)*
interaction	**interacción**	*(een-tehr-ahk-see-ohn)*
interpersonal	**interpersonal**	*(een-tehr-pehr-soh-nahl)*
loneliness	**soledad**	*(soh-leh-dahd)*
loss	**pérdida**	*(pehr-dee-dah)*
manifestation	**manifestación**	*(mahn-ee-fehs-tah-see-ohn)*
manipulation	**manipulación**	*(mahn-ee-poo-lah-see-ohn)*
personality	**personalidad**	*(pehr-soh-nah-lee-dahd)*
planning	**planificación**	*(plah-nee-fee-kah-see-ohn)*
purpose	**propósito**	*(proh-poh-see-toh)*
relation	**relación**	*(reh-lah-see-ohn)*

(Trah-tah deh ah-blahr kohn soo ehs-poh-sah ah-sehr-kah deh soo trah-bah-hoh)

Do you have her support in everything?

¿Tiene apoyo de ella en todo?
(Tee-eh-neh ah-poh-yoh deh eh-yah ehn toh-doh)

Do you have insomnia?

¿Tiene insomnio?
(Tee-eh-neh een-sohm-nee-oh)

Do you try to relax to forget your anxiety?

¿Procura distraerse para olvidar su ansiedad?
(Proh-koo-rah dees-trah-ehr-seh pah-rah ohl-bee-dahr soo ahn-see-eh-dahd)

If your behavior changes you must go to a specialist.

Si continúa con cambios en su persona debe acudir con un especialista.
(See kohn-tee-noo-ah kohn kahm-bee-ohs ehn soo pehr-soh-nah deh-beh ah-koo-deer kohn oon ehs-peh-see-ah-lees-tah)

For now, follow these recommendations:

Por ahora, siga estas recomendaciones:
(Pohr ah-oh-rah, see-gah ehs-tahs reh-koh-mehn-dah-see-oh-nehs)

1. Take 30 minutes every day to examine your feelings. Think about what makes you depressed.

1. **Tome treinta minutos diariamente para examinar sus sentimientos. Piense qué le causa depresión.**
(Toh-meh treh-een-tah mee-noo-tohs dee-ah-ree-ah-mehn-teh pah-rah ehx-ah-mee-nahr soos sehn-tee-mee-ehn-tohs. Pee-ehn-seh keh leh kah-oo-sah deh-preh-see-ohn.

2. Do not deny your feelings.

2. **No niegue sus sentimientos.**
(Noh nee-eh-geh soos sehn-tee-mee-ehn-tohs)

3. If it is something you cannot control, ignore it!

3. **Si es algo que no puede controlar, ¡ignórelo!**
(See ehs ahl-goh keh noh poo-eh-deh kohn-troh-lahr, eeg-noh-reh-loh)

TABLE 14–3 Selected Words | **TABLA 14–3 Palabras selectas**

English	Spanish	Pronunciation
cognitive	**cognoscitivo**	*(kohg-noh-see-tee-boh)*
concepts	**conceptos**	*(kohn-sehp-tohs)*
coping	**sobrellevando**	*(soh-breh-yeh-bahn-doh)*
flexibility	**flexibilidad**	*(flehx-ee-bee-lee-dahd)*
grieving	**afligir**	*(ah-flee-heer)*
guilt	**culpa**	*(kool-pah)*
mechanisms	**mecanismos**	*(meh-kah-nees-mohs)*
methodology	**metodología**	*(meh-toh-doh-loh-hee-ah)*
mistrust	**desconfianza**	*(dehs-kohn-fee-ahn-sah)*
response	**contestación**	*(kohn-tehs-tah-see-ohn)*
rigidity	**rigidez**	*(ree-hee-dehs)*
sample	**muestra**	*(moo-ehs-trah)*
sociocultural	**sociocultural**	*(soh-see-oh-kool-too-rahl)*
somatization	**somatización**	*(soh-mah-tee-sah-see-ohn)*
theories	**teorías**	*(teh-oh-ree-ahs)*
trust	**confianza**	*(kohn-fee-ahn-sah)*
victims	**víctimas**	*(beek-tee-mahs)*

4. Share your feelings with your wife and one friend.

4. Comparta sus sentimientos con su esposa y un amigo.
(Kohm-pahr-tah soos sehn-tee-mee-ehn-tohs kohn soo ehs-poh-sah ee oon ah-mee-goh)

5. Every day, spend time in exercise or a hobby.

5. Diariamente, tome tiempo para hacer ejercicio o una actividad favorita.
(Dee-ah-ree-ah-mehn-teh, toh-meh tee-ehm-poh pah-rah ah-sehr eh-hehr-see-see-oh, oh oo-nah ahk-tee-bee-dahd fah-boh-ree-tah)

6. Make your home pleasant and cheerful.

6. Haga su hogar placentero y alegre.
(Ah-gah soo oh-gahr plah-sehn-teh-roh ee ah-leh-greh)

7. Treat everyone with affection.

7. Trate a todos con afecto.
(Trah-teh ah toh-dohs kohn ah-fehk-toh)

8. Do not isolate yourself.
8. No se aparte.
(Noh seh ah-pahr-teh)

9. When you feel depressed, go for a walk.
9. Cuando se deprima, salga de paseo.
(Koo-ahn-doh seh deh-pree-mah, sahl-gah deh pah-seh-oh)

10. Eat and sleep well.
10. Aliméntese y duerma bien.
(Ah-lee-mehn-teh-seh ee doo-ehr-mah bee-ehn)

11. Do not assume others don't understand what you are feeling.
11. No presuma que otros no entienden lo que está sintiendo.
(Noh preh-soo-mah keh oh-trohs noh ehn-tee-ehn-dehn loh keh ehs-tah seen-tee-ehn-doh)

Roger is hospitalized in a psychiatric unit. Part of the milieu therapy requires that he participate in activities.

Roger está hospitalizado en una unidad de psiquiatría. Parte de la terapia de medio ambiente requiere que participe en actividades.

Roger, it is time to go to your O. T. appointment.
Roger, es la hora de ir a su cita de terapia ocupacional (OT).
(Roger, ehs lah oh-rah deh eer ah soo see-tah deh teh-rah-pee-ah oh-koo-pah-see-oh-nahl [OT])

—I'm not going today.
—Hoy no voy a ir.
(Oh-ee noh boh-ee ah eer)

You are not going?
¿Usted no va?
(Oos-tehd noh bah)

—No.
—No.
(Noh)

You enjoyed working on your house yesterday.
Disfrutó de trabajar en su casa ayer.
(Dees-froo-toh deh trah-bah-hahr ehn soo kah-sah ah-yehr)

—No, I did not enjoy working on my house.
—No, no disfruté el trabajar en mi casa.
(Noh, noh dees-froo-teh ehl trah-bah-hahr ehn mee kah-sah)

It looked as if a professional had made it.
Parece como si un profesional lo hubiera hecho.
(Pah-reh-seh koh-moh see oon proh-feh-see-oh-nahl loh oo-bee-eh-rah heh-choh)

—I don't like it.	**—No me gusta.** *(Noh meh goos-tah)*
Please keep your appointment.	**Por favor, acuda a la cita.** *(Pohr fah-bohr, ah-koo-dah ah lah see-tah)*
Activities are part of the plan while you are here.	**Las actividades son parte del plan de tratamiento mientras esté aquí.** *(Lahs ahk-tee-bee-dah-dehs sohn pahr-teh dehl plahn deh trah-tah-mee-ehn-toh mee-ehn-trahs ehs-tee ah-kee)*
I will return in ten minutes and we can walk down together.	**Volveré en diez minutos y podremos caminar juntos.** *(Bohl-beh-reh ehn dee-ehs mee-noo-tohs ee poh-dreh-mohs kah-mee-nahr hoon-tohs)*

TABLE 14–4
Selected Phrases

TABLA 14–4
Frases selectas

English	Spanish and Pronunciation
certain anxiety	**cierta ansiedad** *(see-ehr-tah ahn-see-eh-dahd)*
I changed jobs recently.	**Cambié de trabajo recientemente.** *(Kahm-bee-eh deh trah-bah-hoh reh-see-ehn-teh-mehn-teh)*
I feel uneasy constantly.	**Me siento abatido constantemente.** *(Meh see-ehn-toh ah-bah-tee-doh kohns-tahn-teh-mehn-teh)*
identification of the problem	**identificación del problema** *(ee-dehn-tee-fee-kah-see-ohn dehl proh-bleh-mah)*
incapable of having fun	**incapacidad de gozar** *(een-kah-pah-see-dah deh goh-sahr)*
increase the level	**incrementar el nivel** *(een-kreh-mehn-tahr ehl nee-behl)*
our society	**nuestra sociedad** *(noo-ehs-trah soh-see-eh-dahd)*
psychosocial evaluation	**asesoría psicosocial** *(ah-seh-soh-ree-ah see-koh-soh-see-ahl)*
responsibilities and activities	**responsabilidades y actividades** *(rehs-pohn-sah-bee-lee-dah-dehs ee ahk-tee-bee-dah-dehs)*
stressful factors	**factores estresantes** *(fahk-tohr-ehs ehs-trah-sahn-tehs)*

TABLE 14–5 Selected Phrases | **TABLA 14–5 Frases selectas**

English	Spanish	Pronunciation
crisis intervention	**intervención de la crisis**	*(ehn-tehr-behn-see-ohn deh lah kree-sees)*
difficulties at work	**dificultades en su trabajo**	*(dee-fee-kool-tah-dehs ehn soo trah-bah-hoh)*
family therapy	**terapia familiar**	*(teh-rah-pee-ah fah-mee-lee-ahr)*
group therapy	**terapia de grupo**	*(teh-rah-pee-ah deh groo-poh)*
mental health	**salud mental**	*(sah-lood mehn-tahl)*
mental patient	**enfermo mental**	*(ehn-fehr-moh mehn-tahl)*
milieu therapy	**terapia de medio ambiente**	*(teh-rah-pee-ah deh meh-dee-oh ahm-bee-ehn-teh)*
nutritional disorders	**desórdenes alimenticios**	*(dehs-ohr-deh-nehs ah-lee-mehn-tee-see-ohs)*
therapy for couples	**terapia de parejas**	*(teh-rah-pee-ah deh pah-reh-hahs)*
try to have a good time	**procure divertirse**	*(proh-koo-reh dee-behr-teer-seh)*
try to talk	**trate de conversar**	*(trah-teh deh kohn-behr-sahr)*

Ten minutes pass and the nurse returns.
Diez minutos pasaron y la enfermera regresa.

It is time to go, Roger.
Es tiempo de ir, Roger.
(Ehs tee-ehm-poh deh eer, Roger)

Roger gets up and moves to the door.
Roger se levanta y va a a puerta.

—Why do you make me do things I don't want to do?
—¿Por qué me haces hacer cosas que no quiero?
(Pohr-keh meh ah-sehs ah-sehr koh-sahs keh noh kee-eh-roh?

—I wish all of you would leave me alone.
—Deseo que todos ustedes me dejen solo.
(Deh-seh-oh keh toh-dohs oos-teh-dehs meh deh-hehn soh-loh)

Are you mad because you are going to O.T.?
¿Está enojado porque va a O.T.?
(Ehs-tah eh-noh-hah-doh pohr-keh bah ah O.T.)

—No, I just don't want to go. It's not helping me.

—No, sólo que no quiero ir. No me está ayudando.
(Noh, soh-loh keh noh kee-eh-roh eer. Noh meh ehs-tah ah-yoo-dahn-doh)

Roger, age 26, was involved in the preparation for exams when he experienced a profound depression. He tried to commit suicide by slashing his wrists. He was hospitalized for observation.

Roger estaba ocupado preparando para exámenes cuando se deprimió profundamente. Trató de suicidarse cortándose las muñecas. Se le hospitalizó para observarlo.

Roger states:
—Failure in the exams represents a disappointment for my family.

Roger dice:
—La falla en los exámenes representa una desilusión para mi familia.
(Roger dee-seh: Lah fah-yah ehn lohs ehx-ah-meh-nehs reh-preh-sehn-tah oo-nah deh-see-loo-see-ohn pah-rah mee fah-mee-lee-ah)

He sees failure as disgrace, an obstacle to future plans, and a blow to his self-esteem. Roger is now undergoing assessment by the psychiatrist who asks him a number of questions.

El ve el fracaso como una desgracia, un obstáculo para sus planes futuros y un golpe a su autoestima. Roger se somete a una asesoría por el psiquiatra quien le hace varias preguntas.

How long have you felt depressed?

¿Desde cuándo se siente deprimido?
(Dehs-deh koo-ahn-doh seh see-ehn-teh deh-pree-mee-doh)

Is this your first suicide attempt?

¿Es éste su primer intento de suicidio?
(Ehs ehs-teh soo pree-mehr een-tehn-toh deh soo-ee-see-dee-oh)

What kind of weapons have you used?

¿Qué clase de armas ha usado?
(Keh klah-seh deh ahr-mahs ah oo-sah-doh)

Did you call anyone?

¿Llamó a alguien?
(Yah-moh ah ahl-ghee-ehn)

What triggered your depression?

¿Qué precipitó su depresión?
(Keh preh-see-pee-toh soo deh-preh-see-ohn)

TABLE 14–6 Selected Phobias | **TABLA 14–6 Fobias selectas**

English	Spanish	Pronunciation
acrophobia	**acrofobia**	*(ah-kroh-foh-bee-ah)*
[height]	**[altura]**	*[ahl-too-rah]*
agoraphobia	**agorafobia**	*(ah-goh-rah-foh-bee-ah)*
[open spaces]	**[espacios abiertos]**	*[ehs-pah-see-ohs ah-bee-ehr-tohs]*
anthropophobia	**antropofobia**	*(ahn-troh-poh-foh-bee-ah)*
[people]	**[personas]**	*[pehr-soh-nahs]*
claustrophobia	**claustrofobia**	*(klah-oos-troh-foh-bee-ah)*
[closed spaces]	**[espacios cerrados]**	*[ehs-pah-see-ohs seh-rah-dohs]*
hydrophobia	**hidrofobia**	*(ee-droh-foh-bee-ah)*
[water]	**[agua]**	*[ah-goo-ah]*
mikophobia	**micofobia**	*(mee-koh-foh-bee-ah)*
[germs]	**[gérmenes]**	*[gehr-meh-nehs]*
mysophobia	**misofobia**	*(mee-soh-foh-bee-ah)*
[dirt]	**[tierra]**	*[tee-eh-rah]*
[contamination]	**[contaminación]**	*[kohn-tah-mee-nah-see-ohn]*
nuctophobia	**nuctofobia**	*(nook-toh-foh-bee-ah)*
[darkness]	**[oscuridad]**	*[ohs-koo-ree-dahd]*
thanatophobia	**tanatofobia**	*(tah-nah-toh-foh-bee-ah)*
[death]	**[muerte]**	*[moo-ehr-teh]*
zoophobia	**zoofobia**	*(soh-oh-foh-bee-ah)*
[animals]	**[animales]**	*[ah-nee-mah-lehs]*

Do you take any drugs? — **¿Toma drogas?**
(Toh-mah droh-gahs)

What kind? — **¿Qué clase?**
(Keh klah-seh)

How do you feel now? — **¿Cómo se siente ahora?**
(Koh-moh seh see-ehn-teh ah-oh-rah)

When was the last time you ate? — **¿Cuándo fue la última vez que comió?**
(Koo-ahn-doh foo-eh lah ool-tee-mah behs keh koh-mee-oh)

Is your family in the city? — **¿Está su familia en la ciudad?**
(Ehs-tah soo fah-mee-lee-ah ehn lah see-oo-dahd)

I will talk to you every day. — **Hablaré con usted todos los días.**
(Ah-blah-reh kohn oos-tehd toh-dohs lohs dee-ahs)

The nurse will complete the assessment.	**La enfermera completará la evaluación.** *(Lah ehn-fehr-meh-rah kohm-pleh-tah-rah lah eh-bah-loo-ah-see-ohn)*

The nurse initiates the following interventions.
La enfermera inicia las intervenciones siguientes.

Mental status examination.	**Exámen del estado mental.** *(Ehx-ah-mehn dehl ehs-tah-doh mehn-tahl)*
Includes: appearance, activity level, mood and affect, speech, thought content, memory, and intellectual level.	**Incluye: la apariencia, el nivel de actividad, disposición de ánimo y afecto, conversación, contenido de los pensamientos, memoria y nivel intelectual.** *(Een-kloo-yeh: lah ah-pah-ree-ehn-see-ah, ehl nee-behl deh ahk-tee-bee-dahd, dees-poh-see-see-ohn deh ah-nee-moh ee ah-fehk-toh, kohn-behr-sah-see-ohn, kohn-teh-nee-doh deh lohs pehn-sah-mee-ehn-tohs, meh-moh-ree-ah ee nee-behl een-teh-lehk-too-ahl)*
Establish a contract so he does not harm himself.	**Establecer un contrato para que no se cause daño.** *(Ehs-tah-bleh-sehr oon kohn-trah-toh pah-rah keh noh seh kah-oo-seh dah-nyoh)*
Help the patient to identify positive aspects.	**Ayudar al paciente a identificar aspectos positivos.** *(Ah-yoo-dahr ahl pah-see-ehn-teh ah ee-dehn-tee-fee-kahr ahs-pehk-tohs poh-see-tee-bohs)*
Plan an adequate diet.	**Planear alimentos adecuados.** *(Plah-neh-ahr ah-lee-mehn-tohs ah-deh-koo-ah-dohs)*
Encourage relaxation exercises.	**Estimular los ejercicios de relajamiento.** *(Ehs-tee-moo-lahr lohs eh-hehr-see-see-ohs deh reh-lah-hah-mee-ehn-toh)*

Chapter Fifteen — Capítulo quince

A Visit to the Dentist — Una visita al dentista

Care of the mounth requires frequent visits to the dentist. The condition of the teeth allows for proper chewing and thus assists in digestion of foods. A healthy mouth will always be considered a sign of good health.

El cuidado general de la boca requiere visitas frecuentes al dentista. El buen estado de los dientes permite una buena masticación y por lo tanto la buena digestión de los alimentos. Una boca sana será siempre un signo del buen cuidado personal.

Patient Medical History — *La historia médica del paciente*

Are you under the care of a doctor?

¿Está bajo tratamiento de un doctor?
(Ehs-tah bah-hoh trah-tah-mee-ehn-toh deh oon dohk-tohr)

Are you allergic to penicillin or other medications?

¿Tiene alergias a la penicilina u otros medicamentos?
(Tee-eh-neh ah-lehr-hee-ahs ah lah peh-nee-see-lee-nah oo oh-trohs meh-dee-kah-mehn-tohs)

Have you ever had a heart attack or pains in your heart?

¿Ha tenido ataque al corazón o dolor en el pecho?
(Hah teh-nee-doh ah-tah-keh ahl koh-rah-sohn oh doh-lohr ehn ehl peh-cho)

rheumatic fever?

¿fiebre reumática?
(fee-eh-breh reh-oo-mah-tee-kah)

joint replacement?

¿le han reemplazado alguna articulación?
(leh ahn rehm-plah-sah-doh ahl-goo-nah ahr-tee-koo-lah-see-ohn)

Do you have a pacemaker?

¿Tiene marcapasos?
(Tee-eh-neh mahr-kah-pah-sohs)

Have you ever had:	**Ha tenido:** *(Ah teh-nee-doh)*
cancer?	**¿cáncer?** *(kahn-sehr)*
chemotherapy treatment?	**¿tratamiento de quimioterapia?** *(trah-tah-mee-ehn-toh deh kee-mee-oh-tehr-ah-pee-ah)*
allergic reaction to a local anesthetic?	**¿alergia a la anestesia local?** *(ah-lehr-hee-ah ah lah ah-nehs-teh-see-ah loh-kahl)*
tuberculosis/lung problems?	**¿tuberculosis/problemas con los pulmones?** *(too-behr-koo-lohs-ees/proh-bleh-mahs kohn lohs pool-moh-nehs)*
hepatitis or cirrhosis?	**¿hepatitis o cirrosis?** *(eh-pah-tee-tees oh see-roh-sees)*
a sexually transmitted disease?	**¿enfermedades transmitidas sexualmente?** *(ehn-fehr-meh-dah-dehs trahns-mee-tee-dahs sehx-oo-ahl-mehn-teh)*
Do you have:	**Tiene:** *(Tee-eh-neh)*
diabetes?	**¿diabetes?** *(dee-ah-beh-tehs)*
convulsions?	**¿convulsiones?** *(kohn-bool-see-oh-nehs)*
any blood disorders such as anemia or leukemia?	**¿problemas de sangre como anemia o leucemia?** *(proh-bleh-mahs deh sahn-greh koh-moh ah-neh-mee-ah oh loo-seh-mee-ah)*
Are you taking:	**Está tomando:** *(Ehs-tah toh-mahn-doh)*
any medications?	**¿algunas medicinas?** *(ahl-goo-nahs meh-dee-see-nahs)*
steroids?	**¿esteroides?** *(ehs-teh-roh-ee-dehs)*
anticoagulants?	**¿anticoagulantes?** *(ahn-tee-koo-ah-goo-lahn-tehs)*
antidepressants?	**¿antidepresivos?** *(ahn-tee-deh-preh-see-bohs)*
nitroglycerin?	**¿nitroglicerina?** *(nee-troh-glee-seh-ree-nah)*

Are you pregnant?	**¿Está embarazada?** *(Ehs-tah ehm-bah-rah-sah-dah)*
(If yes) When is your due date?	**[Si es así] ¿Cuándo se alivia?** *([See ehs ah-see] Koo-ahn-doh seh ah-lee-bee-ah)*
Do you smoke or drink alcohol?	**¿Fuma o toma alcohol?** *(Foo-mah oh toh-mah ahl-kohl)*
Do you have any condition or disease not listed in this questionnaire?	**¿Tiene problemas o condiciones de salud que no están en este cuestionario?** *(Tee-eh-neh proh-bleh-mahs oh kohn-dee-see-ohn-ehs deh sahl-ood keh noh ehs-tahn ehn ehs-teh koo-ehs-tee-oh-nah-ree-oh)*
Oral examination:	**Examinación oral:** *(Ehx-ah-mee-nah-see-ohn oh-rahl)*
Good afternoon, Miss Gonzalez.	**Buenas tardes, señorita González.** *(Boo-eh-nahs tahr-dehs, seh-nyoh-ree-tah Gohn-sah-lehs)*
Come in.	**Pase./Entre.** *(Pah-seh/Ehn-treh)*
Sit down, please.	**Siéntese, por favor.** *(See-ehn-teh-seh, pohr fah-bohr)*
What is the matter?	**¿Qué le pasa/sucede?** *(Keh leh pah-sah/soo-seh-deh)*
When did you see the dentist last?	**¿Cuándo vió al dentista la última vez?** *(Koo-ahn-doh bee-oh ahl dehn-tees-tah lah ool-tee-mah behs)*
Open your mouth, please.	**Abra la boca, por favor.** *(Ah-brah lah boh-kah, pohr fah-bohr)*
I will check your teeth.	**Revisaré sus dientes.** *(Reh-bee-sah-reh soos dee-ehn-tehs)*
I am going to hit gently.	**Voy a darle golpecitos.** *(Boh-ee ah dahr-leh gohl-peh-see-tohs)*
Point when it hurts.	**Señale cuando duela.** *(Seh-nyah-leh koo-ahn-doh doo-eh-lah)*
Bite!	**¡Muerda!** *(Moo-ehr-dah)*
Please open your mouth some more.	**Por favor, abra más la boca.** *(Pohr fah-bohr, ah-brah mahs lah boh-kah)*

TABLE 15–1
Common Words

TABLA 15–1
Palabras comunes

English	Spanish	Pronunciation
air	**aire**	*(ah-ee-reh)*
anesthesia	**anestesia**	*(ah-nehs-teh-see-ah)*
antibiotic	**antibiótico**	*(ahn-tee-bee-oh-tee-koh)*
anticoagulant	**anticoagulante**	*(ahn-tee-koh-ah-goo-lahn-teh)*
baby tooth	**diente de leche**	*(dee-ehn-teh deh leh-cheh)*
Bite!	**¡Muerda!**	*(Moo-ehr-dah)*
caries	**caries**	*(kah-ree-ehs)*
cavity	**cavidad**	*(kah-bee-dahd)*
cement	**cemento**	*(seh-mehn-toh)*
chemotherapy	**quimioterapia**	*(kee-mee-oh-teh-rah-pee-ah)*

I am going to clean your teeth.
Voy a limpiarle los dientes.
(Boy ah leem-pee-ahr-leh lohs dee-ehn-tehs)

Do your gums bleed?
¿Le sangran las encías?
(Leh sahn-grahn lahs ehn-see-ahs)

Are your teeth sensitive to cold?
¿Tiene sensibilidad al tomar frío?
(Tee-eh-neh sehn-see-bee-lee-dahd ahl toh-mahr free-oh)

shock?
¿toques?
(toh-kehs)

pain?
¿dolor?
(doh-lohr)

Do you have bad breath?
¿Tiene mal aliento?
(Tee-eh-neh mahl ah-lee-ehn-toh)

frequent blisters/ulcerations?
¿ulceraciones frecuentes?
(ool-seh-rah-see-oh-nehs freh-koo-ehn-tehs)

Does the wind hurt your teeth?
¿Le molesta el aire?
(Leh moh-lehs-tah ehl ah-ee-reh)

Does it hurt when you chew very hard?
¿Le duele al masticar con fuerza?
(Leh doo-eh-leh ahl mahs-tee-kahr kohn foo-ehr-sah)

Rinse your mouth.
Enjuague su boca.
(Ehn-hoo-ah-geh soo boh-kah)

I am going to take X-rays.
Le tomaré radiografías.
(Leh toh-mah-reh rah-dee-oh-grah-fee-ahs)

I will return shortly.
Regreso en seguida.
(Reh-greh-soh ehn seh-ghee-dah)

I checked your X-rays.	**Revisé sus radiografías.** *(Reh-bee-seh soos rah-dee-oh-grah-fee-ahs)*
I have to take out your tooth.	**Tengo que extraer/sacar el diente.** *(Tehn-goh keh ehx-trah-ehr/sah-kahr ehl dee-ehn-teh)*
I am going to use local anesthetic.	**Voy a usar anestesia local.** *(Boh-ee ah oo-sahr ah-nehs-teh-see-ah loh-kahl)*
Tell me when it feels numb.	**Avíseme cuando sienta dormido.** *(Ah-bee-seh-meh koo-ahn-doh see-ehn-tah dohr-mee-doh)*
Are you okay?	**¿Se siente bien?** *(Seh see-ehn-teh bee-ehn)*
Does it still hurt?	**¿Todavía le duele?** *(Toh-dah-bee-ah leh doo-eh-leh)*
I pulled your tooth.	**Le saqué el diente.** *(Leh sah-keh ehl dee-ehn-teh)*
I am putting in a temporary filling.	**Le aplicaré empaste temporal.** *(Leh ah-plee-kah-reh ehm-pahs-teh tehm-poh-rahl)*
I will use resins.	**Usaré resinas.** *(Oo-sah-reh reh-see-nahs)*

TABLE 15–2
Proper Vocabulary

TABLA 15–2
Vocabulario apropiado

English	Spanish	Pronunciation
dental floss	**hilo dental**	*(ee-loh dehn-tahl)*
dental surgeon	**cirujano dentista**	*(see-roo-hah-noh dehn-tees-tah)*
dentifrice	**dentífrico**	*(dehn-tree-fee-koh)*
dentist	**dentista**	*(dehn-tees-tah)*
disclosing solution	**solución reveladora**	*(soh-loo-see-ohn reh-beh-lah-doh-rah)*
enamel	**esmalte**	*(ehs-mahl-teh)*
extract	**extraer/sacar**	*(ehx-trah-ehr/sah-kahr)*
eyetooth	**diente canino/colmillo**	*(dee-ehn-teh kah-nee-noh/kohl-mee-yoh)*
fluoride	**fluoruro**	*(floh-roo-roh)*
to fill	**empastar/rellenar**	*(ehm-pahs-tahr/reh-yeh-nahr)*

I'm going to polish your teeth.	**Ahora voy a pulír sus dientes.** *(Ah-oh-rah boy a poo-leer soos dee-ehn-tehs)*
You need to brush your teeth better.	**Necesita cepillar mejor sus dientes.** *(Neh-seh-see-tah seh-pee-yahr meh-hohr soos dee-ehn-tehs)*
Use dental floss.	**Use hilo dental.** *(Oo-seh ee-loh dehn-tahl)*
Return in 10 days.	**Regrese en diez días.** *(Reh-greh-seh ehn dee-ehs dee-ahs)*
Please return as needed.	**En caso necesario, puede regresar.** *(Ehn kah-soh neh-seh-sah-ree-oh, poo-eh-deh reh-greh-sahr)*
I hope you do well.	**Qué siga bien.** *(Keh see-gah bee-ehn)*

It is very important to give oral hygiene instructions to all patients receiving dental care. This prevents future damage and helps preserve the teeth.

Es de suma importancia el dar instrucciones a todos los pacientes que reciben tratamiento dental. Esto evita daños futuros y ayuda a conservar los dientes.

I want to talk about bacterial plaque.	**Quiero platicar acerca de la placa bacteriana.** *(Kee-eh-roh plah-tee-kahr ah-sehr-kah deh lah plah-kah bahk-teh-ree-ah-nah)*
Plaque is a sticky, colorless layer of bacteria.	**La placa es una capa pegajosa sin color y con bacterias.** *(Lah plah-kah ehs oo-nah kah-pah peh-gah-hoh-sah seen koh-lohr ee kohn bahk-teh-ree-ahs)*
It causes dental caries.	**Causa caries dental.** *(Kah-oo-sah kah-ree-ehs dehn-tahl)*
It also causes pyorrhea and tooth loss.	**Causa también pérdida de dientes y piorrea.** *(Kah-oo-sah tahm-bee-ehn pehr-dee-dah deh dee-ehn-tehs ee pee-oh-reh-ah)*
Plaque can be prevented by brushing and flossing.	**La placa se evita usando hilo dental y cepillo.** *(Lah plah-kah seh eh-bee-tah oo-sahn-doh ee-loh dehn-tahl ee seh-pee-yoh)*

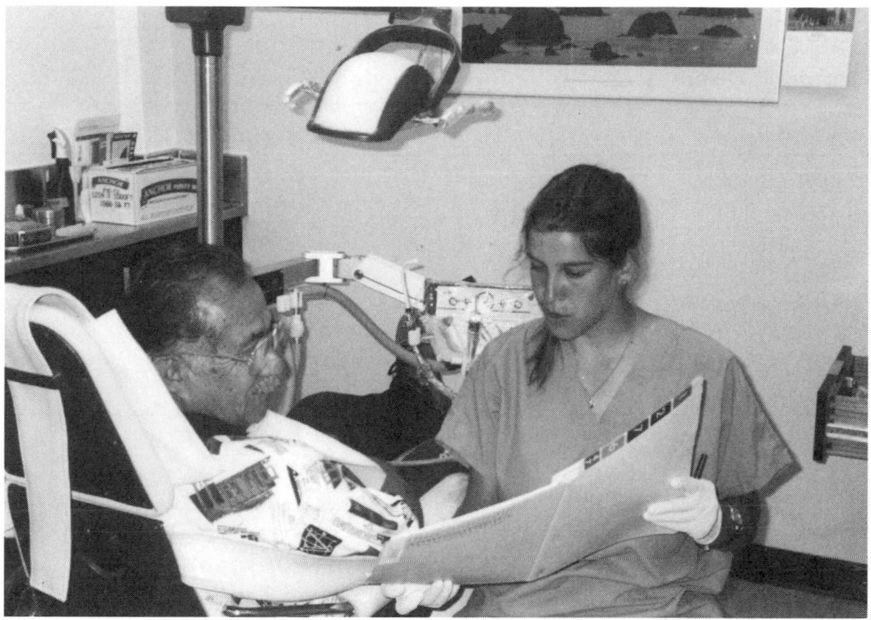

Figure 15–1 It is important to give written instructions to patients.

The only way we can see plaque is by using a solution that stains the teeth.

La única manera de ver la placa es al usar una solución que mancha los dientes.

(Lah oo-nee-kah mah-neh-rah deh behr lah plah-kah ehs ahl oo-sahr oo-nah soh-loo-see-ohn keh mahn-chah lohs dee-ehn-tehs)

I am going to put some solution around all your teeth.

Voy a poner una solución alrededor de todos sus dientes.

(Boy ah poh-nehr oo-nah soh-loo-see-ohn ahl-reh-deh-dohr deh toh-dohs soos dee-ehn-tehs)

Here is a glass of water to rinse with.

Aquí está un vaso de agua para que se enjuague.

(Ah-kee ehs-tah oon bah-soh deh ah-goo-ah pah-rah keh seh ehn-hoo-ah-geh)

Give the patient a hand mirror and toothbrush.

Déle al paciente un espejo de mano y un cepillo de dientes.

(Deh-leh ahl pah-see-ehn-teh oon ehs-peh-hoh deh mah-noh ee oon seh-pee-yoh deh dee-ehn-tehs)

TABLE 15–3 Common Diseases	**TABLA 15–3 Enfermedades comunes**	
English	**Spanish**	**Pronunciation**
dental plaque	**placa**	*(plah-kah)*
gingivitis	**gingivitis**	*(heen-hee-bee-tees)*
gumboil	**flemón/absceso**	*(fleh-mohn/ahb-seh-soh)*
lesions	**lesiones**	*(leh-see-oh-nehs)*
odontalgia/tooth ache	**odontalgia/dolor de muela**	*(oh-dohn-tahl-ee-ah/doh-lohr deh moo-eh-lah)*
phyorrhea	**piorrea**	*(pee-oh-reh-ah)*
tumor	**tumor**	*(too-mohr)*

If any plaque is present point to the areas saying:

Si hay placa apunte a las áreas y diga:
(See ah-ee plah-kah ah-poon-teh ah lahs ah-reh-ahs ee dee-gah)

Can you see the places that are stained?

¿Puede ver los lugares que están dañados?
(Poo-eh-deh behr lohs loo-gah-rehs keh ehs-tahn dah-nyah-dohs)

That is plaque.

Esa es la placa.
(Eh-sah ehs lah plah-kah)

You will need to brush a little better in these areas.

Necesitará cepillarse mejor en estas áreas.
(Neh-seh-see-tah-rah seh-pee-yahr-seh meh-hohr ehn ehs-tahs ah-reh-ahs)

Let me show you with your toothbrush a way that will help you remove the plaque.

Déjeme enseñarle con su cepillo una manera que le ayudará a quitar la placa.
(Deh-heh-meh ehn-seh-nyahr-leh kohn soo seh-pee-yoh oo-nah mah-neh-rah keh leh ah-yoo-dahr-ah ah kee-tahr lah plah-kah)

Demonstrate the basic technique first on yourself, making sure the patient can see exactly what you are doing. Next have the patient practice the technique on himself.

Demuestre la técnica básica primero, asegurando que el paciente vea exactamente lo que hace. Luego, haga que el paciente practique la técnica.

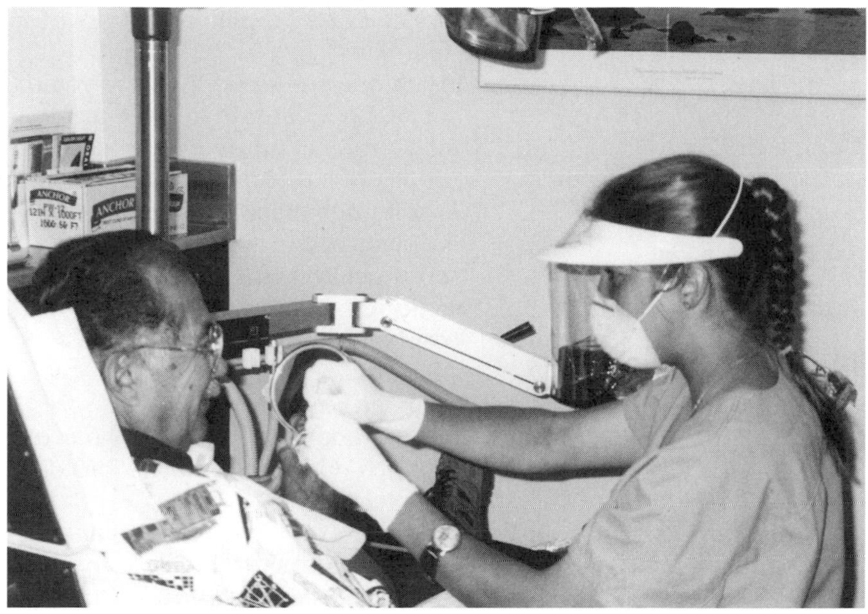

Figure 15–2 Explain to the patient what you are about to do.

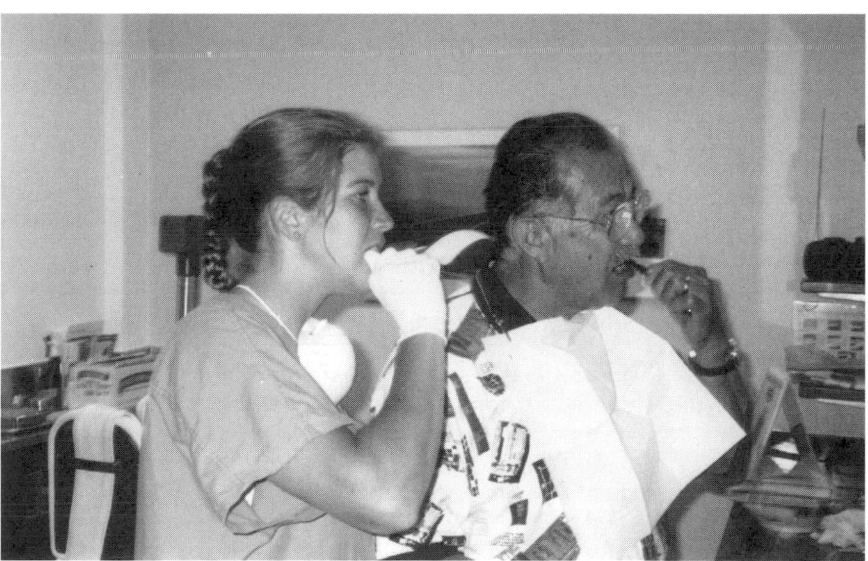

Figure 15–3 Demonstrate the procedure to the patient and then have him demonstrate to assure understanding.

Make sure that you point the toothbrush toward the gumline.	**Asegure que el cepillo apunte contra la encía.** *(Ah-seh-goo-reh keh ehl seh-pee-yoh ah-poon-teh kohn-trah lah ehn-see-ah)*
Using a circular motion, brush one to two teeth at a time.	**Usando movimiento circular, cepille uno o dos dientes a la vez.** *(Oo-sahn-doh moh-bee-mee-ehn-toh seer-koo-lahr, seh-pee-yeh oo-noh oh dohs dee-ehn-tehs ah lah behs)*
Practice with the brush; make sure you go around all the teeth.	**Practique con el cepillo; asegure de cepillar alrededor de todos los dientes.** *(Prahk-tee-keh kohn ehl seh-pee-yoh; ah-seh-goo-reh deh seh-pee-yahr ahl-reh-deh-dohr deh toh-dohs lohs dee-ehn-tehs)*
After you finish brushing, we will practice flossing.	**Después de terminar de cepillar practicaremos usando el hilo dental.** *(Dehs-poo-ehs deh tehr-mee-nahr deh seh-pee-yahr prahk-tee-kah-reh-mohs oo-sahn-doh ehl ee-loh dehn-tahl)*
Plaque gets in between the teeth where the brush cannot reach.	**La placa entra en medio de los dientes donde no alcanza el cepillo.** *(Lah plah-kah ehn-trah ehn meh-dee-oh deh lohs dee-ehn-tehs dohn-deh noh ahl-kahn-zah ehl seh-pee-yoh)*

TABLE 15–4
Dental Appliances

TABLA 15–4
Aditamentos dentales

English	Spanish	Pronunciation
braces	**abrazaderas**	*(ah-brah-sah-deh-rahs)*
complete dentures	**dentadura completa**	*(dehn-tah-doo-rah kohm-pleh-tah)*
crowns	**coronas**	*(koh-roh-nahs)*
fixed bridge	**puente fijo**	*(poo-ehn-teh fee-hoh)*
gold tooth	**diente de oro**	*(dee-ehn-teh deh oh-roh)*
implant	**implante**	*(eem-plahn-teh)*
movable bridge	**puente móvil**	*(poo-ehn-teh moh-beel)*
partial denture	**dentadura parcial**	*(dehn-tah-doo-rah pahr-see-ahl)*
sealant	**placa protectora**	*(plah-kah proh-tehk-toh-rah)*

That is why it is important to clean these areas.
Por ello es importante limpiar estas áreas.
(Pohr eh-yoh ehs eem-pohr-tahn-teh leem-pee-ahr ehs-tahs ah-reh-ahs)

Let me show you the correct way to floss.
Déjeme enseñarle la manera correcta de usar el hilo.
(Deh-heh-meh ehn-seh-nyahr-leh lah mah-neh-rah koh-rehk-tah deh oo-sahr ehl ee-loh)

Begin demonstration, explaining each step to the patient.
Empieze la demostración, explicando cada paso al paciente.

Wind 18 inches of floss around one middle finger.
Enrede dieciocho pulgadas de hilo alrededor del tercer dedo.
(Ehn-reh-deh dee-eh-see-oh-choh pool-gah-dahs deh ee-loh ahl-reh-deh-dohr dehl tehr-sehr deh-doh)

Wind the rest around the middle finger of the other hand.
Enrede el resto alrededor del dedo medio de la otra mano.
(Ehn-reh-deh ehl rehs-toh ahl-reh-deh-dohr dehl deh-doh meh-dee-oh deh lah oh-trah mah-noh)

Use thumbs and forefingers to guide the floss.
Use el dedo gordo y el índice para guiar el hilo.
(Oo-seh ehl deh-doh gohr-doh ee ehl een-dee-seh pah-rah gee-ahr ehl ee-loh)

Insert the floss gently between the teeth.
Meta el hilo suavemente en medio de los dientes.
(Meh-tah ehl ee-loh soo-ah-beh-mehn-teh ehn meh-dee-oh deh lohs dee-ehn-tehs)

Curve the floss into a "C."
Ponga el hilo en forma de "C".
(Pohn-gah ehl ee-loh ehn fohr-mah deh "C")

Fluoride makes teeth stronger and healthy. It also helps with sensitivity.

El fluoruro ayuda a que los dientes sean fuertes y sanos. También evita la sensibilidad.

Now I am going to give you some fluoride.	**Ahora voy a darle fluoruro.** *(Ah-oh-rah boh-ee ah dahr-leh floh-roo-roh)*
This is to help your teeth become stronger, and if cavities are present it will help slow the process.	**Esto ayudará a hacer que los dientes sean más fuertes y si tiene cavidades, ayudará a retardar el proceso.** *(Ehs-toh ah-yoo-dahr-ah ah ah-sehr keh lohs dee-ehn-tehs seh-ahn mahs foo-ehr-tehs ee see tee-ehn-eh kah-bee-dah-dehs, ah-yoo-dahr-ah ah reh-tahr-dahr ehl proh-seh-soh)*
It will also help if you have any teeth that are sensitive.	**Ayudará también si los dientes están sensibles.** *(Ah-yoo-dah-rah tahm-bee-ehn see-lohs dee-ehn-tehs ehs-tahn sehn-see-blehs)*
I will place the trays over the teeth.	**Pondré las bandejas sobre los dientes.** *(Pohn-dreh lahs bahn-deh-hahs soh-breh lohs dee-ehn-tehs)*
I want you to chew on them for four minutes.	**Quiero que las muerda por cuatro minutos.** *(Kee-eh-roh keh lahs moo-ehr-dah pohr koo-ah-troh mee-noo-tohs)*
I will place the saliva ejector in between the trays so that you will not swallow any of the fluoride.	**Pondré el extractor de saliva en medio de las bandejas, para que no se trague el fluoruro.** *(Pohn-dreh ehl ehx-trahk-tohr deh sah-lee-bah ehn meh-dee-oh deh lahs bahn-deh-hahs, pah-rah keh noh seh trah-geh ehl floh-roo-roh)*
Do not eat or drink anything for thirty minutes.	**No coma o beba nada por treinta minutos.** *(Noh koh-mah oh beh-bah nah-dah pohr treh-een-tah mee-noo-tohs)*
Please return in six months.	**Por favor regrese en seis meses.** *(Pohr fah-bohr reh-greh-seh ehn seh-ees meh-sehs)*

Chapter Sixteen | **Capítulo dieciséis**

A Home Visit | Una visita al hogar

A home visit gives you the opportunity to assess several members of the family. It is also a convenient time to assess the home environment and to determine how the family members are coping with their needs. The community worker approaches Mr. Ríos, the grandfather. Mr. Ríos suffered a stroke 5 months ago and is recuperating.

Una visita al hogar proporciona la oportunidad de asesorar a varios miembros de la familia. También es una ocasión conveniente para evaluar el ambiente familiar y determinar cómo se están dando abasto con sus necesidades. El trabajador comunitario se dirige al señor Ríos, el abuelo. El señor Ríos sufrió un ataque de apoplejía hace cinco meses y se está recuperando.

Mr. Ríos, how are you?	**Señor Ríos, ¿cómo está?** *(Seh-nyohr Ree-ohs, koh-moh ehs-tah)*
Good afternoon!	**¡Buenas tardes!** *(Boo-eh-nahs tahr-dehs)*
Do you remember me?	**¿Se acuerda de mí?** *(Seh ah-koo-ehr-dah deh mee)*
I am:	**Yo soy:** *(Yo soh-ee)*
the medical student.	**el/la estudiante de medicina.** *(ehl/lah ehs-too-dee-ahn-teh deh meh-dee-see-nah)*
the nurse.	**el/la enfermero(a).** *(ehl/lah ehn-fehr-meh-roh[ah])*
the therapist.	**el/la terapista.** *(ehl/lah teh-rah-pees-tah)*
I want to talk to you.	**Quiero hablar con usted.** *(Kee-eh-roh ah-blahr kohn oos-tehd)*
Can you get out of bed?	**¿Puede salir de la cama?** *(Poo-eh-deh sah-leer deh lah kah-mah)*

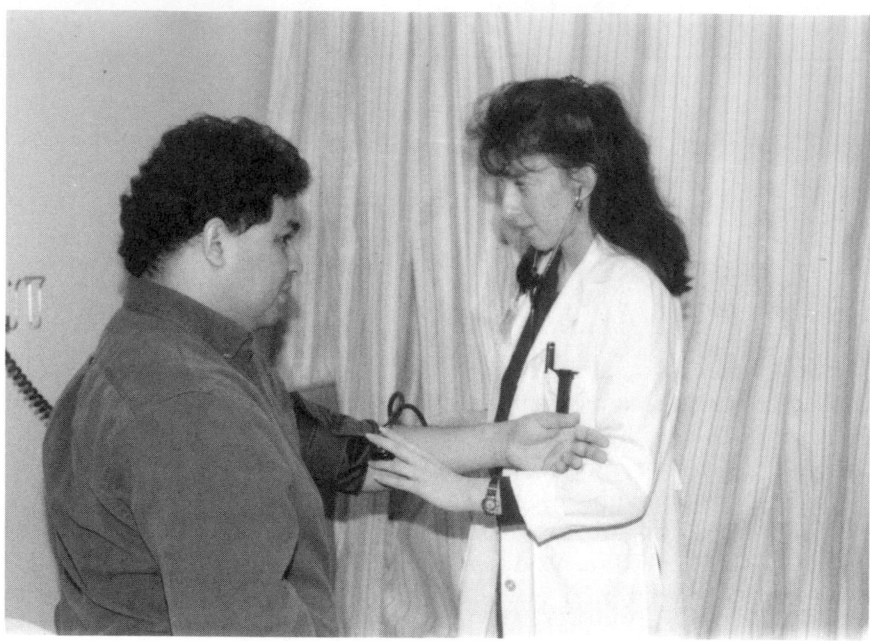

Figure 16–1 Vital signs are taken routinely during a home visit.

Please raise this arm.	**Por favor, levante este brazo.** *(Pohr fah-bohr, leh-bahn-teh ehs-teh brah-soh)*
Now raise the left arm.	**Ahora levante el brazo izquierdo.** *(Ah-oh-rah leh-bahn-teh ehl brah-soh ees-kee-ehr-doh)*
I will help you sit.	**Le ayudaré a sentarse.** *(Leh ah-yoo-dah-reh ah sehn-tahr-seh)*
Stay sitting.	**Quédese sentado.** *(Keh-deh-seh sehn-tah-doh)*
I have some paper.	**Tengo papel.** *(Tehn-goh pah-pehl)*
I want you to write your name and today's date.	**Quiero que escriba su nombre y la fecha de hoy.** *(Kee-eh-roh keh ehs-kree-bah soo nohm-breh ee lah feh-chah deh oh-ee)*
Now, stand up and walk.	**Ahora, levántese y camine.** *(Ah-oh-rah, leh-bahn-teh-seh ee kah-mee-neh)*

Walk six paces.	**Camine seis pasos.** *(Kah-mee-neh seh-ees pah-sohs)*
Do not hold on to the wall.	**No se agarre de la pared.** *(Noh seh ah-gah-reh deh lah pah-rehd)*
Sit in the chair.	**Siéntese en la silla.** *(See-ehn-teh-seh ehn lah see-yah)*
Please cross your leg.	**Por favor, cruce la pierna.** *(Pohr fah-bohr, kroo-seh lah pee-ehr-nah)*
Lift your right foot.	**Levante el pie derecho.** *(Leh-bahn-teh ehl pee-eh deh-reh-choh)*
Have you had swelling?	**¿Ha tenido hinchazón?** *(Ah teh-nee-doh een-chah-sohn)*
on your feet?	**¿en los pies?** *(ehn lohs pee-ehs)*
ankles?	**¿tobillos?** *(toh-bee-yohs)*
eyelids?	**¿párpados?** *(pahr-pah-dohs)*
Are you taking your medicines?	**¿Está tomando sus medicinas?** *(Ehs-tah toh-mahn-doh soos meh-dee-see-nahs)*

TABLE 16–1
Personal Pronouns

TABLA 16–1
Pronombres personales

English	Spanish	Pronunciation
I	**Yo**	*(yoh)*
You (*familiar*)	**Tú**	*(too)*
You (*formal*)	**Usted**	*(oos-tehd)*
He	**Él**	*(ehl)*
She	**Ella**	*(eh-yah)*
We (*masculine*)	**Nosotros**	*(noh-soh-trohs)*
We (*feminine*)	**Nosotras**	*(noh-soh-trahs)*
They (*masculine*)	**Ellos**	*(eh-yohs)*
They (*feminine*)	**Ellas**	*(eh-yahs)*

How many times a day?	**¿Cuántas veces al día?** *(Koo-ahn-tahs beh-sehs ahl dee-ah)*
Do you sleep during the day?	**¿Duerme durante el día?** *(Doo-ehr-meh doo-rahn-teh ehl dee-ah)*
At what time do you go to sleep?	**¿A qué hora se acuesta a dormir?** *(Ah keh oh-rah seh ah-koo-ehs-tah ah dohr-meer)*
At what time do you get up?	**¿A qué hora se levanta?** *(Ah keh oh-rah seh leh-bahn-tah)*
Do you wake up at night?	**¿Se despierta en la noche?** *(Seh dehs-pee-ehr-tah ehn lah noh-cheh)*
Your appetite is good?	**¿Tiene buen apetito?** *(Tee-eh-neh boo-ehn ah-peh-tee-toh)*
Is your appetite bad?	**¿Tiene mal apetito?** *(Tee-eh-neh mahl ah-peh-tee-toh)*
How many times do you eat per day?	**¿Cuántas veces come por día?** *(Koo-ahn-tahs beh-sehs koh-meh pohr dee-ah)*
What did you eat for breakfast?	**¿Qué comió en el desayuno?** *(Keh koh-mee-oh ehn ehl deh-sah-yoo-noh)*
Tell me what foods.	**Dígame qué alimentos.** *(Dee-gah-meh keh ah-lee-mehn-tohs)*
Do you drink coffee?	**¿Toma café?** *(Toh-mah kah-feh)*
How many cups per day?	**¿Cuántas tazas diarias?** *(Koo-ahn-tahs tah-sahs dee-ah-ree-ahs)*
How many glasses of water do you drink?	**¿Cuántos vasos de agua toma?** *(Koo-ahn-tohs bah-sohs deh ah-goo-ah toh-mah)*
When was the last time you used the toilet?	**¿Cuándo fue la última vez que hizo del baño/que obró?** *(Koo-ahn-doh foo-eh lah ool-tee-mah behs keh ee-soh dehl bah-nyoh/keh oh-broh)*
Are you constipated?	**¿Está estreñido?** *(Ehs-tah ehs-treh-nyee-doh)*
Do you have diarrhea?	**¿Tiene diarrea?** *(Tee-eh-neh dee-ah-reh-ah)*
How often do you urinate?	**¿Cuántas veces orina?** *(Koo-ahn-tahs beh-sehs oh-ree-nah)*

What was the color of the urine?	**¿Cuál era el color de la orina?** *(Koo-ahl eh-rah ehl koh-lohr deh lah oh-ree-nah)*
Did you see blood in the urine?	**¿Vio sangre en la orina?** *(Bee-oh sahn-greh ehn lah oh-ree-nah)*
Do you dribble?	**¿Se orina sin sentir?** *(Seh oh-ree-nah seen sehn-teer)*
Do you have problems with starting to urinate?	**¿Tiene dificultad para empezar a orinar?** *(Tee-eh-neh dee-fee-kool-tahd pah-rah ehm-peh-sahr ah oh-ree-nahr)*
Do you have hesitancy?	**¿Se corta el chorro de la orina?** *(Seh kohr-tah ehl choh-roh deh lah oh-ree-nah)*
Do you have questions?	**¿Tiene preguntas que hacerme?** *(Tee-eh-neh preh-goon-tahs keh ah-sehr-meh)*
Thank you for the information.	**Gracias por la información.** *(Grah-see-ahs pohr lah een-fohr-mah-see-ohn)*

Unit 3

Unidad 3

Chapter Seventeen **Capítulo diecisiete**

The Patient's Room / El cuarto del paciente

Mr. González has been admitted to room 569 (five hundred sixty-nine), of the surgery floor.

Al señor González lo admitieron en el cuarto cinco, seis, nueve, (quinientos sesenta y nueve) del piso de cirugía.

Hello, Mr. González. I am the nurse in charge.

Hola, señor González. Yo soy la enfermera encargada/el enfermero encargado.
(Oh-lah, seh-nyohr Gohn-sah-lehs. Yoh soh-ee lah ehn-fehr-meh-rah ehn-kahr-gah-dah/ehl ehn-fehr-meh-roh ehn-kahr-gah-doh)

This is a handout that deals with the hospital's guidelines.

Este es un folleto que trata de las reglas/guías del hospital.
(Ehs-teh ehs oon foh-yeh-toh keh trah-tah deh lahs reh-glahs/gee-ahs dehl ohs-pee-tahl)

I am going to give you a tour of the floor.

Voy a darle un recorrido por el piso.
(Boy ah dahr-leh oon reh-koh-ree-doh pohr ehl pee-soh)

This is the lobby.

Esta es la sala de espera.
(Ehs-tah ehs lah sah-lah deh ehs-peh-rah)

You can bring your family here.

Puede traer a su familia aquí.
(Poo-eh-deh trah-ehr ah soo fah-mee-lee-ah ah-kee)

This is the service area.

Esta es el área de servicio.
(Ehs-tah ehs ehl ah-reh-ah deh sehr-bee-see-oh)

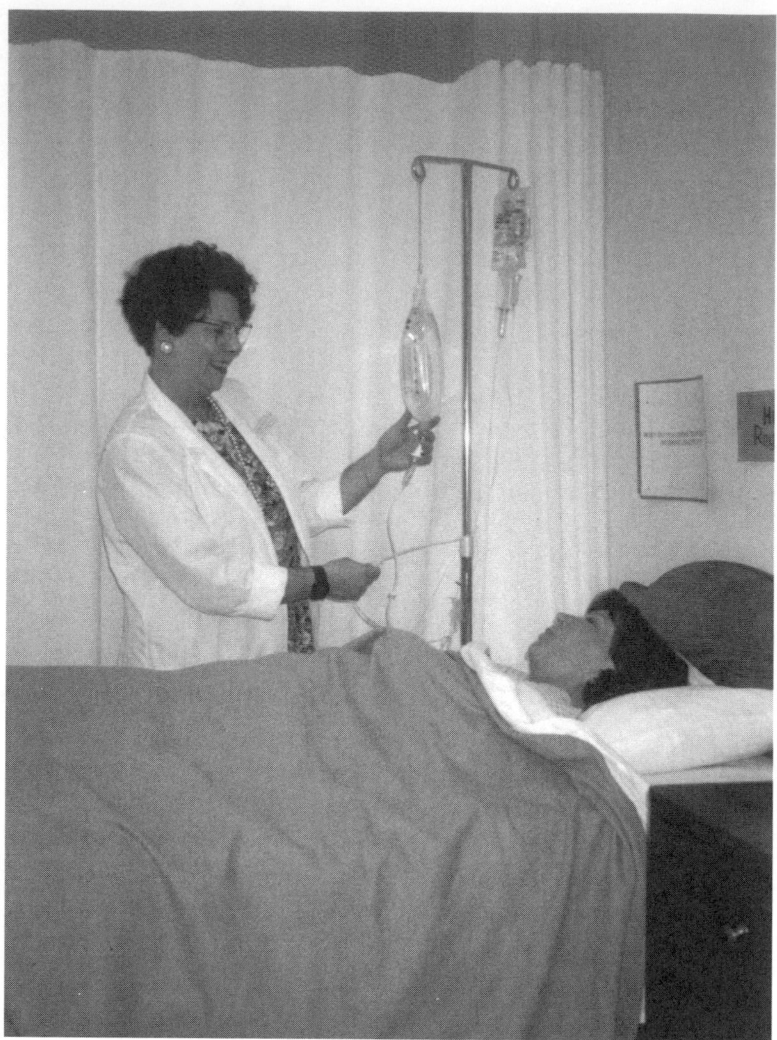

Figure 17–1 There are hospital expectations for the patient.

You can order coffee here.	**Puede ordenar café aquí.** *(Poo-eh-deh ohr-deh-nahr kah-feh ah-kee)*
The stairs are at the end of the hallway.	**La escalera está al final del pasillo.** *(Lah ehs-kah-leh-rah ehs-tah ahl feen-ahl dehl pah-see-yoh)*

TABLE 17–1 Pronunciation of Selected Words

TABLA 17–1 Pronunciación de palabras selectas

English	Spanish	Pronunciation
bathroom	**baño**	*(bah-nyoh)*
bell	**campana/timbre**	*(kahm-pah-nah/teem-breh)*
button	**botón**	*(boh-tohn)*
corner	**esquina**	*(ehs-kee-nah)*
patient	**paciente**	*(pah-see-ehn-teh)*
room	**cuarto**	*(koo-ahr-toh)*
stairs	**escalera**	*(ehs-kah-leh-rah)*
table	**mesa**	*(meh-sah)*
wall	**pared**	*(pah-rehd)*
window	**ventana**	*(behn-tah-nah)*

The elevators work twenty-four hours.

Los elevadores funcionan las veinticuatro horas.
(Lohs eh-leh-bah-doh-rehs foon-see-oh-nahn lahs beh-een-tee-koo-ah-troh oh-rahs)

In case of fire, take the stairs.

En caso de fuego, use la escalera.
(Ehn kah-soh deh foo-eh-goh, oo-seh lah ehs-kah-leh-rah)

There are bathrooms for guests in the corner.

Hay baños para las visitas en la esquina.
(Hay bah-nyohs pah-rah lahs bee-see-tahs ehn lah ehs-kee-nah)

This is your room.

Este es su cuarto.
(Ehs-teh ehs soo koo-ahr-toh)

You cannot hang anything from the ceiling.

No puede colgar nada del techo.
(Noh poo-eh-deh kohl-gahr nah-dah dehl teh-choh)

You cannot hang anything from the door.

No puede colgar nada en la puerta.
(Noh poo-eh-deh kohl-gahr nah-dah ehn lah poo-ehr-tah)

You can tape pictures to the wall.

Puede pegar retratos en la pared.
(Poo-eh-deh peh-gahr reh-trah-tohs ehn lah pah-rehd)

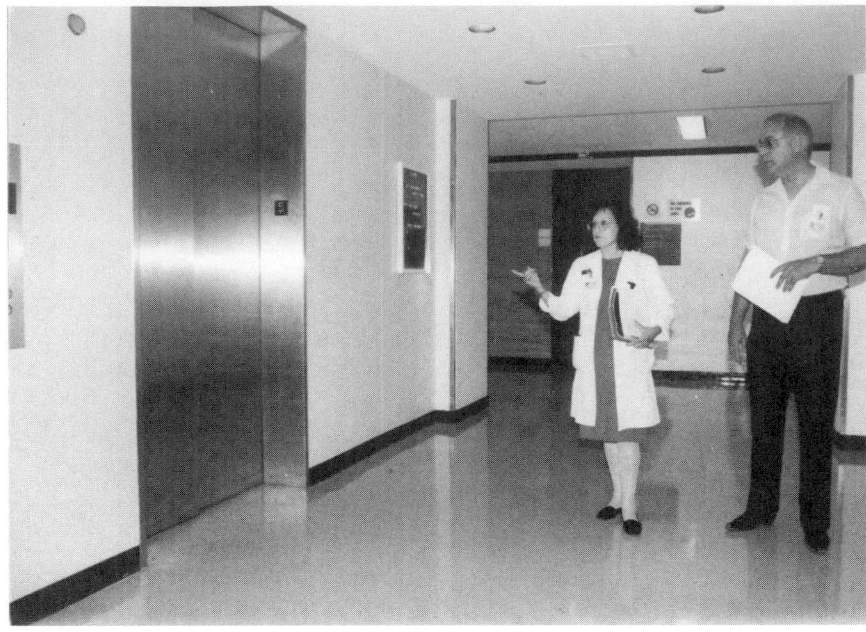

Figure 17–2 The restroom for visitors is across the lobby next to the elevators.

You can put cards on the shelf.	**Puede poner tarjetas en el estante.** *(Poo-eh-deh poh-nehr tahr-heh-tahs ehn ehl ehs-tahn-teh)*
You can have flowers.	**Puede tener flores.** *(Poo-eh-deh teh-nehr floh-rehs)*
This chair turns into a bed.	**Esta silla se hace cama.** *(Ehs-tah see-yah seh ah-seh kah-mah)*
This is the call bell/buzzer.	**Esta es la campana/el timbre.** *(Ehs-tah ehs lah kahm-pah-nah/ehl teem-breh)*
This button lowers (raises) the headboard.	**Este botón baja (sube) la cabecera de la cama.** *(Ehs-teh boh-tohn bah-hah [soo-beh] lah kah-beh-seh-rah deh lah kah-mah)*
Do you need the headboard up?	**¿Necesita levantar más la cabecera?** *(Neh-seh-see-tah leh-bahn-tahr mahs lah kah-beh-seh-rah)*
The bed has one blanket.	**La cama tiene una frazada/colcha.** *(Lah kah-mah tee-eh-neh oo-nah frah-sah-dah/kohl-chah)*

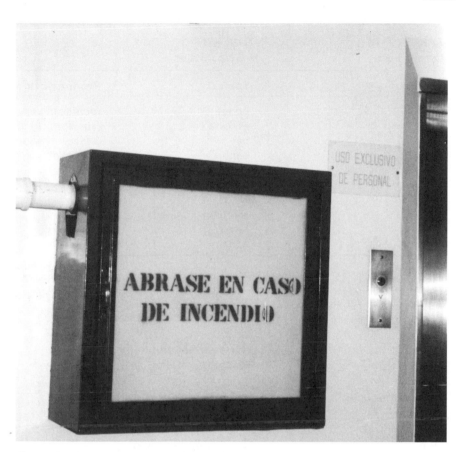

Figure 17–3 It is important to know where emergency equipment is located.

If you need more sheets, call the assistant.	**Si necesita más sábanas, llame a la/al asistente.** *(See neh-seh-see-tah mahs sah-bah-nahs, yah-meh ah lah/ahl ah-sees-tehn-teh)*
Do you need more pillows?	**¿Necesita más almohadas?** *(Neh-seh-see-tah mahs ahl-moh-ah-dahs)*
Keep the siderails up at night.	**Mantenga los barandales levantados durante la noche.** *(Mahn-tehn-gah lohs bah-rahn-dah-lehs leh-bahn-tah-dohs doo-rahn-teh lah noh-cheh)*
You have a private bathroom.	**Tiene un baño/inodoro privado.** *(Tee-eh-neh oon bah-nyoh/ee-noh-doh-roh pree-bah-doh)*

TABLE 17–2 Useful Verbs	**TABLA 17–1 Verbos útiles**	
English	**Spanish**	**Pronunciation**
can, to be able to	**poder**	*(poh-dehr)*
is	**es/está**	*(ehs/ehs-tah)*
there is/are	**hay**	*(ah-ee)*
to bathe	**bañar**	*(bah-nyahr)*
to close	**cerrar**	*(seh-rahr)*
to cry	**llorar**	*(yoh-rahr)*
to go	**ir**	*(eer)*
to hang	**colgar**	*(kohl-gahr)*
to have	**tener**	*(teh-nehr)*
to speak	**hablar**	*(ah-blahr)*

There is a shower.	**Hay una ducha/regadera.** *(Ah-ee oo-nah doo-chah/reh-gah-deh-rah)*
There is also a bathub/tub.	**También hay una bañera/tina.** *(Tahm-bee-ehn ah-ee oo-nah bah-nyeh-rah/tee-nah)*
Your clothes go in the closet.	**Su ropa va en el closet/ropero.** *(Soo roh-pah bah ehn ehl kloh-seht/roh-peh-roh)*
Don't walk barefoot.	**No camine descalzo.** *(No kah-mee-neh dehs-kahl-soh)*
Use the house shoes; the floor is cold.	**Use las pantunflas/chanclas; el piso está frío.** *(Oo-seh lahs pahn-toon-flahs/chahn-klahs; ehl pee-soh ehs-tah free-oh)*
You can make local phone calls.	**Puede hacer llamadas locales.** *(Poo-eh-deh ah-sehr yah-mah-dahs loh-kah-lehs)*
Dial 9, wait for the tone, then dial the number you want to call.	**Marque el nueve, espere el tono, luego marque el número que quiera llamar.** *(Mahr-keh ehl noo-eh-beh, ehs-peh-reh ehl toh-noh, loo-eh-goh mahr-keh ehl noo-meh-roh keh kee-eh-rah yah-mahr)*
You can call collect.	**Puede llamar por cobrar.** *(Poo-eh-deh yah-mahr pohr koh-brahr)*

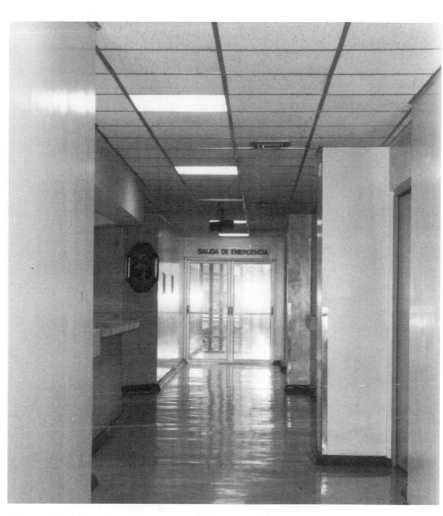

Figure 17–4 Use the emergency exit in case of fire.

If you want to watch TV, you have to pay a fee.	**Si quiere ver la televisión, tiene que pagar una cuota.** *(See kee-eh-reh behr lah teh-leh-bee-see-ohn, tee-eh-neh keh pah-gahr oo-nah koo-oh-tah)*
You cannot smoke in your room.	**No puede fumar en el cuarto.** *(Noh poo-eh-deh foo-mahr ehn ehl koo-ahr-toh)*
You can smoke in the patio.	**Puede fumar en el patio.** *(Poo-eh-deh foo-mahr ehn ehl pah-tee-oh)*

TABLE 17–3 Useful Items | **TABLA 17–3 Artículos útiles**

English	Spanish	Pronunciation
comb	**peine**	*(peh-ee-neh)*
cosmetics	**cosméticos**	*(kohs-meh-tee-kohs)*
(drinking) glass	**vaso**	*(bah-soh)*
lipstick	**lápiz de labios**	*(lah-pees deh lah-bee-ohs)*
nightgown	**camisa de dormir/bata**	*(kah-mee-sah deh dohr-meer/ bah-tah)*
perfume	**perfume**	*(pehr-foo-meh)*
razor	**navaja/máquina de afeitar**	*(nah-bah-hah/mah-kee-nah deh ah-feh-ee-tahr)*
toothbrush	**cepillo de dientes**	*(seh-pee-yoh deh dee-ehn-tehs)*
toothpaste	**pasta de dientes**	*(pahs-tah deh dee-ehn-tehs)*

TABLE 17–4 Clothing Items | **TABLA 17–4 Artículos de vestir**

English	Spanish	Pronunciation
blouse	**blusa**	*(bloo-sah)*
coat	**abrigo**	*(ah-bree-goh)*
dress	**vestido**	*(behs-tee-doh)*
gown	**bata/vestido**	*(bah-tah/behs-tee-doh)*
hose/stockings	**medias**	*(meh-dee-ahs)*
jacket	**chaqueta**	*(chah-keh-tah)*
pants/slacks	**pantalones**	*(pahn-tah-loh-nehs)*
shoes	**zapatos**	*(sah-pah-tohs)*
skirt	**falda**	*(fahl-dah)*
socks	**calcetines/calcetas**	*(kahl-seh-tee-nehs/kahl-seh-tahs)*
suit	**traje**	*(trah-heh)*
sweater	**chamarra/suéter**	*(chah-mah-rah/soo-eh-tehr)*
tie	**corbata**	*(kohr-bah-tah)*
underwear	**ropa interior**	*(roh-pah een-teh-ree-ohr)*

You cannot open the windows.

No puede abrir las ventanas.
(Noh poo-eh-deh ah-breer lahs behn-tah-nahs)

Visiting hours are from nine in the morning to nine at night.

Las horas de visita son de las nueve de la mañana a las nueve de la noche.
(Lahs oh-rahs deh bee-see-tah sohn deh lahs noo-eh-beh deh lah mah-nyah-nah ah lahs noo-eh-beh deh lah noh-cheh)

Chapter Eighteen — Capítulo dieciocho

The Laboratory — El laboratorio

Mrs. Garza is going to have blood drawn in preparation for 24-hour urine collection. The nurse explains the laboratory procedure and the hospital routine.

A la señora Garza le van a tomar muestras de sangre y se prepara para colectar/juntar su orina por veinticuatro horas. La enfermera le explica el procedimiento y la rutina del laboratorio del hospital.

Mrs. Garza, the doctor ordered blood samples.	**Señora Garza, el doctor/la doctora ordenó muestras de sangre.** *(Seh-nyoh-rah Gahr-sah, ehl dohk-tohr/ lah dohk-toh-rah ohr-deh-noh moo-ehs-trahs deh sahn-greh)*
Almost always the technician comes at six in the morning.	**Casi siempre el laboratorista viene a las seis de la mañana.** *(Kah-see see-ehm-preh ehl lah-boh-rah-toh-rees-tah bee-eh-neh ah lahs seh-ees deh lah mah-nyah-nah)*
Please do not eat after midnight.	**Por favor, no coma después de medianoche.** *(Pohr fah-bohr, noh koh-mah dehs-poo-ehs deh meh-dee-ah-noh-cheh)*
In your case, eat nothing after 8 o'clock.	**En su caso, no coma nada después de las ocho de la noche.** *(Ehn soo kah-soh, noh koh-mah nah-dah dehs-poo-ehs deh lahs oh-choh deh lah noh-cheh)*
Tomorrow they will give you a special test.	**Mañana le harán un examen especial.** *(Mah-nyah-nah leh ah-rahn oon ehx-ah-mehn ehs-peh-see-ahl)*
I am going to explain how to collect the urine.	**Le voy a explicar cómo juntar la orina.** *(Leh boy ah ehx-plee-kahr koh-moh hoon-tahr lah oh-ree-nah)*

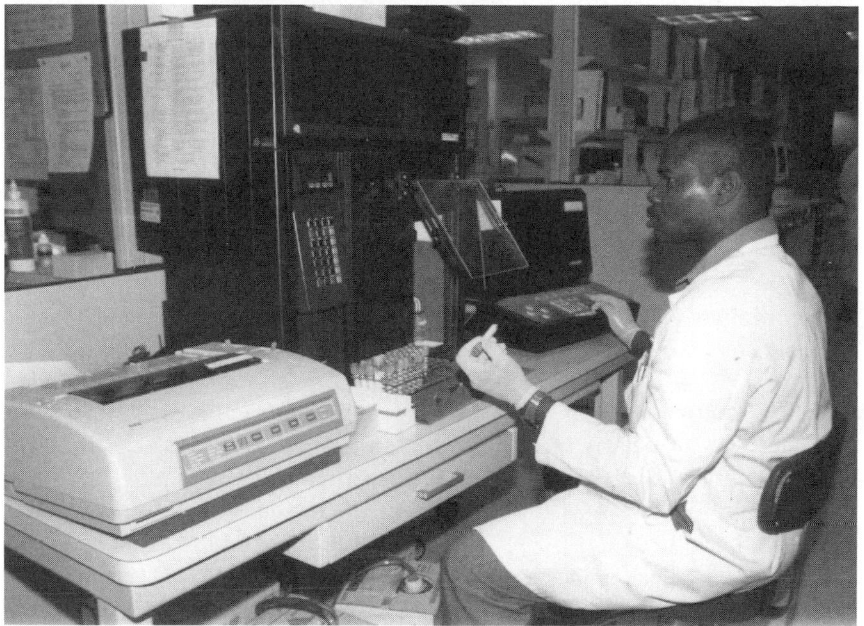

Figure 18–1 Many blood tests are run in the laboratory.

TABLE 18–1 Pronunciation of Selected Words

TABLA 18–1 Pronunciación de palabras selectas

English	Spanish	Pronunciation
after	**después**	*(dehs-poo-ehs)*
blood	**sangre**	*(sahn-greh)*
bottle	**botella**	*(boh-teh-yah)*
every time	**cada vez**	*(kah-dah behs)*
explain	**explique**	*(ehx-plee-keh)*
in the morning	**en la mañana**	*(ehn lah mah-nyah-nah)*
laboratory	**laboratorio**	*(lah-boh-rah-toh-ree-oh)*
next	**siguiente**	*(see-gee-ehn-teh)*
pin prick	**picadura**	*(pee-kah-doo-rah)*
remain	**quédese**	*(keh-deh-seh)*
sample	**muestra**	*(moo-ehs-trah)*
technician	**técnico**	*(tehk-nee-koh)*
tomorrow	**mañana**	*(mah-nyah-nah)*
tubes	**tubos**	*(too-bohs)*

I will wake you up in the morning.	**La voy a despertar en la mañana.** *(Lah boy ah dehs-pehr-tahr ehn lah mah-nyah-nah)*
I will ask you to urinate.	**Le diré que orine.** *(Leh dee-reh keh oh-ree-neh)*
Every time you urinate, put it in the container.	**Cada vez que orine, póngala en el frasco.** *(Kah-dah behs keh oh-ree-neh, pohn-gah-lah ehn ehl frahs-koh)*
The container will be kept in a bucket with ice.	**El frasco se mantendrá en una tina con hielo.** *(Ehl frahs-koh seh mahn-tehn-drah ehn oo-nah tee-nah kohn ee-eh-loh)*
The next day, it will be sent to the laboratory.	**Al día siguiente, se mandará al laboratorio.** *(Ahl dee-ah see-gee-ehn-teh, seh mahn-dah-rah ahl lah-boh-rah-toh-ree-oh)*
Hello, Mrs. Garza.	**Hola, señora Garza.** *(Oh-lah, seh-nyoh-rah Gahr-sah)*

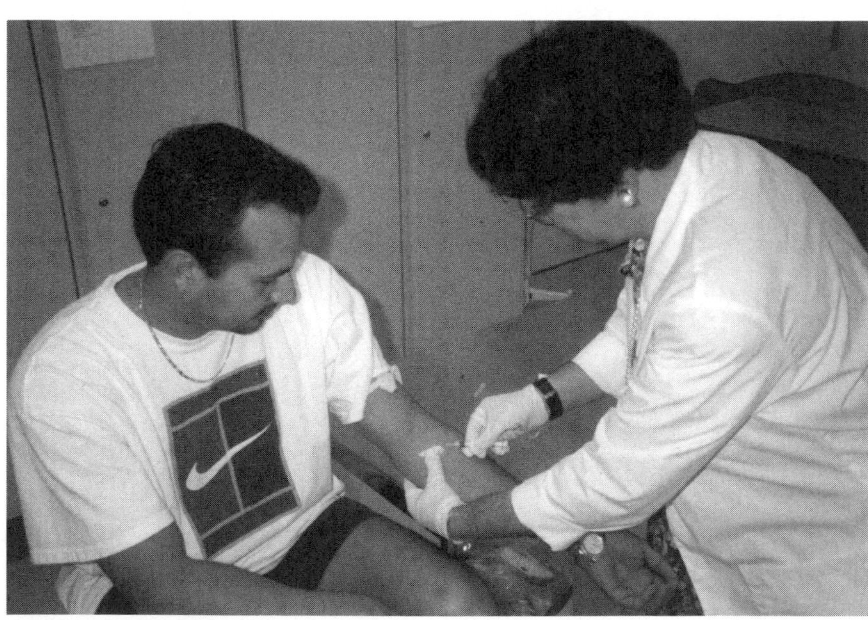

Figure 18–2 Having blood drawn may be a scary situation.

I am here to draw your blood.	**Estoy aquí para tomarle una muestra de sangre.** *(Ehs-toh-ee ah-kee pah-rah toh-mahr-leh oo-nah moo-ehs-trah deh sahn-greh)*
Please stay/remain in bed.	**Por favor, quédese en la cama.** *(Pohr fah-bohr, keh-deh-seh ehn lah kah-mah)*
I am going to lift your sleeve.	**Voy a levantar la manga.** *(Boy ah leh-bahn-tahr lah mahn-gah)*
Make a fist.	**Cierre la mano./Haga un puño.** *(See-eh-reh lah mah-noh/Ah-gah oon poo-nyoh)*
Relax, it will not hurt.	**Relájese, no le va a doler.** *(Reh-lah-heh-seh, no leh bah ah doh-lehr)*
Open your hand.	**Abra la mano.** *(Ah-brah lah mah-noh)*
I want to take a sample from your finger.	**Quiero tomar una muestra del dedo.** *(Kee-eh-roh toh-mahr oo-nah moo-ehs-trah dehl deh-doh)*
I want to see the sugar level.	**Quiero ver el nivel de azúcar.** *(Kee-eh-roh behr ehl nee-behl deh ah-soo-kahr)*
Do not move.	**No se mueva.** *(Noh seh moo-eh-bah)*
This is done quickly.	**Esto se hace rápido.** *(Ehs-toh seh ah-seh rah-pee-doh)*
Have you had blood drawn before?	**¿Le han tomado muestras antes?** *(Leh ahn toh-mah-doh moo-ehs-trahs ahn-tehs)*
You will feel pain like a pin prick.	**Sentirá dolor como una picadura.** *(Sehn-tee-rah doh-lohr koh-moh oo-nah pee-kah-doo-rah)*
I need two tubes of blood:	**Necesito dos tubos de sangre:** *(Neh-seh-see-toh dohs too-bohs deh sahn-greh)*
one tube for a blood count.	**un tubo para una biometría hemática.** *(oon too-boh pah-rah oo-nah bee-oh-meh-tree-ah eh-mah-tee-kah)*

TABLE 18–2
Common Lab Words

TABLA 18–2
Palabras comunes en el laboratorio

English	Spanish	Pronunciation
alcohol	**alcohol**	*(ahl-kohl)*
complete blood count	**biometría hemática* complete**	*(bee-oh-meh-tree-ah heh-mah-tee-kah kohm-pleh-tah)*
fasting	**en ayunas**	*(ehn ah-yoo-nahs)*
gloves	**guantes**	*(goo-ahn-tehs)*
needle	**aguja**	*(ah-goo-hah)*
pathology	**patología**	*(pah-toh-loh-hee-ah)*
procedure	**procedimiento**	*(proh-seh-dee-mee-ehn-toh)*
reports	**reportes**	*(reh-pohr-tehs)*
specimen	**muestra**	*(moo-ehs-trah)*
STAT/emergency	**STAT/emergencia**	*(ehs-taht)/(eh-mehr-hehn-see-ah)*
syringe	**jeringa**	*(heh-reen-gah)*

*In Spanish, the letter **h** is always silent.

another for a serology test.	**otro para una prueba serológica.** *(Oh-troh pah-rah oo-nah proo-eh-bah seh-roh-loh-hee-kah)*
Take a deep breath.	**Respire hondo.** *(Rehs-pee-reh ohn-doh)*
Relax, calm down.	**Relájese, cálmese.** *(Reh-lah-heh-seh, kahl-meh-seh)*
I need to use a tourniquette.	**Necesito usar un torniquete.** *(Neh-seh-see-toh oo-sahr oon tohr-nee-keh-teh)*
That is all!	**¡Es todo!** *(Ehs toh-doh)*

Please note that many products' brand names are often not translated, but their pronunciation changes a bit.

Favor de notar que hay muchas marcas de productos que no se traducen, pero la pronunciación cambia un poco.

I am going to put a Band-Aid on you.	**Voy a ponerle una cinta adhesiva/un curita/un bandaid.** *(Boy ah poh-nehr-leh oo-nah seen-tah ah-deh-see-bah/oon koo-ree-tah/oon bahn-dah-eed).*

TABLE 18–3
Helpful Verbs

TABLA 18–3
Verbos útiles

English	Spanish	Pronunciation
to ask	**preguntar**	*(preh-goon-tahr)*
to bend	**doblar**	*(doh-blahr)*
to come	**venir**	*(beh-neer)*
to draw	**sacar/tirar/dibujar**	*(sah-kahr/tee-rahr/dee-boo-hahr)*
to drink	**beber/tomar**	*(beh-behr/toh-mahr)*
to eat	**comer**	*(koh-mehr)*
to go	**ir**	*(eer)*
to keep	**guardar/mantener**	*(goo-ahr-dahr/mahn-teh-nehr)*
to lift	**levantar/elevar**	*(leh-bahn-tahr/eh-leh-bahr)*
to place	**poner/colocar**	*(poh-nehr/koh-loh-kahr)*
to wake	**despertar**	*(dehs-pehr-tahr)*

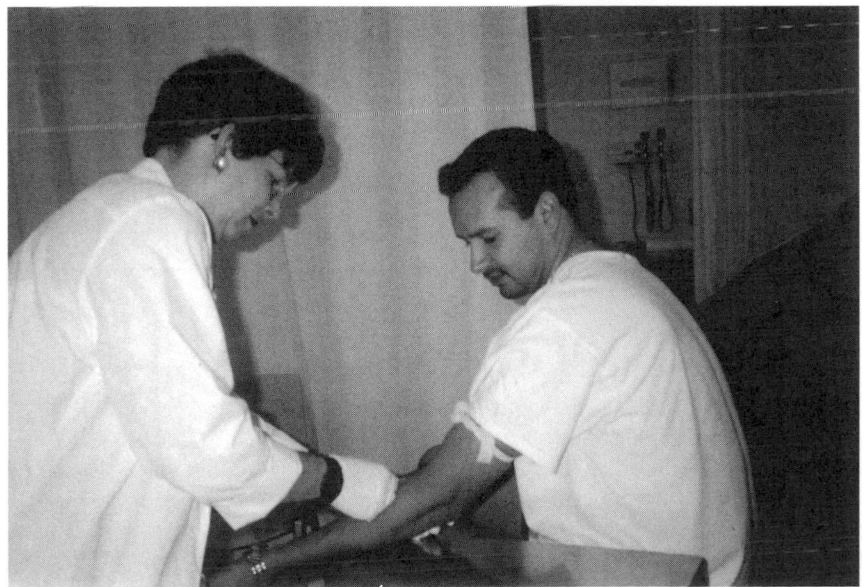

Figure 18–3 Precautions must be observed when drawing blood.

Please bend your arm for about five minutes.	**Por favor, doble el brazo por cinco minutos.** *(Pohr fah-bohr, doh-bleh ehl brah-soh pohr seen-koh mee-noo-tohs)*
I am through!	**¡Ya terminé!** *(Yah tehr-mee-neh)*
The nurse wants to talk to you.	**La enfermera quiere hablarle.** *(Lah ehn-fehr-meh-rah kee-eh-reh ah-blahr-leh)*
Mrs. Garza, I want you to get up and go to urinate.	**Señora Garza, quiero que se levante y vaya a orinar.** *(Seh-nyoh-rah Gahr-sah, kee-eh-roh keh seh leh-bahn-teh ee bah-yah ah oh-ree-nahr)*
Void a little, then put urine in this cup.	**Orine un poco, luego ponga la orina en esta taza.** *(Oh-ree-neh oon poh-koh, loo-eh-goh pohn-gah lah oh-ree-nah ehn ehs-tah tah-sah)*
Remember that you are to urinate and put it in the container.	**Recuerde que debe orinar y poner la orina en el frasco.** *(Reh-koo-ehr-deh keh deh-beh oh-ree-nahr ee poh-nehr lah oh-ree-nah ehn ehl frahs-koh)*

TABLE 18–4
Pronunciation of Selected Words

TABLA 18–4
Pronunciación de palabras selectas

English	Spanish	Pronunciation
additive	**aditivo**	*(ah-dee-tee-boh)*
adhesive	**adhesivo**	*(ah-deh-see-boh)*
blood bank	**banco de sangre**	*(bahn-koh deh sahn-greh)*
coagulated	**coagulado**	*(koh-ah-goo-lah-doh)*
hematology	**hematología***	*(eh-mah-toh-loh-hee-ah)*
limitations	**limitaciones**	*(lee-mee-tah-see-ohn-ehs)*
package	**paquete**	*(pah-keh-teh)*
puncture	**pinchazo/picadura**	*(peen-chah-soh/pee-kah-doo-rah)*
rub	**frotar/restregar**	*(froh-tahr/rehs-treh-gahr)*
spread	**untar/extender**	*(oohn-tahr/ehx-tehn-dehr)*
sterile	**estéril**	*(ehs-teh-reel)*

*In Spanish, the letter **h** is always silent.

Remember that you will do this for 24 hours.
Recuerde que hará esto por veinticuatro horas.
(Reh-koo-ehr-deh keh ah-rah ehs-toh pohr beh-een-tee-koo-ah-troh oh-rahs)

If there is no ice in the bucket, call me.
Si no hay hielo en la tina, llámeme.
(See noh ah-ee ee-eh-loh ehn lah tee-nah, yah-meh-meh)

I will remind you during the day.
Le recordaré durante el día.
(Leh reh-kohr-dah-reh doo-rahn-teh ehl dee-ah)

Do you feel all right?
¿Se siente bien?
(Seh see-ehn-teh bee-ehn)

Are you hungry?
¿Tiene hambre?
(Tee-eh-neh ahm-breh)

Do you want a cup of coffee?
¿Quiere una taza de café?
(Kee-eh-reh oo-nah tah-sah deh kah-feh)

Did you understand?
¿Entendió?
(Ehn-tehn-dee-oh)

Tomorrow, bring a specimen of your stool in this container.
Mañana, traiga una muestra de su excremento en este frasco.
(Mah-nyah-nah, trah-ee-gah oo-nah moo-ehs-trah deh soo ehx-kreh-mehn-toh ehn ehs-teh frahs-koh)

Chapter Nineteen | Capítulo diecinueve

The Pharmacy | La farmacia

The pharmacy provides services as an integral part of total patient care. Drugs are dispensed only upon the order of a physician. The nurse orders the medication from the pharmacy after the doctor has prescribed the treatment for the patient.

La farmacia provee servicios como parte integral del cuidado total del paciente. Los medicamentos son distribuidos solamente por órdenes

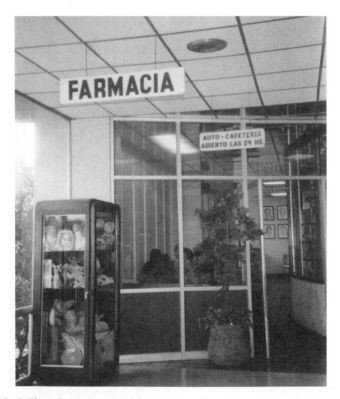

Figure 19–1 The pharmacy provides services for patients.

del doctor. La/el enfermera(o) ordena la medicina a la farmacia después de que el doctor dejó la receta con el tratamiento para el paciente.

The inpatient pharmacy	**La farmacia para pacientes que están internados** *(Lah fahr-mah-see-ah pah-rah pah-see-ehn-tehs keh ehs-tahn een-tehr-nah-dohs)*
It is open from seven A.M. to one A.M.	**Está abierta de las siete de la mañana a la una de la mañana.** *(Ehs-tah ah-bee-ehr-tah deh lahs see-eh-teh deh lah mah-nyah-nah ah lah oo-nah deh lah mah-nyah-nah)*
The pharmacy is open Monday through Friday.	**La farmacia está abierta de lunes a viernes.** *(Lah fahr-mah-see-ah ehs-tah ah-bee-ehr-tah deh loo-nehs ah bee-ehr-nehs)*

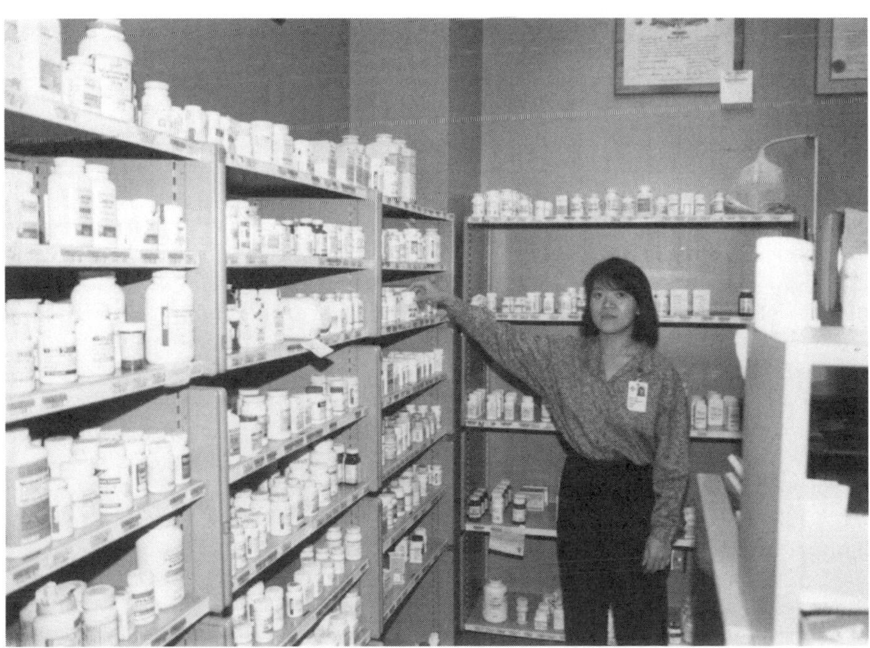

Figure 19–2 The inpatient pharmacy is staffed around the clock.

It is open Saturday, Sunday, and holidays.	**Está abierta los sábados, domingos y días festivos.** *(Ehs-tah ah-bee-ehr-tah lohs sah-bah-dohs, doh-meen-gohs ee dee-ahs fehs-tee-bohs)*
It is open 7:00 A.M. to 12:00 midnight.	**Esta abierta de siete de la mañana a doce de la noche/a medianoche.** *(Ehs-tah ah-bee-ehr-tah deh see-eh-teh deh lah mah-nyah-nah ah doh-seh deh lah noh-cheh/ah meh-dee-ah-noh-cheh)*
The staff delivers and picks up orders every hour from the floors.	**Los empleados recogen y surten órdenes cada hora en los pisos.** *(Los ehm-pleh-ah-dohs reh-koh-hehn ee soor-tehn ohr-deh-nehs kah-dah oh-rah ehn lohs pee-sohs)*
Nursing staff take STAT orders to the pharmacy.	**Las enfermeras llevan órdenes urgentes a la farmacia.** *(Lahs ehn-fehr-meh-rahs yeh-bahn ohr-deh-nehs oor-hehn-tehs ah lah fahr-mah-see-ah)*

TABLE 19–1
Drug Categories

TABLA 19–1
Categorías de los medicamentos

English	Spanish	Pronunciation
analgesic	**analgésicos**	*(ah-nahl-heh-see-kohs)*
antacid	**antiácidos**	*(ahn-tee-ah-see-dohs)*
antianxiety	**contra la ansiedad/ansiolíticos**	*(kohn-trah lah ahn-see-eh-dahd/ahn-see-oh-lee-tee-kohs)*
antiarrhythmic	**antiarritmias**	*(ahn-tee-ah-reet-mee-ahs)*
antibiotics	**antibióticos**	*(ahn-tee-bee-oh-tee-kohs)*
anticonvulsant	**anticonvulsivo/antiepiléptico**	*(ahn-tee-kohn-bool-see-boh/ahn-tee-eh-pee-lehp-tee-koh)*
antiemetic	**antiemético**	*(ahn-tee-eh-meh-tee-koh)*
antiviral	**antivirales**	*(ahn-tee-bee-rah-lehs)*
contraceptives	**contraceptivos**	*(kohn-trah-sehp-tee-bohs)*
decongestants	**descongestionantes**	*(dehs-kohn-hehs-tee-oh-nahn-tehs)*
laxatives	**laxantes/purgantes**	*(lahx-ahn-tehs/poor-gahn-tehs)*
narcotics	**narcóticos**	*(nahr-koh-tee-kohs)*
sedatives	**sedativo/sedantes**	*(seh-dah-tee-boh/seh-dahn-tehs)*

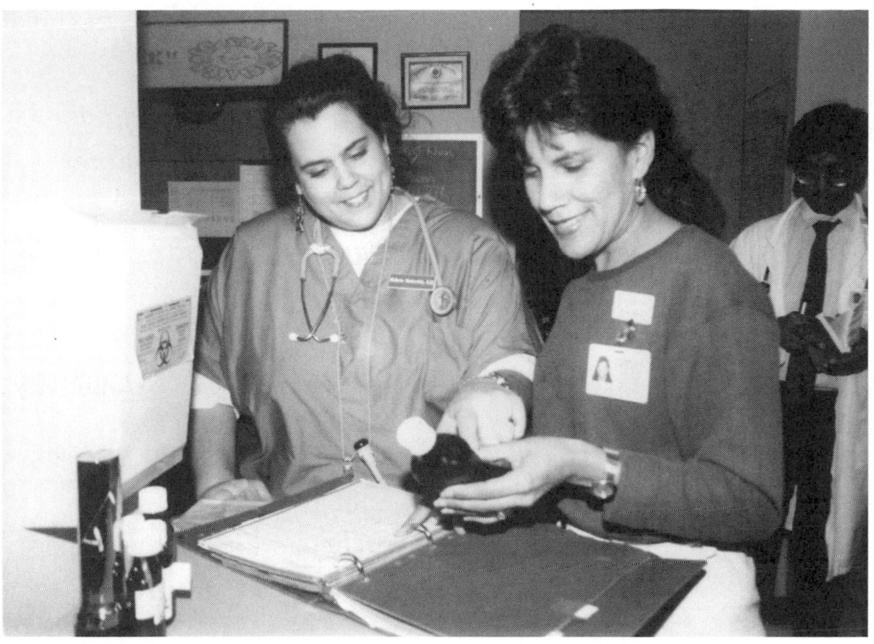

Figure 19–3 Nurses maintain medication records; pharmacists are available to nursing staff for consultation.

Nurses control narcotic records on the unit.	**Las enfermeras controlan archivos de narcóticos en el piso.** *(Lahs ehn-fehr-meh-rahs kohn-troh-lahn ahr-chee-bohs deh nahr-koh-tee-kohs ehn ehl pee-soh)*
Expired items on the unit are returned to the pharmacy.	**Los artículos con fecha vencida se devuelven a la farmacia.** *(Lohs ahr-tee-koo-lohs kohn feh-chah behn-see-dah seh deh-boo-ehl-behn ah lah fahr-mah-see-ah)*
Monthly the medication area is inspected.	**Cada mes se inspecciona el área de medicamentos.** *(Kah-dah mehs seh eens-pehk-see-ohn-ah ehl ah-reh-ah deh meh-dee-kah-mehn-tohs)*

Medication carts are checked for quantity, number, and expiration date on each item.

Los carros con medicamentos se revisan para anotar la cantidad, número y fecha de caducidad en cada artículo.

A standard schedule is used.	**Se usa un horario estándar.** *(Seh oo-sah oon oh-rah-ree-oh ehs-tahn-dahr)*
The pharmacist interprets the physician's order.	**El farmacéutico interpreta la orden del doctor.** *(Ehl fahr-mah-seh-oo-tee-koh een-tehr-preh-tah lah ohr-dehn dehl dohk-tohr)*
Vials, pills, capsules, liquids, and IV fluids are dispensed.	**Frascos, pastillas, cápsulas, líquidos y sueros se surten.** *(Frahs-kohs, pahs-tee-yahs, kahp-soo-lahs, lee-kee-dohs ee soo-eh-rohs seh soor-tehn).*
She assigns a dosage schedule in the computer.	**Ella asigna el horario de dosis en la computadora.** *(Eh-yah ah-seeg-nah ehl oh-rah-ree-oh deh doh-sees ehn lah kohm-poo-tah-doh-rah)*
Four times a day.	**Cuatro veces al día.** *(Koo-ah-troh beh-sehs ahl dee-ah)*

TABLE 19–2
Potential Poisons

TABLA 19–2
Posibilidad de envenenamiento

English	Spanish	Pronunciation
alcohol	**alcohol**	*(ahl-kohl)*
antihistamine	**antihistamínico**	*(ahn-tee-ees-tah-mee-nee-koh)*
ammonia	**amonia/amoníaco**	*(ah-moh-nee-ah/ah-moh-nee-ah-koh)*
aspirin	**aspirina**	*(ahs-pee-ree-nah)*
barbiturates	**barbitúricos**	*(bahr-bee-too-ree-kohs)*
boric acid	**ácido bórico**	*(ah-see-doh boh-ree-koh)*
cocaine	**cocaína**	*(koh-kah-ee-nah)*
digitalis	**digitálicos**	*(dee-hee-tah-lee-kohs)*
lead	**plomo**	*(ploh-moh)*
morphine	**morfina**	*(mohr-fee-nah)*
nicotine	**nicotina**	*(nee-koh-tee-nah)*
nitroglycerin	**nitroglicerina**	*(nee-troh-glee-seh-ree-nah)*

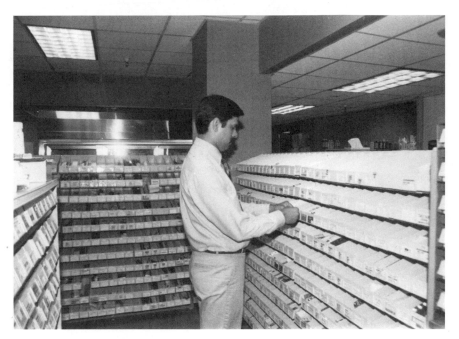

Figure 19–4 Pharmacists interpret doctors' orders.

Three times a day.	**Tres veces al día.** *(Trehs beh-sehs ahl dee-ah)*
Twice a day.	**Dos veces al día.** *(Dohs beh-sehs ahl dee-ah)*
Daily.	**Diariamente./Una por día./Cada día.** *(Dee-ah-ree-ah-mehn-teh/Oo-nah pohr dee-ah/Kah-dah dee-ah)*

TABLE 19–3
Apothecary Measures

TABLA 19–3
Medidas apotecarias

English	Spanish	Pronunciation
gallon	**galón**	*(gah-lohn)*
grains	**granos**	*(grah-nohs)*
ounces	**onzas**	*(ohn-sahs)*
quart	**cuarto**	*(koo-ahr-toh)*
pound	**libra**	*(lee-brah)*

TABLE 19–4 Metric Measures	**TABLA 19–4 Medidas métricas**	
English	**Spanish**	**Pronunciation**
centimeter	**centímetro**	*(sehn-tee-meh-troh)*
cubic centimeter	**centímetro cúbico**	*(sehn-tee-meh-troh koo-bee-koh)*
grams	**gramos**	*(grah-mohs)*
kilogram	**kilogramos/kilo**	*(kee-loh-grah-mohs/kee-loh)*
liter	**litro**	*(lee-troh)*
meter	**metro**	*(meh-troh)*
milligram	**miligramo**	*(mee-lee-grah-moh)*
milliliter	**mililitro**	*(mee-lee-lee-troh)*

Before/after meals. — **Antes/después de las comidas.** *(Ahn-tehs/dehs-poo-ehs deh lahs koh-mee-dahs)*

At bedtime. — **Al acostarse./A la hora de dormir.** *(Ahl ah-kohs-tahr-seh/Ah lah oh-rah deh dohr-meer)*

The pharmacist assists with patient education. — **El farmacéutico/La farmacéutica asiste con la educación del paciente.** *(Ehl fahr-mah-seh-oo-tee-koh/Lah fahr-mah-seh-oo-tee-kah ah-sees-teh kohn lah eh-doo-kah-see-ohn dehl pah-see-ehn-teh)*

TABLE 19–5 Household Measures	**TABLA 19–5 Medidas caseras**	
English	**Spanish**	**Pronunciation**
cup	**taza**	*(tah-sah)*
drop	**gota**	*(goh-tah)*
glass	**vaso**	*(bah-soh)*
tablespoon	**cucharada**	*(koo-chah-rah-dah)*
teaspoon	**cucharadita**	*(koo-chah-rah-dee-tah)*

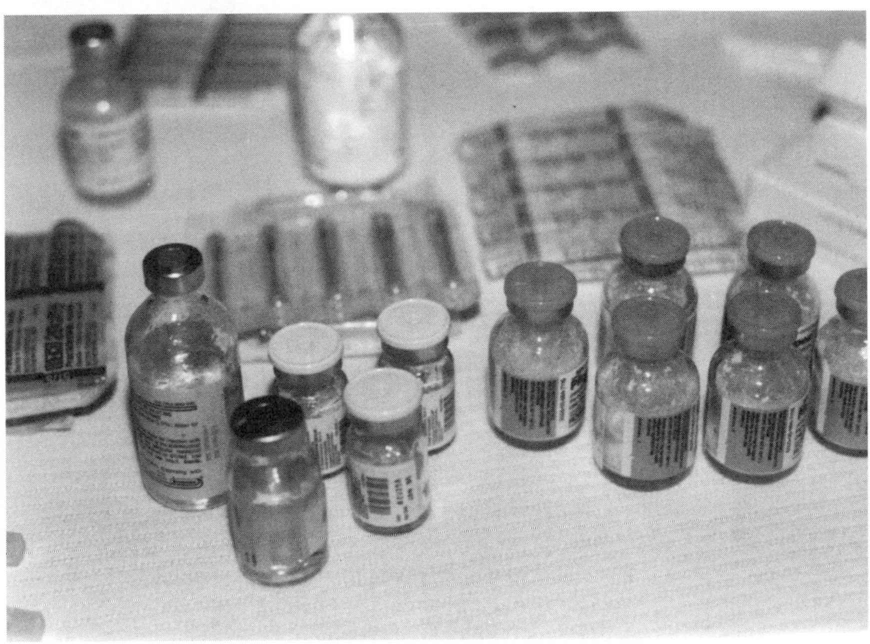

Figure 19–5 Each medication (vials, suppositories) must be labeled.

In case of a medication error, the doctor is notified.	**En caso de error en el medicamento, se notifica al doctor.** ***(Ehn kah-soh deh eh-rohr ehn ehl meh-dee-kah-mehn-toh, seh noh-tee-fee-kah ahl dohk-tohr)***
Outpatient prescriptions are also dispensed.	**Las recetas para pacientes de consulta externa se surten también.** ***(Lahs reh-seh-tahs pah-rah pah-see-ehn-tehs deh kohn-sool-tah ehx-tehr-nah seh soor-tehn tahm-bee-ehn)***
Include in the label:	**Incluya en la etiqueta:** ***(Een-kloo-yah ehn lah eh-tee-keh-tah)***
name of the patient;	**nombre del paciente;** ***(nohm-breh dehl pah-see-ehn-teh)***
date;	**fecha;** ***(feh-chah)***
doctor's name;	**nombre del doctor;** ***(nohm-breh dehl dohk-tohr)***

TABLE 19–6 Medication Forms | **TABLA 19–6 Formas de los medicamentos**

English	Spanish	Pronunciation
capsule	**cápsula**	*(kahp-soo-lah)*
diluent	**diluyente**	*(dee-loo-yehn-teh)*
fluid	**fluido**	*(floo-ee-doh)*
gel	**gelatina**	*(heh-lah-tee-nah)*
inhalant	**inhalante**	*(een-ah-lahn-teh)*
liquid	**líquido**	*(lee-kee-doh)*
lotion	**loción**	*(loh-see-ohn)*
ointment	**ungüento***	*(oon-goo-ehn-toh)*
pill	**píldora**	*(peel-doh-rah)*
rectal suppository	**supositorio rectal**	*(soo-poh-see-toh-ree-oh rehk-tahl)*
semi-solid	**semisólido**	*(seh-mee-soh-lee-doh)*
solid	**sólido**	*(soh-lee-doh)*
solution	**solución**	*(soh-loo-see-ohn)*
syrup	**jarabe/zumo**	*(hah-rah-beh/soo-moh)*
tablet	**tableta**	*(tah-bleh-tah)*
topical	**tópico**	*(toh-pee-koh)*
vaginal suppository	**supositorio vaginal**	*(soo-poh-see-toh-ree-oh bah-hee-nahl)*

*The sign above the ü is used to emphasize it.

name of the drug;	**nombre de la droga/del medicamento;** *(nohm-breh deh lah droh-gah/dehl meh-dee-kah-mehn-toh)*
dosage;	**dosis;** *(doh-sees)*
route;	**vía/ruta;** *(bee-ah/roo-tah)*
volume;	**volumen;** *(boh-loo-mehn)*
total number of pills;	**número total de pastillas;** *(noo-meh-roh toh-tahl deh pahs-tee-yahs)*
lot number;	**número de lote;** *(noo-meh-roh deh loh-teh)*
expiration date.	**caducidad.** *(kah-doo-see-dahd)*

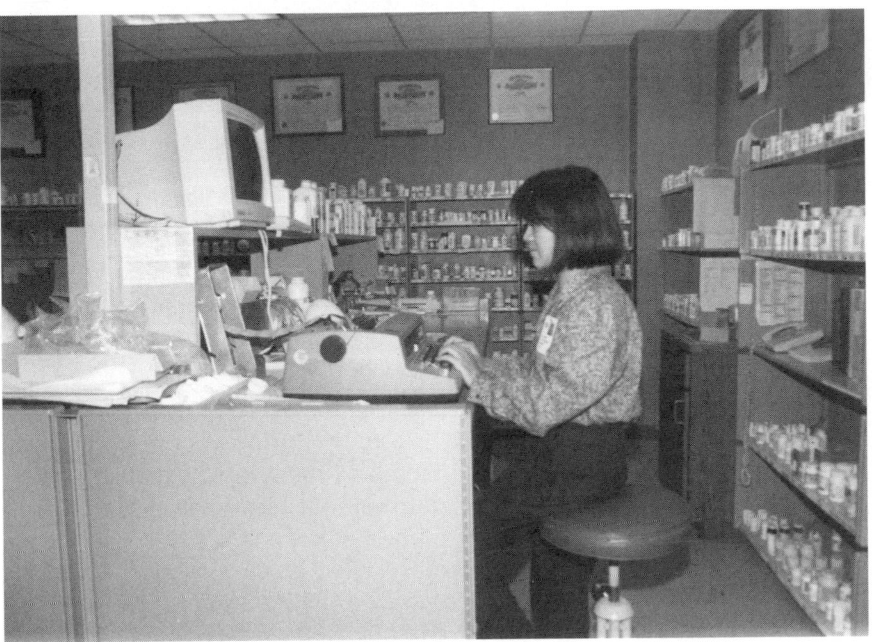

Figure 19–6 The pharmacist logs in the computer the schedules of each medication.

TABLE 19–7
Administration Routes

TABLA 19–7
Vías de administración

English	Spanish	Pronunciation
by mouth	**por la boca**	*(pohr lah boh-kah)*
intramuscular	**intramuscular**	*(een-trah-moos-koo-lahr)*
intravenous	**intravenoso**	*(een-trah-beh-noh-soh)*
nasal	**nasal**	*(nah-sahl)*
ophthalmic	**oftálmico**	*(ohf-tahl-mee-koh)*
oral	**oral**	*(oh-rahl)*
otic	**ótico**	*(oh-tee-koh)*
patch	**parche**	*(pahr-cheh)*
per rectum	**por el recto/rectal**	*(pohr ehl rehk-toh/rehk-tahl)*
subcutaneous	**subcutáneo**	*(soob-koo-tah-neh-oh)*
sublingual	**sublingual**	*(soob-leen-goo-ahl)*
vaginal	**vaginal**	*(bah-hee-nahl)*

TABLE 19–8 Useful Words	TABLA 19–8 Palabras útiles	
English	**Spanish**	**Pronunciation**
induce	**inducir**	*(een-doo-seer)*
lavage	**lavabo**	*(lah-bah-boh)*
lubricant	**lubricante**	*(loo-bree-kahn-teh)*
nausea	**náusea**	*(nah-oo-seh-ah)*
sterile	**estéril**	*(ehs-teh-reel)*
systemic	**sistemático**	*(sees-teh-mah-tee-koh)*
vomiting	**vomitando**	*(boh-mee-tahn-doh)*

The outpatient pharmacy opens daily from 9 A.M. to 6 P.M.	**La farmacia de consulta externa abre diariamente de nueve de la mañana a seis de la tarde todos los días.** *(Lah fahr-mah-see-ah deh kohn-sool-tah ehx-tehr-nah ah-breh dee-ah-ree-ah-mehn-teh deh noo-eh-beh deh lah mah-nyah-nah ah seh-ees deh lah tahr-deh toh-dohs lohs dee-ahs)*
Please come back in a few minutes.	**Por favor, regrese en unos minutos.** *(Pohr fah-bohr, reh-greh-seh ehn oon-ohs mee-noo-tohs)*
Wait your turn.	**Espere su turno.** *(Ehs-peh-reh soo toor-noh)*
You will have to wait.	**Tendrá que esperar.** *(Tehn-drah keh ehs-peh-rahr)*
Wait several minutes!	**¡Espere varios minutos!** *(Ehs-peh-reh bah-ree-ohs mee-noo-tohs)*
At least 30 minutes!	**¡Al menos treinta minutos!** *(Ahl meh-nohs treh-een-tah mee-noo tohs)*
The prescription will be ready at _____.	**La receta estará lista a las _____.** *(Lah reh-seh-tah ehs-tah-rah lees-tah ah lahs _____)*
Take the medicine with juice.	**Tome la medicina con jugo.** *(Toh-meh lah meh-dee-see-nah kohn joo-goh)*
Take it with a full glass of water.	**Tómela con un vaso lleno de agua.** *(Toh-meh-lah kohn oon bah-soh yeh-noh deh ah-goo-ah)*

Do not drink alcohol with this medicine.	**No tome alcohol con esta medicina.** *(Noh toh-meh ahl-kohl kohn ehs-tah meh-dee-see-nah)*
It can cause drowsiness.	**Le puede causar sueño.** *(Leh poo-eh-deh kah-oo-sahr soo-eh-nyoh)*
Do not drive!	**¡No maneje/conduzca!** *(Noh mah-neh-heh/kohn-doos-kah)*
Do not operate machinery!	**¡No maneje/opere una máquina/maquinaria!** *(Noh mah-neh-heh/oh-peh-reh oo-nah mah-kee-nah/mah-kee-nah-ree-ah)*
This is an antacid.	**Este es un antiácido.** *(Ehs-teh ehs oon ahn-tee-ah-see-doh)*
This is a sedative.	**Este es un sedante.** *(Ehs-teh ehs oon seh-dahn-teh)*
This medicine is a pain killer.	**Esta medicina quita/alivia el dolor.** *(Ehs-tah meh-dee-see-nah kee-tah/ah-lee-bee-ah ehl doh-lohr)*

TABLE 19–9
Similar Terms

TABLA 19–9
Términos similares

English	Spanish	Pronunciation
anemia	**anemia**	*(ah-neh-mee-ah)*
angina	**angina**	*(ahn-hee-nah)*
bronchitis	**bronquitis**	*(brohn-kee-tees)*
cataract	**catarata**	*(kah-tah-rah-tah)*
cirrhosis	**cirrosis**	*(see-roh-sees)*
constipation	**constipación/estreñimiento**	*(kohns-tee-pah-see-ohn/ehs-treh-nyee-mee-ehn-toh)*
enteritis	**enteritis**	*(ehn-teh-ree-tees)*
gangrene	**gangrena**	*(gahn-greh-nah)*
hypertension	**hipertensión**	*(ee-pehr-tehn-see-ohn)*
laryngitis	**laringitis**	*(lah-reen-hee-tees)*
pancreatitis	**pancreatitis**	*(pahn-kreh-ah-tee-tees)*
pneumonia	**pulmonía/neumonía**	*(pool-moh-nee-ah/neh-oo-moh-nee-ah)*
rubella	**rubéola**	*(roo-beh-oh-lah)*
tonsillitis	**tonsilitis/amigdalitis**	*(tohn-see-lee-tees/ah-meeg-dah-lee-tees)*
vaginitis	**vaginitis**	*(bah-hee-nee-tees)*

Take on an empty stomach.	**Tómela con el estómago vacío.** *(Toh-meh-lah kohn ehl ehs-toh-mah-goh bah-see-oh)*
Take one hour before eating.	**Tómela una hora antes de comer.** *(Toh-meh-lah oo-nah oh-rah ahn-tehs deh koh-mehr)*
Take the medicine with food.	**Tome la medicina con comida.** *(Toh-meh lah meh-dee-see-nah kohn koh-mee-dah)*
Avoid sunlight.	**Evite asolearse/los rayos del sol.** *(Eh-bee-teh ah-soh-leh-ahr-seh/lohs rah-yohs dehl sohl)*
Follow the instructions carefully.	**Siga las instrucciones con cuidado.** *(See-gah lahs eens-trook-see-ohn-ehs kohn koo-ee-dah-doh)*
Take two aspirins.	**Tome dos aspirinas.** *(Toh-meh dohs ahs-pee-ree-nahs)*
Sleep at least 8 hours.	**Duerma al menos ocho horas.** *(Doo-ehr-mah ahl meh-nohs oh-choh oh-rahs)*
You can refill ____ times.	**Puede surtir ____ veces.** *(Poo-eh-deh soor-teer ____ beh-sehs)*
Take all the medicine in the prescription.	**Tome toda la medicina indicada en la receta.** *(Toh-meh toh-dah lah meh-dee-see-nah een-dee-kah-dah ehn lah reh-seh-tah)*
This prescription may not be refilled.	**Esta receta no se puede surtir de nuevo.** *(Ehs-tah reh-seh-tah noh seh poo-eh-deh soor-teer deh noo-eh-boh)*
If you react to the medicine, call your physician.	**Si reacciona mal al medicamento, llame a su médico.** *(See reh-ahk-see-ohn-ah mahl ahl meh-dee-kah-mehn-toh yah-meh ah soo meh-dee-koh)*
Go immediately to the hospital!	**¡Vaya inmediatamente/en seguida al hospital!** *(Bah-yah een-meh-dee-ah-tah-mehn-teh/ehn seh-gee-dah ahl ohs-pee-tahl)*

Chapter Twenty | Capítulo veinte

The X-Ray Department | El departamento de rayos X

Mr. Martínez, a 60-year-old patient, is going to have X-rays. He is scheduled for abdomen and chest X-rays.

El señor Martínez, paciente de sesenta años, le van a tomar rayos X. Está en el horario para tomarle rayos X del abdomen y del pecho.

Good morning, Mr. Martínez.	**Buenos días, señor Martínez.** *(Boo-eh-nohs dee-ahs, seh-nyohr Mahr-tee-nehs)*
Transportation is here.	**El transporte está aquí.** *(Ehl trahns-pohr-teh ehs-tah ah-kee)*
—Good morning!	**—¡Buenos días!** *(Boo-eh-nohs dee-ahs)*
—Where do I need to go?	**—¿Adónde tengo que ir?** *(Ah-dohn-deh tehn-goh keh eer)*
We are going to X-rays.	**Vamos a rayos X.** *(Bah-mohs ah rah-yohs eh-kees)*
I am going to help you lie on the stretcher.	**Voy a ayudarlo a acostarse en la camilla.** *(Boy ah ah-yoo-dahr-loh ah ah-kohs-tahr-seh ehn lah kah-mee-yah)*
Don't move!	**¡No se mueva!** *(Noh seh moo-eh-bah)*
We are going to pull the sheet at the count of three.	**Vamos a jalar la sábana al contar tres.** *(Bah-mohs ah hah-lahr lah sah-bah-nah ahl kohn-tahr trehs)*
One, two, three . . .	**Uno, dos, tres...** *(Oo-noh, dohs, trehs)*
Very good!	**¡Muy bien!** *(Moo-ee bee-ehn)*
Don't hold the rail.	**No agarre el barandal.** *(Noh ah-gah-reh ehl bah-rahn-dahl)*

I am going to cover you with a sheet.	**Voy a cubrirlo con una sábana.** *(Boy ah koo-breer-loh kohn oo-nah sah-bah-nah)*
Take your medical file.	**Lleve su archivo.** *(Yeh-beh soo ahr-chee-boh)*
Take your hospital card.	**Lleve su tarjeta del hospital.** *(Yeh-beh soo tahr-heh-tah dehl ohs-pee-tahl)*
Remember to bring them back.	**Acuérdese de regresarlos.** *(Ah-koo-ehr-deh-seh deh reh-greh-sahr-lohs)*
It's not very far.	**No está muy lejos.** *(Noh ehs-tah moo-ee leh-hohs)*
We are here!	**¡Ya llegamos!/¡Estamos aquí!** *(Yah yeh-gah-mohs/Ehs-tah-mohs ah-kee)*
Stay as you are.	**Quédese como está.** *(Keh-deh-seh koh-moh ehs-tah)*

Mr. Martínez arrives at the department.
El señor Martínez llega al departamento.

Hello, Mr. Martínez.	**Hola, señor Martínez.** *(Oh-lah, seh-nyohr Mahr-tee-nehs)*
I am the technician.	**Yo soy el técnico/la técnica.** *(Yoh soh-ee ehl tehk-nee-koh/lah tehk-nee-kah)*
Please change clothes.	**Por favor, cámbiese de ropa.** *(Por fah-bohr, kahm-bee-eh-seh deh roh-pah)*
I am going to take X-rays of the abdomen first.	**Voy a tomar rayos X del abdomen primero.** *(Boy ah toh-mahr rah-yohs eh-kees dehl ahb-doh-mehn pree-meh-roh)*
Lie down.	**Acuéstese.** *(Ah-koo-ehs-teh-seh)*
I am putting a cassette under your waist.	**Estoy poniendo una placa abajo de la cintura.** *(Ehs-toh-ee poh-nee-ehn-doh oo-nah plah-kah ah-bah-hoh deh lah seen-too-rah)*

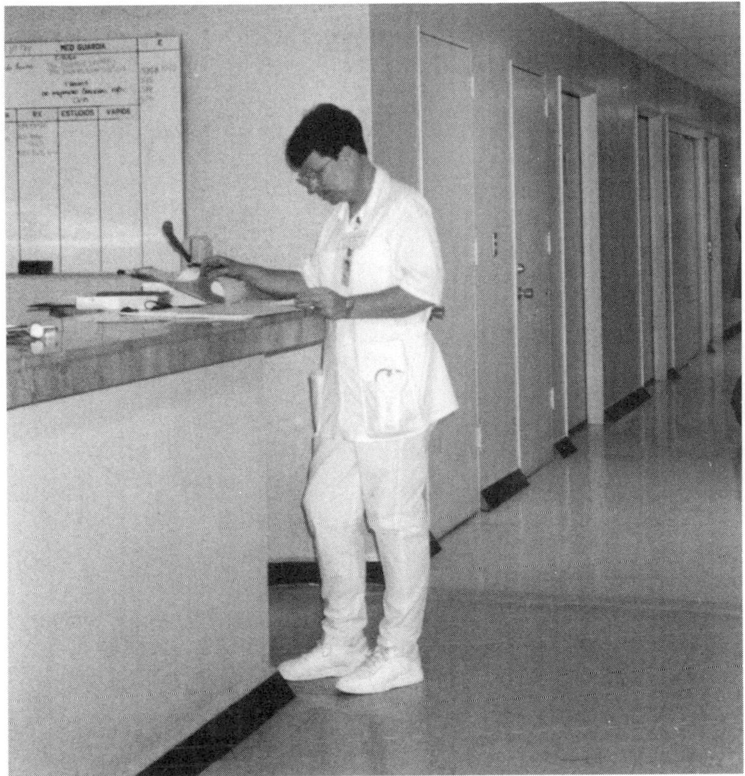

Figure 20–1 Transportation will take the patient's chart and card.

It feels like a board inside.
Se siente como una tabla.
(Seh see-ehn-teh koh-moh oo-nah tah-blah)

It has the film inside.
Tiene la película adentro.
(Tee-eh-neh lah peh-lee-koo-lah ah-dehn-troh)

Don't move!
¡No se mueva!
(Noh seh moo-eh-bah)

When I tell you, hold your breath.
Cuando le avise, no respire.
(Koo-ahn-doh leh ah-bee-seh, noh rehs-pee-reh)

Don't breathe!
¡No respire!
(Noh rehs-pee-reh)

You can breathe now.
Ya puede respirar.
(Yah poo-eh-deh rehs-pee-rahr)

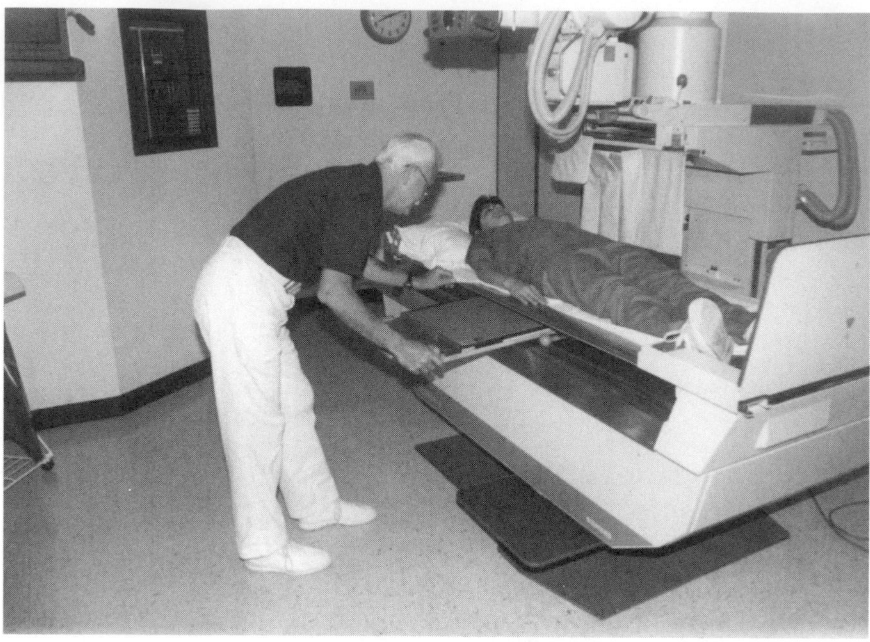

Figure 20–2 Lying supine and keeping quiet helps while taking X-rays.

TABLE 20–1
Common Commands

TABLA 20–1
Órdenes/mandatos comunes

English	**Spanish**	**Pronunciation**
Keep your feet together!	**¡Mantenga los pies juntos!**	*(Mahn-tehn-gah lohs pee-ehs hoon-tohs)*
Lift your arms!	**¡Levante los brazos!**	*(Leh-bahn-teh lohs brah-sohs)*
Stand straight!	**¡Párese derecho!**	*(Pah-reh-seh deh-reh-choh)*
Stay as you are!	**¡Quédese como está!**	*(Keh-deh-seh koh-moh ehs-tah)*
Tighten your muscle!	**¡Apriete el músculo!**	*(Ah-pree-eh-teh ehl moos-koo-loh)*
Turn on your side!	**¡Voltéese de lado!**	*(Bohl-teh-eh-seh deh lah-doh)*
Turn to the right!	**¡Voltee a la derecha!**	*(Bohl-teh-eh ah lah deh-reh-chah)*
Walk straight ahead!	**¡Camine derecho!**	*(Kah-mee-neh deh-reh-choh)*

Breathe out.	**Exhale./Respire.** *(Ehx-ah-leh/Rehs-pee-reh)*
Turn on your side.	**Voltéese de lado.** *(Bohl-teh-eh-seh deh lah-doh)*
Turn to the right.	**Voltee a la derecha.** *(Bohl-teh-eh ah lah deh-reh-chah)*
One more time.	**Una vez más.** *(Oo-nah behs mahs)*
Hold your breath.	**No respire.** *(Noh rehs-pee-reh)*
Breathe!	**¡Respire!** *(Rehs-pee-reh)*
Now I need to X-ray the chest.	**Ahora necesito tomar radiografía del pecho.** *(Ah-oh-rah neh-seh-see-toh toh-mahr rah-dee-oh-grah-fee-ah dehl peh-choh)*

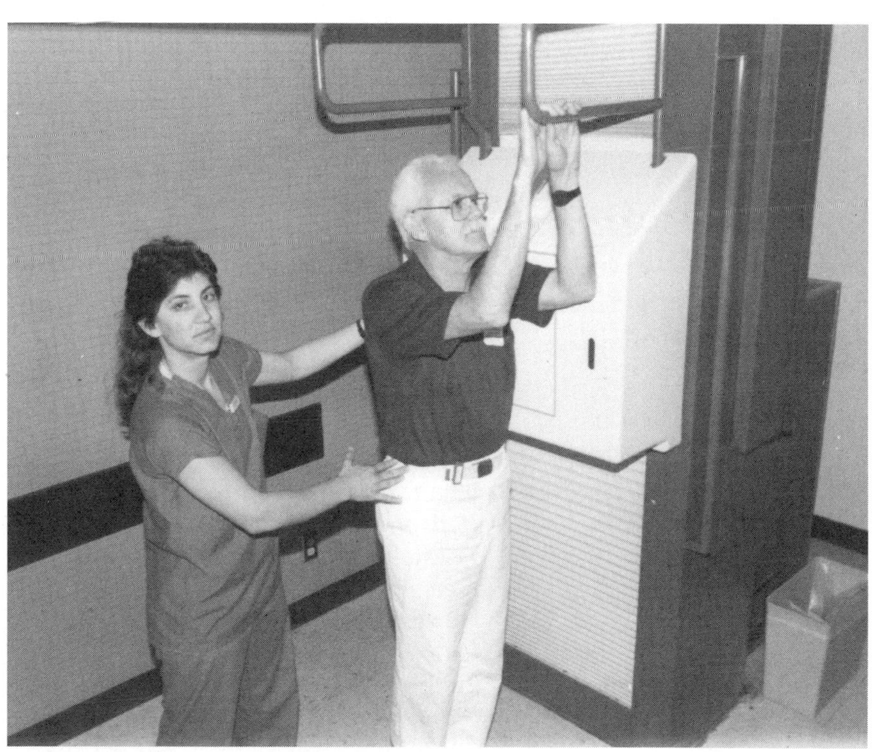

Figure 20–3 Raise your arms and don't breathe!

TABLE 20–2 Commands | **TABLA 20–2 Órdenes/mandatos**

English	Spanish	Pronunciation
Breathe!	**¡Respire!**	*(Rehs-pee-reh)*
Don't breathe!	**¡No respire!**	*(Noh rehs-pee-reh)*
Don't hold on!	**¡No se agarre!**	*(Noh seh ah-gahr-reh)*
Don't laugh!	**¡No se ría!**	*(Noh seh ree-ah)*
Don't lie down!	**¡No se acueste!**	*(Noh seh ah-koo-ehs-teh)*
Don't move!	**¡No se mueva!**	*(Noh seh moo-eh-bah)*
Hold your breath!	**¡No respire!**	*(Noh rehs-pee-reh)*
Keep quiet!	**¡Estése quieto!/ ¡No se mueva!**	*(Ehs-teh-seh kee-eh-toh/Noh seh moo-eh-bah)*
Lie down!	**¡Acuéstese!**	*(Ah-koo-ehs-teh-seh)*
Press hard!	**¡Presione fuerte!**	*(Preh-see-oh-neh foo-ehr-teh)*
Sit down!	**¡Siéntese!**	*(See-ehn-teh-seh)*
Stay still!	**¡Quédese quieto!**	*(Keh-deh-seh kee-eh-toh)*
Talk!	**¡Hable!**	*(Ah-bleh)*

Stand straight.	**Párese derecho.** *(Pah-reh-seh deh-reh-choh)*
Keep your feet together.	**Ponga los pies juntos.** *(Pohn-gah lohs pee-ehs hoon-tohs)*
Lift your arms.	**Levante los brazos.** *(Leh-bahn-teh lohs brah-sohs)*
Stay like this for a while.	**Quédese así por un rato.** *(Keh-deh-seh ah-see pohr oon rah-toh)*
Now, turn to the screen.	**Ahora, voltee hacia la placa.** *(Ah-oh-rah, bohl-teh-eh ah-see-ah lah plah-kah)*
This will feel cold.	**Esto se sentirá frío.** *(Ehs-toh seh sehn-tee-rah free-oh)*
It will take a minute.	**Va a tomar un minuto.** *(Bah ah toh-mahr oon mee-noo-toh)*
Are you hurting?	**¿Tiene dolor?** *(Tee-eh-neh doh-lohr)*
Stop breathing.	**No respire.** *(Noh rehs-pee-reh)*
You can breathe.	**Puede respirar.** *(Poo-eh-deh rehs-pee-rahr)*
I am through.	**Ya terminé.** *(Yah tehr-mee-neh)*

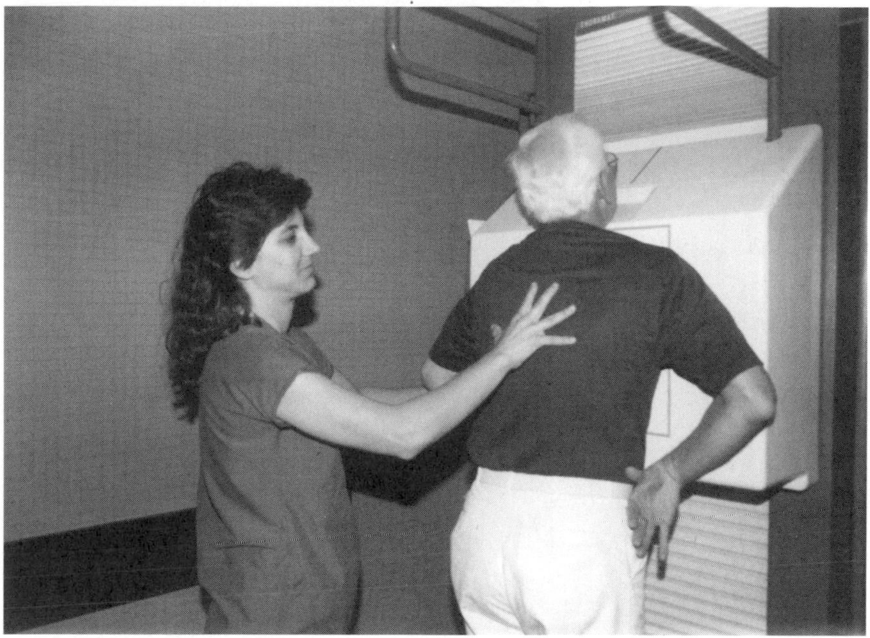

Figure 20–4 Give clear directions to your patient.

I will return shortly.	**Regresaré en seguida.** *(Reh-greh-sah-reh ehn seh-gee-dah)*
Please sit down.	**Siéntese, por favor.** *(See-ehn-teh-seh, pohr fah-bohr)*
Don't change clothes.	**No se cambie de ropa.** *(Noh seh kahm-bee-eh deh roh-pah)*
I want to see if the X-rays are good.	**Quiero ver si las radiografías salieron bien.** *(Kee-eh-roh behr see lahs rah-dee-oh-grah-fee-ahs sah-lee-eh-rohn bee-ehn)*
I am back.	**Ya regresé.** *(Yah reh-greh-seh)*
Now you can change clothes.	**Ahora se puede cambiar de ropa.** *(Ah-oh-rah seh poo-eh-deh kahm-bee-ahr deh roh-pah)*
Do you need help?	**¿Necesita ayuda?** *(Neh-seh-see-tah ah-yoo-dah)*
I am going to call the radiologist.	**Voy a llamar al radiólogo.** *(Boy ah yah-mahr ahl rah-dee-oh-loh-goh)*

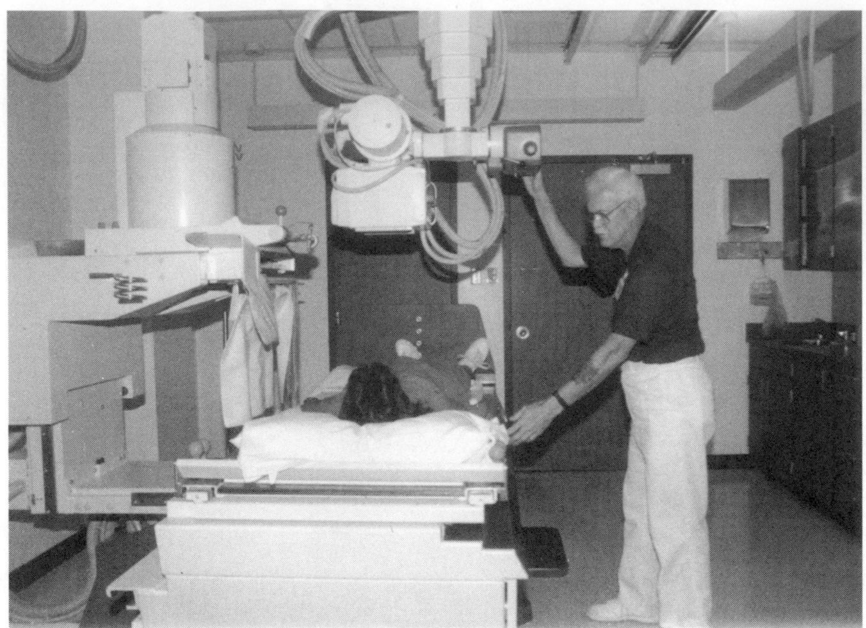

Figure 20–5 You must be perfectly still!

He will talk to you.	**El hablará con usted.** *(Ehl ah-blah-rah kohn oos-tehd)*

Dr. Blanco, the radiologist, stands by the door and greets the patient.
El doctor Blanco, radiólogo, se para en la puerta y saluda al paciente.

Good morning!	**¡Buenos días!** *(Boo-eh-nohs dee-ahs)*
I am Dr. Blanco.	**Yo soy el doctor Blanco.** *(Yo soh-ee ehl dohk-tohr Blahn-koh)*
We need to bring you back.	**Necesitamos que regrese.** *(Neh-seh-see-tah-mohs keh reh-greh-seh)*
But we will give you something to drink.	**Pero le daremos algo que tomar.** *(Peh-roh leh dah-reh-mohs ahl-goh keh toh-mahr)*

TABLE 20–3
Common Questions

TABLA 20–3
Preguntas comunes

English	Spanish	Pronunciation
Where do I need to go?	**¿Adónde necesito ir?**	*(Ah-dohn-deh neh-seh-see-toh eer)*
Do you need help?	**¿Necesita ayuda?**	*(Neh-seh-see-tah ah-yoo-dah)*
Have you had X-rays?	**¿Le han tomado rayos X?**	*(Leh ahn toh-mah-doh rah-yohs eh-kees)*
When was the last time?	**¿Cuándo fue la última vez?**	*(Koo-ahn-doh foo-eh lah ool-tee-mah behs)*
Do you know why?	**¿Sabe por qué?**	*(Sah-beh pohr keh)*
How old are you?	**¿Cuántos años tiene?**	*(Koo-ahn-tohs ah-nyohs tee-eh-neh)*
Are you pregnant?	**¿Está embarazada?**	*(Ehs-tah ehm-bah-rah-sah-dah)*
Have you had cancer?	**¿Ha tenido cáncer?**	*(Ah teh-nee-doh kahn-sehr)*
Family history of cancer?	**¿Hay historia de cáncer en la familia?**	*(Ah-ee ees-toh-ree-ah deh kahn-sehr ehn lah fah-mee-lee-ah)*

We will X-ray the abdomen again, at the same time that we take the X-rays.

Vamos a tomar otras radiografías del abdomen, al mismo tiempo que tomamos los rayos X

(Bah-mohs ah toh-mahr oh-trahs rah-dee-oh-grah-fee-ahs dehl ahb-doh-mehn ahl mees-moh tee-ehm-poh keh toh-mah-mohs lohs rah-yohs eh-kees)

Tonight, eat lightly.

Esta noche coma ligero.

(Ehs-tah noh-cheh koh-mah lee-heh-roh)

Take these pills after your meal.

Tómese estas pastillas después de la cena.

(Toh-meh-seh ehs-tahs pahs-tee-yahs dehs-poo-ehs deh lah seh-nah)

You can drink water.

Puede tomar agua.

(Poo-eh-deh toh-mahr ah-goo-ah)

Please tell the nurse to call me.

Por favor, dígale a la enfermera que me llame.

(Por fah-bohr, dee-gah-leh ah lah ehn-fehr-meh-rah keh meh yah-meh)

TABLE 20–4 Phrases | **TABLA 20–4 Frases**

English	Spanish	Pronunciation
I am going to help you.	**Voy a ayudarlo.**	*(Boy ah ah-yoo-dahr-loh)*
We are going to pull.	**Vamos a jalar.**	*(Bah-mohs ah hah-lahr)*
Very good!	**¡Muy bien!**	*(Moo-ee bee-ehn)*
Take your medical file.	**Lleve su archivo.**	*(Yeh-beh soo ahr-chee-boh)*
Take your hospital card.	**Lleve su tarjeta.**	*(Yeh-beh soo tahr-heh-tah)*
It's not very far.	**No está muy lejos.**	*(Noh ehs-tah moo-ee leh-hohs)*
We are here.	**Estamos aquí.**	*(Ehs-tah-mohs ah-kee)*
Please put this gown on.	**Por favor, póngase esta bata.**	*(Pohr fah-bohr, pohn-gah-seh ehs-tah bah-tah)*

TABLE 20–5 Helpful Phrases | **TABLA 20–5 Frases útiles**

English	Spanish	Pronunciation
It feels like a board.	**Se siente como una tabla.**	*(Seh see-ehn-teh koh-moh oo-nah tah-blah)*
One more time.	**Una vez más.**	*(Oo-nah behs mahs)*
It will take a minute.	**Va a tomar un minuto.**	*(Bah ah toh-mahr oon mee-noo-toh)*
I am through.	**Ya terminé.**	*(Yah tehr-mee-neh)*
I will return!	**¡Regresaré!**	*(Reh-greh-sah-reh)*
You need to return.	**Necesita regresar.**	*(Neh-seh-see-tah reh-greh-sahr)*
You need to drink water.	**Necesita tomar agua.**	*(Neh-seh-see-tah toh-mahr ah-goo-ah)*
When I tell you . . .	**Cuando le diga...**	*(Koo-ahn-doh leh dee-gah)*

TABLE 20–6
Common Words

TABLA 20–6
Palabras comunes

English	Spanish	Pronunciation
arteriogram	**arteriograma**	*(ahr-teh-ree-oh-grah-mah)*
bowel	**intestino**	*(een-tehs-tee-noh)*
contrast	**contraste**	*(kohn-trahs-teh)*
division	**división**	*(dee-bee-see-ohn)*
enema	**enema/sonda**	*(eh-neh-mah/sohn-dah)*
irradiate	**irradiar**	*(ee-rah-dee-ahr)*
gallbladder	**vesícula biliar/hiel**	*(beh-see-koo-lah bee-lee-ahr/ee-ehl)*
laxative	**laxante/purgante**	*(lahx-ahn-teh/poor-gahn-teh)*
liver	**hígado**	*(ee-gah-doh)*
nuclear medicine	**medicina nuclear**	*(meh-dee-see-nah noo-kleh-ahr)*
thyroid	**tiróide/tiroidea**	*(tee-roh-ee-deh/tee-roh-ee-deh-ah)*
ultrasound	**ultrasonido**	*(ool-trah-soh-nee-doh)*
ventilation	**ventilación**	*(behn-tee-lah-see-ohn)*

Do you have any questions?
¿Tiene preguntas?
(Tee-eh-neh preh-goon-tahs)

I will see you tomorrow at nine.
Lo veré mañana a las nueve.
(Loh beh-reh mah-nyah-nah ah lahs noo-eh-beh)

Have a good day!
¡Pase un buen día!
(Pah-seh oon boo-ehn dee-ah)

Transportation will take you back to your room
Transportación lo regresará a su cuarto.
(Trahns-pohr-tah-see-ohn loh reh-greh-sah-rah ah soo koo-ahr-toh)

Chapter Twenty-one / Capítulo veintiuno

The Meals / Las comidas

For many patients, meals served in the hospital are not very appetizing. Hispanic patients, in general, prefer foods that are spicy and juicy. They are quite attached to special **"bocadillos"** (*appetizers*) that may not be available in the hospital. Please explain to patients what foods they are able to bring from home and assist them with selections that they can make from their menus. Table 21–1 has a list of some diets available in the hospital.

Para muchos pacientes las comidas que se sirven en el hospital no son apetitosas. Los hispanos, en general, prefieren comidas condimentadas y jugosas. Están acostumbrados a comer bocadillos especiales (aperitivos)

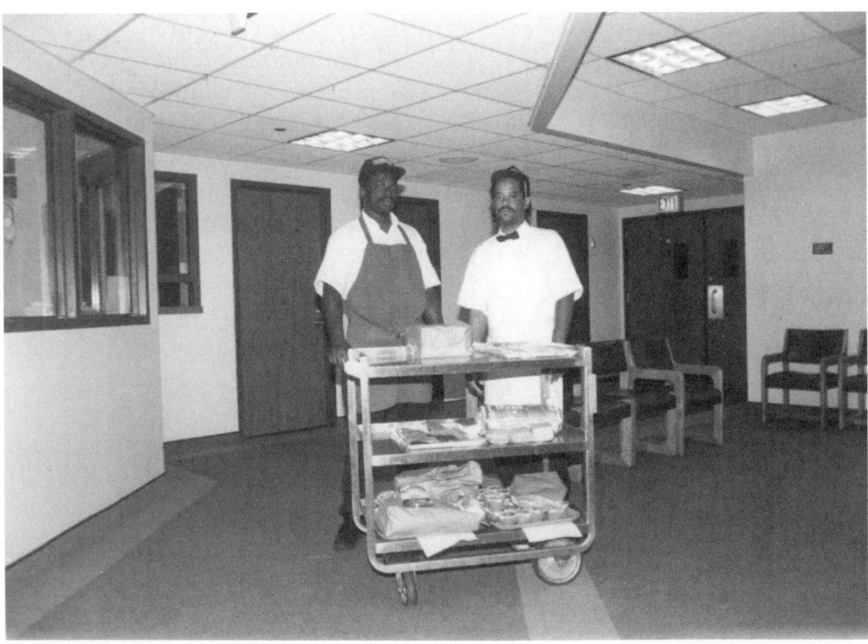

Figure 21–1 Serving foods in the hospital is a complex activity.

que a veces no se pueden encontrar en los hospitales. Por favor explíqueles a los pacientes si pueden traer comida de su casa y ayúdeles con las selecciones que pueden hacer en sus menús. La Tabla 21–1 tiene una lista de algunas de las dietas que se ofrecen en el hospital.

There are many diets available to patients.	**Hay muchas dietas para los pacientes.** *(Ah-ee moo-chahs dee-eh-tahs pah-rah lohs pah-see-ehn-tehs)*
The doctor has to prescribe it.	**El/la doctor(a) debe de recetarla.** *(Ehl dohk-tohr/Lah dohk-toh-rah deh-beh deh reh-seh-tahr-lah)*
Can you tell me what kind of diet you have?	**¿Puede decirme qué dieta tiene?** *(Poo-eh-deh deh-seer-meh keh dee-eh-tah tee-eh-neh)*
What foods do you like?	**¿Qué comidas le gustan?** *(Keh koh-mee-dahs leh goos-tahn)*

Many patients do not follow a balanced diet because they do not eat a variety of needed foods.

Muchos pacientes no llevan una dieta balanceada porque no comen una variedad de alimentos necesarios.

The following should be included in your diet every day:	**Lo siguiente se debe incluir en su dieta todos los días:** *(Loh see-gee-ehn-teh seh deh-beh een-kloo-eer ehn soo dee-eh-tah toh-dohs lohs dee-ahs)*
2 to 4 servings of milk;	**dos a cuatro porciones de leche;** *(dohs ah koo-ah-troh pohr-see-ohn-ehs deh leh-cheh)*
2 to 3 servings of meat, fish, or poultry;	**dos a tres porciones de carne, pescado o aves de corral;** *(dohs ah trehs pohr-see-oh-nehs deh kahr-neh, pehs-kah-doh oh ah-behs deh ko-rahl)*
2 to 4 servings of fruit;	**dos a cuatro porciones de fruta;** *(dohs ah koo-ah-troh pohr-see-ohn-ehs deh froo-tah)*
6 to 11 servings of starches;	**seis a once porciones de almidones/féculas;** *(seh-ees ah ohn-seh pohr-see-oh-nehs deh ahl-mee-doh-nehs/feh-koo-lahs)*

TABLE 21–1
Types of Diets

TABLA 21–1
Tipos de dietas

English	Spanish	Pronunciation
diabetic	**para diabético**	*(pah-rah dee-ah-beh-tee-koh)*
liquid	**líquida**	*(lee-kee-dah)*
low cholesterol	**colesterol bajo**	*(koh-lehs-teh-rohl bah-hoh)*
low fat	**poca grasa**	*(poh-kah grah-sah)*
no salt	**sin sal**	*(seen sahl)*
regular	**regular**	*(reh-goo-lahr)*
soft	**suave**	*(soo-ah-beh)*

wheat bread and cereals;	**pan de trigo y cereales;** *(pahn deh tree-goh ee seh-reh-ah-lehs)*
3 to 5 servings of vegetables.	**tres a cinco porciones de vegetales.** *(trehs ah seen-koh pohr-see-oh-nehs deh beh-heh-tah-lehs)*
I am going to give you a list.	**Voy a darle una lista.** *(Boy ah dahr-leh oo-nah lees-tah)*
For breakfast:	**Para el desayuno:** *(Pah-rah ehl deh-sah-yoo-noh)*
eggs	**huevos** *(oo-eh-bohs)*
toast	**pan tostado** *(pahn tohs-tah-doh)*
coffee	**café** *(kah-feh)*
milk	**leche** *(leh-cheh)*
juice	**jugo** *(joo-goh)*
fruit	**fruta** *(froo-tah)*
How do you like your coffee?	**¿Cómo le gusta el café?** *(Koh-moh leh goos-tah ehl kah-feh)*
black	**negro** *(neh-groh)*

with cream	**con crema** *(kohn kreh-mah)*
with sugar	**con azúcar** *(kohn ah-soo-kahr)*
What kind of coffee?	**¿Qué clase de café?** *(Keh klah-seh deh kah-feh)*
regular	**regular** *(reh-goo-lahr)*
decaffeinated	**descafeinado** *(dehs-kah-feh-ee-nah-doh)*
instant	**instantáneo** *(eens-tahn-tah-neh-oh)*
What kind of juices?	**¿Qué clase de jugos?** *(Keh klah-seh deh joo-gohs)*
orange	**naranja** *(nah-rahn-hah)*
grape	**uva** *(oo-bah)*
apple	**manzana** *(mahn-sah-nah)*
grapefruit	**toronja** *(toh-rohn-hah)*
prune	**ciruela** *(see-roo-eh-lah)*
tomato	**tomate** *(toh-mah-teh)*
How do you like the eggs fixed?	**¿Cómo le gustan los huevos?** *(Koh-moh leh goos-tahn lohs oo-eh-bohs)*
scrambled	**revueltos** *(reh-boo-ehl-tohs)*
over-easy	**volteados** *(bohl-teh-ah-dohs)*
fried	**fritos** *(free-tohs)*
hard-boiled	**duros** *(doo-rohs)*
with ham	**con jamón** *(kohn hah-mohn)*
We have cereals.	**Tenemos cereales.** *(Teh-neh-mohs seh-reh-ah-lehs)*
Do you like them hot/cold?	**¿Le gustan calientes/fríos?** *(Leh goos-tahn kah-lee-ehn-tehs/free-ohs)*

oatmeal	**avena** *(ah-beh-nah)*
cream of wheat	**crema de trigo** *(kreh-mah deh tree-goh)*
corn flakes	**hojitas de maíz/corn flakes** *(oh-hee-tahs deh mah-ees/kohrn fleh-ee-ks)*
We serve lunch at twelve noon.	**Servimos la comida al mediodía.** *(Sehr-bee-mohs lah koh-mee-dah ahl meh-dee-oh-dee-ah)*
Kitchen personnel bring the food trays.	**Los empleados de la cocina traen las bandejas con comida.** *(Lohs ehm-pleh-ah-dohs deh lah koh-see-nah trah-ehn lahs bahn-deh-hahs kohn koh-mee-dah)*
We have meats:	**Tenemos carnes:** *(Teh-neh-mohs kahr-nehs)*
beef	**res** *(rehs)*
hamburger	**hamburguesa** *(ahm-boor-geh-sah)*

TABLE 21–2
Common Foods

TABLA 21–2
Comidas comunes

English	Spanish	Pronunciation
cereals	**cereales**	*(seh-reh-ah-lehs)*
coffee	**café**	*(kah-feh)*
crab	**cangrejos**	*(kahn-greh-hohs)*
crackers	**galletas saladas**	*(gah-yeh-tahs sah-lah-dahs)*
custard	**flan**	*(flahn)*
desserts	**postres**	*(pohs-trehs)*
eggs	**huevos**	*(oo-eh-bohs)*
enchiladas	**enchiladas**	*(ehn-chee-lah-dahs)*
gelatin	**gelatina**	*(geh-lah-tee-nah)*
lamb	**cordero**	*(kohr-deh-roh)*
shrimp	**camarones**	*(kah-mah-roh-nehs)*
tamales	**tamales**	*(tah-mah-lehs)*
tuna	**atún**	*(ah-toon)*
turkey	**pavo/guajolote**	*(pah-boh/goo-ah-hoh-loh-teh)*
vegetables	**vegetales**	*(beh-heh-tah-lehs)*
vinegar	**vinagre**	*(bee-nah-greh)*

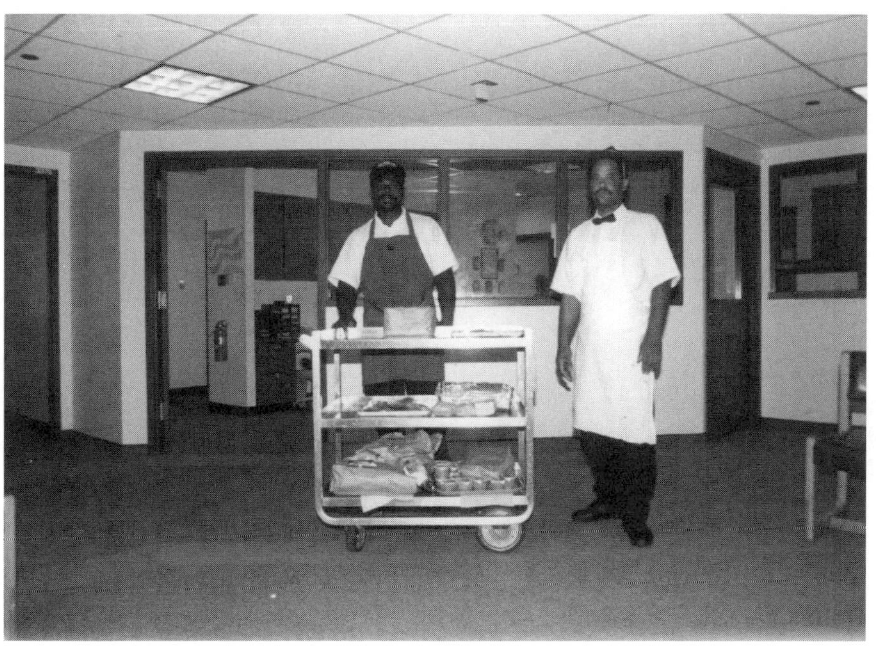

Figure 21–2 Kitchen staff delivers nourishment several times a day.

steak	**bistec** *(bees-tehk)*
roast	**rostizado** *(rohs-tee-sah-doh)*
pork	**puerco** *(poo-ehr-koh)*
chops	**chuletas** *(choo-leh-tahs)*
ribs	**costillas** *(kohs-tee-yahs)*
chicken	**pollo** *(poh-yoh)*
fried chicken	**pollo frito** *(poh-yoh free-toh)*
baked chicken	**pollo asado** *(poh-yoh ah-sah-doh)*
breast	**pechuga** *(peh-choo-gah)*
leg	**pierna** *(pee-ehr-nah)*

wings	**alas** *(ah-lahs)*
fish	**pescado** *(pehs-kah-doh)*
breaded	**empanizado** *(ehm-pah-nee-sah-doh)*
broiled fish	**pescado al horno** *(pehs-kah-doh ahl ohr-noh)*
These meats can be substituted.	**Estas carnes se pueden substituir.** *(Ehs-tahs kahr-nehs seh poo-eh-dehn soobs-tee-too-eer)*
Among the vegetables that we serve are:	**Entre los vegetales que servimos hay:** *(Ehn-treh lohs beh-heh-tah-lehs keh sehr-bee-mohs ah-ee)*
potatoes	**papas** *(pah-pahs)*
baked potatoes	**papas asadas** *(pah-pahs ah-sah-dahs)*
french fries	**papas fritas** *(pah-pahs free-tahs)*
mashed potatoes	**puré de papas** *(poo-reh deh pah-pahs)*

TABLE 21–3 Pronunciation of Selected Words

TABLA 21–3 Pronunciación de palabras selectas

English	Spanish	Pronunciation
alcoholic beverages	**bebidas alcohólicas**	*(beh-bee-dahs ahl-koh-lee-kahs)*
carbonated drinks	**bebidas gaseosas**	*(beh-bee-dahs gah-seh-oh-sahs)*
cottage cheese	**requesón**	*(reh-keh-sohn)*
frozen	**helado/congelado**	*(eh-lah-doh/kohn-heh-lah-doh)*
minerals	**minerales**	*(mee-neh-rah-lehs)*
miscellaneous	**miscelánea**	*(mee-seh-lah-neh-ah)*
raw	**crudo**	*(kroo-doh)*
roast beef	**rosbif**	*(rohs-beef)*
saccharin	**sacarina**	*(sah-kah-ree-nah)*
soups	**sopas**	*(soh-pahs)*
substitutes	**substitutos**	*(soobs-tee-too-tohs)*
toothpick	**palillo**	*(pah-lee-yoh)*
vitamins	**vitaminas**	*(bee-tah-mee-nahs)*

green beans	**ejotes/habichuelas** *(eh-hoh-tehs/ah-bee-choo-eh-lahs)*
peas	**chícharos** *(chee-chah-rohs)*
corn	**maíz/elote** *(mah-ees/eh-loh-teh)*
beans	**frijoles/habas** *(free-hoh-lehs/ah-bahs)*
pinto beans	**frijol pinto** *(free-hohl peen-toh)*
refried	**refritos** *(reh-free-tohs)*
rice	**arroz** *(ah-rohs)*
salad	**ensalada** *(ehn-sah-lah-dah)*
lettuce	**lechuga** *(leh-choo-gah)*
We also have desserts:	**También tenemos postres:** *(Tahm-bee-ehn teh-neh-mohs pohs-trehs)*
ice cream	**nieve/helado** *(nee-eh-beh/eh-lah-doh)*
vanilla	**vainilla** *(bah-ee-nee-yah)*
chocolate	**chocolate** *(choh-koh-lah-teh)*
strawberry	**fresa** *(freh-sah)*
pies	**pasteles** *(pahs-teh-lehs)*
pecan	**nuez** *(noo-ehs)*
apple	**manzana** *(mahn-sah-nah)*
cookies	**galletas** *(gah-yeh-tahs)*
candy	**dulces** *(dool-sehs)*
You can buy canned drinks in the cafeteria.	**Puede comprar bebidas envasadas en la cafetería.** *(Poo-eh-deh kohm-prahr beh-bee-dahs ehn-bah-sah-dahs ehn lah kah-feh-teh-ree-ah)*

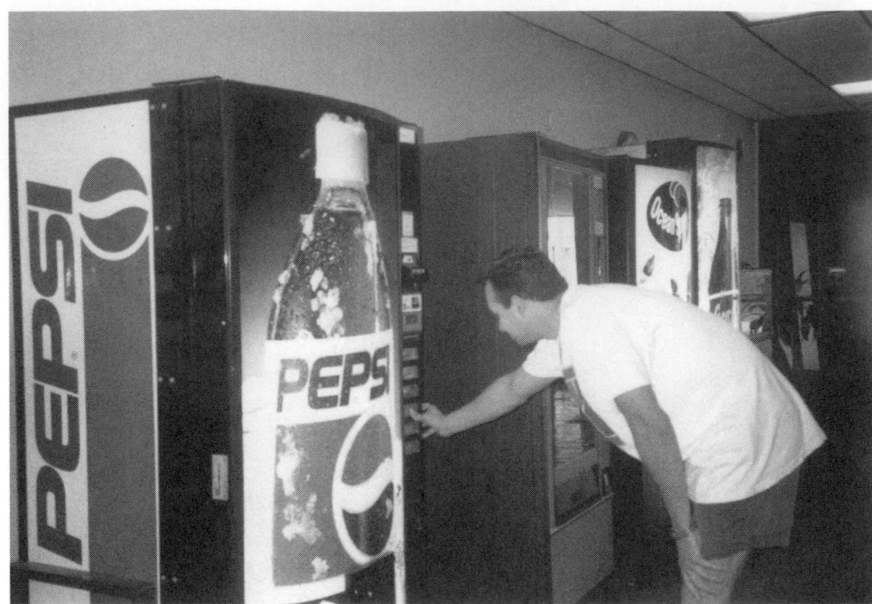

Figure 21–3 Carbonated drinks are sold in the hospital cafeteria.

We don't serve drinks like Cokes or any canned drinks.	**No servimos refrescos como Coca-cola o bebidas envasadas.** *(Noh sehr-bee-mohs reh-frehs-kohs koh-moh Koh-kah-koh-lah oh beh-bee-dahs ehn-bah-sah-dahs)*
You can also ask for snacks:	**También puede pedir aperitivos:** *(Tahm-bee-ehn poo-eh-deh peh-deer ah-peh-ree-tee-bohs)*
juices	**jugos** *(joo-gohs)*
fruit	**fruta** *(froo-tah)*
yogurt	**yogurt** *(yoh-goor)*
peanut butter sandwich	**lonche de crema de cacahuate** *(lohn-cheh deh kreh-mah deh kah-kah-oo-ah-teh)*
milk	**leche** *(leh-cheh)*

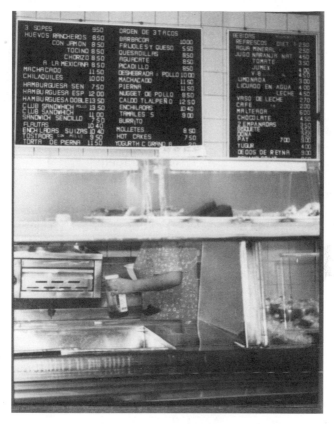

Figure 21–4 Prices are usually posted on the wall in the cafeteria.

variety of breads	**variedad de panes** *(bah-ree-eh-dahd deh pah-nehs)*
corn	**maíz** *(mah-ees)*
wheat	**trigo** *(tree-goh)*
white	**blanco** *(blahn-koh)*
condiments	**condimentos** *(kohn-dee-mehn-tohs)*
spices	**especias** *(ehs-peh-see-ahs)*
butter	**mantequilla** *(mahn-teh-kee-yah)*
mustard	**mostaza** *(mohs-tah-sah)*

hot sauce	**salsa picante** *(sahl-sah pee-kahn-teh)*
mayonnaise	**mayonesa** *(mah-yoh-neh-sah)*
The water is in the glass/pitcher.	**El agua está en el vaso/la jarra.** *(Ehl ah-goo-ah ehs-tah ehn ehl bah-soh/lah hah-rah)*
Do you want water?	**¿Quere agua?** *(Kee-eh-reh ah-goo-ah)*
Do you need ice?	**¿Necesita hielo?** *(Neh-seh-see-tah ee-eh-loh)*
This is the tray.	**Esta es la bandeja.** *(Ehs-tah ehs lah bahn-deh-hah)*
The fork, spoon, and knife are wrapped in the napkin.	**El tenedor, cuchara y cuchillo están envueltos en la servilleta.** *(Ehl teh-neh-dohr, koo-chah-rah ee koo-chee-yoh ehs-tahn ehn-boo-ehl-tohs ehn lah sehr-bee-yeh-tah)*
There is a straw.	**Hay un popote.** *(Ah-ee oon poh-poh-teh)*
The salt and pepper are in these packets.	**La sal y pimienta están en estos paquetes.** *(Lah sahl ee pee-mee-ehn-tah ehs-tahn ehn ehs-tohs pah-keh-tehs)*
Sorry, no toothpicks.	**Lo siento, no hay palillos.** *(Loh see-ehn-toh, noh ah-ee pah-lee-yohs)*
The plates are plastic.	**Los platos son de plástico.** *(Lohs plah-tohs sohn deh plahs-tee-koh)*
They can't break.	**No se pueden romper.** *(Noh seh poo-eh-dehn rohm-pehr)*
The cover is hot.	**La cubierta está caliente.** *(Lah koo-bee-ehr-tah ehs-tah kah-lee-ehn-teh)*
It keeps the food warm.	**Guarda la comida tibia.** *(Goo-ahr-dah lah koh-mee-dah tee-bee-ah)*
You can eat in your room or in the visitors' room.	**Puede comer en su cuarto o en el cuarto para visitas.** *(Poo-eh-deh koh-mehr ehn soo koo-ahr-toh oh ehn ehl koo-ahr-toh pah-rah bee-see-tahs)*

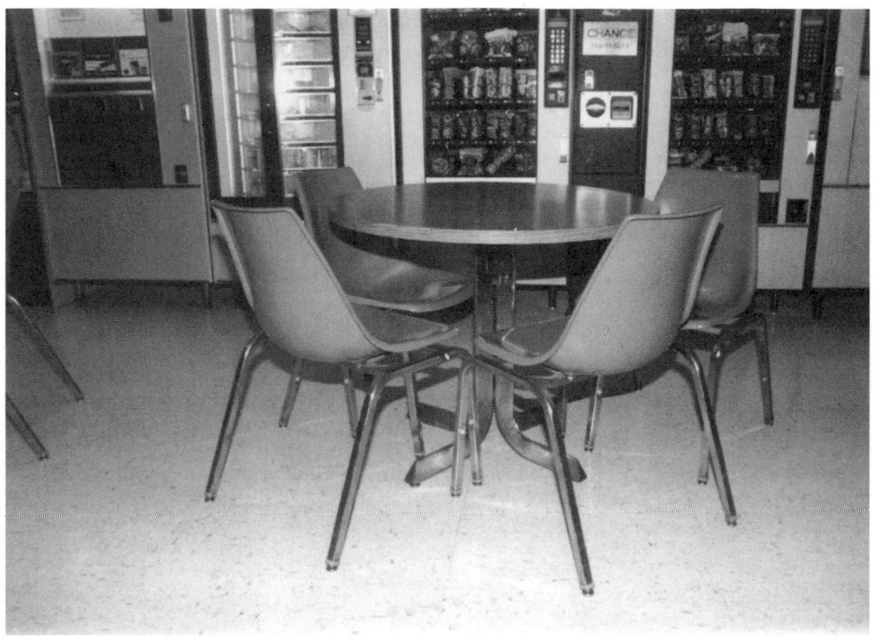

Figure 21–5 Visitors may eat in the lounge.

TABLE 21–4
List of Fruits

TABLA 21–4
Lista de frutas

English	Spanish	Pronunciation
banana	**plátano**	*(plah-tah-noh)*
canteloupe	**melón**	*(meh-lohn)*
cherries	**cerezas**	*(seh-reh-sahs)*
grapefruit	**toronja**	*(toh-rohn-hah)*
lime	**lima**	*(lee-mah)*
orange	**naranja**	*(nah-rahn-hah)*
pears	**peras**	*(peh-rahs)*
pineapple	**piña**	*(pee-nyah)*
plum	**ciruelo**	*(see-roo-eh-loh)*
strawberry	**fresa**	*(freh-sah)*
watermelon	**sandía**	*(sahn-dee-ah)*

Select your foods from the menu after breakfast.	**Seleccione las comidas del menú después del desayuno.** *(Seh-lehk-see-oh-neh lahs koh-mee-dahs dehl meh-noo dehs-poo-ehs dehl deh-sah-yoo-noh)*
You have to choose three meals a day.	**Tiene que escoger tres comidas diarias.** *(Tee-eh-neh keh ehs-koh-hehr trehs koh-mee-dahs dee-ah-ree-ahs)*
You can order one or two portions.	**Puede ordenar una o dos porciones.** *(Poo-eh-deh ohr-deh-nahr oo-nah oh dohs pohr-see-oh-nehs)*
We send the menu to the kitchen.	**Mandamos el menú a la cocina.** *(Mahn-dah-mohs ehl meh-noo ah lah koh-see-nah)*

Some people cannot tolerate gas-producing foods and should avoid eating them.

Algunas personas no toleran comidas que producen gas y deben evitar comerlas.

Gas-producing foods:	**Comidas que producen gas:** *(Koh-mee-dahs keh proh-doo-sehn gahs)*
onions	**cebolla** *(seh-boh-yah)*
beans	**frijoles** *(free-hoh-lehs)*
celery	**apio** *(ah-pee-oh)*
carrots	**zanahoria** *(sah-nah-oh-ree-ah)*
cabbage	**col/repollo** *(kohl/reh-poh-yoh)*
raisins	**pasas** *(pah-sahs)*
bananas	**plátanos** *(plah-tah-nohs)*
prunes	**ciruelas** *(see-roo-eh-lahs)*

Cholesterol is a type of fat found in the blood. A low cholesterol diet may help to lower your blood cholesterol level if it is too high. Cut down on foods that have high cholesterol content. The following list gives you a general idea of foods you should avoid.

El colesterol es un tipo de grasa en la sangre. Una dieta baja en colesterol le puede ayudar a rebajar el nivel si está muy alto. Reduzca las comidas que tienen contenido muy alto de colesterol. La siguiente lista le da una idea en general de las comidas que debe de evitar.

Foods you may not eat:	**Comidas que no debe comer:** *(Koh-mee-dahs keh noh deh-beh koh-mehr)*
butter	**mantequilla** *(mahn-teh-kee-yah)*
shortening	**manteca** *(mahn-teh-kah)*
egg yolks	**yema de huevos** *(yeh-mah deh oo-eh-bohs)*
biscuits	**bisquetes/bizcocho** *(bees-keh-tehs/bees-koh-choh)*
pancakes	**panqué** *(pahn-keh)*
avocados	**aguacates** *(ah-goo-ah-kah-tehs)*
bacon	**tocino** *(toh-see-noh)*
sausage	**salchicha/chorizo** *(sahl-chee-chah/choh-ree-soh)*
hot dog	**perro caliente/emparedado de salchicha** *(peh-roh kah-lee-ehn-teh/ehm-pah-reh-dah-doh deh sahl-chee-chah)*
whole milk	**leche entera** *(leh-cheh ehn-teh-rah)*
ice cream	**nieve/helado** *(nee-eh-beh/eh-lah-doh)*
chocolate	**chocolate** *(choh-koh-lah-teh)*
liver	**hígado** *(ee-gah-doh)*
most red meat	**la mayoría de las carnes rojas** *(lah mah-yoh-ree-ah deh lahs kahr-nehs roh-hahs)*
most cookies	**la mayoría de las galletas** *(lah mah-yoh-ree-ah deh lahs gah-yeh-tahs)*

Unit 4 Unidad 4

Chapter Twenty-two | Capítulo veintidós

Physical Exam | Examen físico

The physical exam is very important. From the moment that we see a person, we start to assess and to note the patient's general well-being. A good review of the body allows us to make a primary diagnosis. With assistance from the laboratory and the X-rays, we are able to make a final diagnosis. The physical exam must be done carefully, since it provides a fundamental base for further decision making. The mental exam is part of the physical exam. It gives us the oportunity to see if the patient is nervous, tense, aggressive, vulnerable, restless, or depressed. We are able to assess whether the patient is oriented to time, person, or place.

El examen físico es muy importante. Desde el momento en que vemos a la persona, podemos darnos cuenta de su estado general. Una buena revisión o exploración del cuerpo nos permitirá hacer un primer diagnóstico. Ayudados por el laboratorio y las radiografías podremos hacer un diagnóstico final. El examen físico debe hacerse con el mayor cuidado posible, ya que es una base fundamental para tomar decisiones posteriores. El examen mental es parte del examen físico; nos permite saber si el paciente está nervioso, tenso, agresivo, vulnerable, inquieto o deprimido. Podremos ver si está orientado en persona, tiempo, lugar y espacio.

Useful commands and phrases that facilitate the physical exam.

Mandatos y frases útiles que facilitan el examen físico.
(Mahn-dah-tohs ee frah-sehs oo-tee-lehs keh fah-see-lee-tahn ehl ehx-ah-mehn fee-see-koh)

Note that the familiar **tú** is being used.
Note que se está usando la forma familiar "tú".

I am going to examine you.

Voy a examinarte.
(Boy ah ehx-ah-mee-nahr-teh)

Please sit up in the bed.

Por favor, siéntate en la cama.
(Pohr fah-bohr, see-ehn-tah-teh ehn lah kah-mah)

TABLE 22–1 Patient's Moods | **TABLA 22–1 Actitud del paciente**

English	Spanish	Pronunciation
aggressive	**agresivo**	*(ah-greh-see-boh)*
anxious	**ansioso**	*(ahn-see-oh-soh)*
depressed	**deprimido**	*(deh-pree-mee-doh)*
euphoric	**eufórico**	*(eh-oo-foh-ree-koh)*
flat	**indiferente**	*(een-dee-feh-rehn-teh)*
irritable	**irritable**	*(ee-ree-tah-bleh)*
nervous	**nervioso**	*(nehr-bee-oh-soh)*
restless	**inquieto**	*(een-kee-eh-toh)*
tense	**tenso**	*(tehn-soh)*

I am going to check your head.	**Voy a revisar tu cabeza.** *(Boy ah reh-bee-sahr too kah-beh-sah)*
Lift your head.	**Levanta la cabeza.** *(Leh-bahn-tah lah kah-beh-sah)*
Lower your head.	**Baja la cabeza.** *(Bah-hah lah kah-beh-sah)*
Move it side to side.	**Muévela de lado a lado.** *(Moo-eh-beh-lah deh lah-doh ah lah-doh)*
I am going to check your eyes.	**Voy a revisar tus ojos.** *(Boy ah reh-bee-sahr toosh oh-hohs)*
Look straight ahead.	**Mira hacia adelante.** *(Mee-rah ah-see-ah ah-deh-lahn-teh)*
Look up.	**Mira hacia arriba.** *(Mee-rah ah-see-ah ah-ree-bah)*
Look down.	**Mira hacia abajo.** *(Mee-rah ah-see-ah ah-bah-hoh)*
Follow my finger.	**Sigue mi dedo.** *(See-geh mee deh-doh)*
Look straight at the light.	**Mira directo a la luz.** *(Mee-rah dee-rehk-toh ah lah loos)*
I am going to check your ears.	**Voy a revisar tus orejas.** *(Boy ah reh-bee-sahr toohs oh-reh-hahs)*
Turn your head to the left.	**Voltea la cabeza a la izquierda.** *(Bohl-teh-ah lah kah-beh-sah ah lah ees-kee-ehr-dah)*

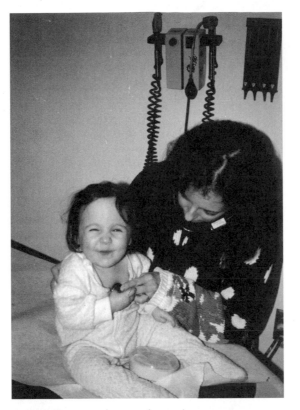

Figure 22–1 It is important to observe the patient.

Turn your head to the right.	**Voltea la cabeza a la derecha.** *(Bohl-teh-ah lah kah-beh-sah ah lah deh-reh-chah)*
I am going to check your nose.	**Voy a revisar la nariz.** *(Boy ah reh-bee-sahr lah nah-rees)*
Wrinkle your nose.	**Arruga la nariz.** *(Ah-roo-gah lah nah-rees)*
I am going to check your throat.	**Voy a revisar la garganta.** *(Boy ah reh-bee-sahr lah gahr-gahn-tah)*
Open your mouth.	**Abre la boca.** *(Ah-breh lah boh-kah)*
Close your mouth.	**Cierra la boca.** *(See-eh-rah lah boh-kah)*

Open again.	**Abrela otra vez.** *(Ah-breh-lah oh-trah behs)*
Say, "ahh."	**Di "aaa".** *(Dee ah-ah-ah)*
Please swallow.	**Traga, por favor.** *(Trah-gah pohr fah-bohr)*
Smile.	**Sonríe.** *(Sohn-ree-eh)*
I am going to check your mouth.	**Voy a revisar tu boca.** *(Boy ah reh-bee-sahr too boh-kah)*

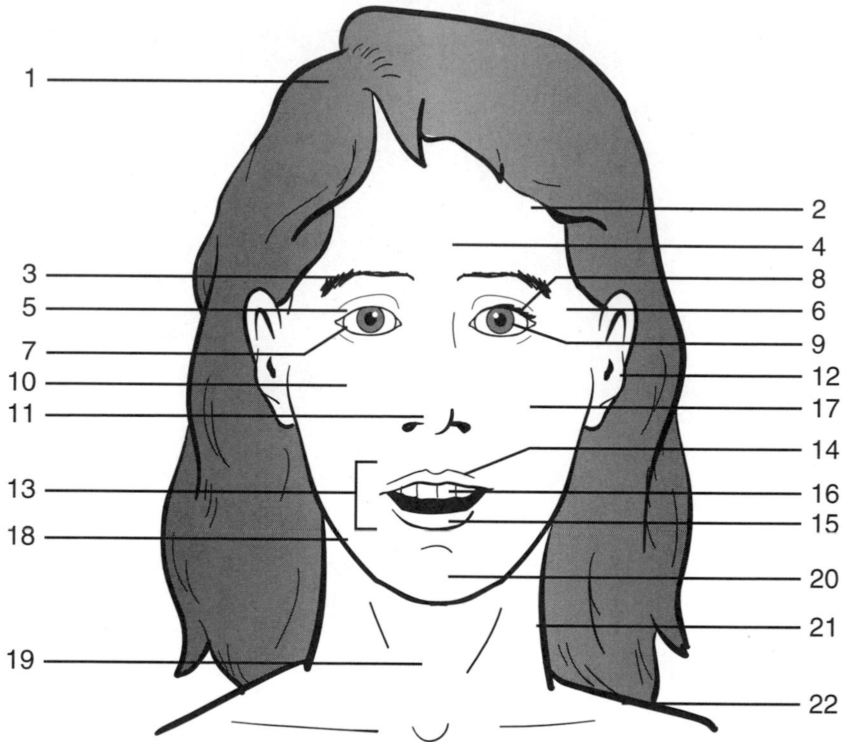

Figure 22–2 The head and neck. (1) El cabello/el pelo (*hair*), (2) el cráneo (*skull*), (3) la ceja (*eyebrow*), (4) la frente (*forehead*), (5) el párpado (*eyelid*), (6) la sien (*temple*), (7) la esclerótica (*sclera*), (8) la pestaña (*eyelash*), (9) el ojo (*eye*), (10) el pómulo (*cheekbone*), (11) la nariz (*nose*), (12) la oreja/el oído (*ear*), (13) la boca (*mouth*), (14) el labio superior (*upper lip*), (15) el labio inferior (*lower lip*), (16) los dientes (*teeth*), (17) la mejilla (*cheek*), (18) la mandíbula (*mandible*), (19) la manzanilla/la nuez de Adán (*Adam's apple*), (20) la barbilla (*chin*), (21) el cuello (*neck*), (22) la piel (*skin*).

Your lips should not be dry.	**Tus labios no deben estar secos.** *(Toos lah-bee-ohs noh deh-behn ehs-tahr seh-kohs)*
Stick out your tongue.	**Saca la lengua.** *(Sah-kah lah lehn-goo-ah)*
I am going to check your gums.	**Voy a revisar tus encías.** *(Boy ah reh-bee-sahr toos ehn-see-ahs)*
I am going to check your teeth.	**Voy a revisar tus dientes.** *(Boy ah reh-bee-sahr toos dee-ehn-tehs)*
Upper extremities:	**Extremidades superiores:** *(ehx-treh-mee-dah-dehs soo-peh-ree-oh-rehs)*
I am going to check your arm.	**Voy a revisar tu brazo.** *(Boy ah reh-bee-sahr too brah-soh)*
Lift your arm.	**Levanta tu brazo.** *(Leh-bahn-tah too brah-soh)*
Extend it.	**Extiéndelo.** *(Ehx-tee-ehn-deh-loh)*
Flex it.	**Dóblalo.** *(Doh-blah-loh)*
Don't let me extend it.	**No me dejes extenderlo.** *(Noh meh deh-hehs ehx-tehn-dehr-loh)*
Rotate it.	**Gíralo./Dale vuelta.** *(Hee-rah-loh/Dah-leh boo-ehl-tah)*
Bend your elbow.	**Dobla el codo.** *(Doh-blah ehl koh-doh)*
I am going to palpate your elbow.	**Voy a palpar tu codo.** *(Boy ah pahl-pahr too koh-doh)*
I am going to palpate your nodes.	**Voy a palpar tus nodos.** *(Boy ah pahl-pahr toos noh-dohs)*
Turn your forearm.	**Voltea el antebrazo.** *(Bohl-teh-ah ehl ahn-teh brah-soh)*
I am going to palpate your shoulder.	**Voy a palpar tu hombro.** *(Boy ah pahl-pahr too ohm-broh)*
Place your arms behind your back.	**Pon los brazos atrás.** *(Pohn lohs brah-sohs ah-trahs)*
Place your hands behind your head.	**Pon tus manos atrás de tu cabeza.** *(Pohn toos mah-nohs ah-trahs deh too kah-beh-sah)*
I am going to check your hand.	**Voy a revisar tu mano.** *(Boy ah reh-bee-sahr too mah-noh)*
I am going to palpate it.	**Voy a palparla.** *(Boy ah pahl-pahr-lah)*

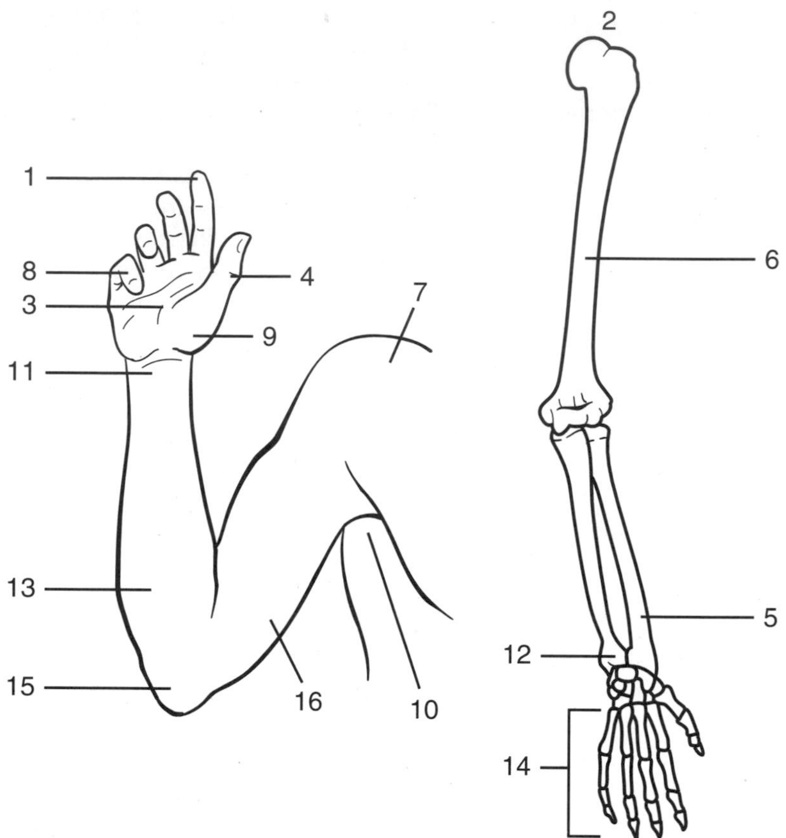

Figure 22–3 The arm and hand. (1) El dedo índice (*index finger*), (2) los huesos (*bones*), (3) la palma de la mano (*palm of the hand*), (4) el dedo pulgar (*thumb*), (5) el radio (*radius*), (6) el húmero (*humerus*), (7) el hombro (*shoulder*), (8) el dedo meñique (*little finger*), (9) la mano derecha (*right hand*), (10) la axila/el sobaco (*armpit/axilla*), (11) la muñeca (*wrist*), (12) la ulna (*ulna*), (13) el antebrazo (*forearm*), (14) los falanges (*phalanges*), (15) el codo (*elbow*), (16) el brazo (*arm*).

Open your hand.	**Abre tu mano.** ***(Ah-breh too mah-noh)***
Close it.	**Ciérrala.** ***(See-eh-rah-lah)***
Open the fingers wide.	**Separa bien los dedos.** ***(Seh-pah-rah bee-ehn lohs deh-dohs)***
Don't let me close them.	**No me dejes cerrarlos.** ***(Noh meh deh-hehs seh-rahr-lohs)***

Make a fist.	**Haz un puño.** *(Ahs oon poo-nyoh)*
Hold my finger.	**Agarra mi dedo.** *(Ah-gah-rah meeh deh-doh)*
Tighten!	**¡Aprieta!** *(Ah-pree-eh-tah)*
Lift your hand.	**Levanta tu mano.** *(Leh-bahn-tah too mah-noh)*
Bend the wrist.	**Dobla la muñeca.** *(Doh-blah lah moo-nyeh-kah)*
Extend your wrist.	**Extiende tu muñeca.** *(Ehx-tee-ehn-deh too moo-nyeh-kah)*
I am going to examine your nailbeds.	**Voy a examinar la base de tus uñas.** *(Boy ah ehx-ah-mee-nahr lah bah-seh deh toos oo-nyans)*
Lower extremities:	**Extremidades inferiores:** *(Ehx-treh-mee-dah-dehs een-feh-ree-oh-rehs)*
I am going to examine your leg.	**Voy a examinar tu pierna.** *(Boy ah ehx-ah-mee-nahr too pee-ehr-nah)*
Lift your leg.	**Levanta la pierna.** *(Leh-bahn-tah lah pee-ehr-nah)*
Bend it.	**Dóblala.** *(Doh-blah-lah)*
Bend your hip.	**Dobla tu cadera.** *(Doh-blah too kah-deh-rah)*
Straighten your knee.	**Endereza la rodilla.** *(Ehn-deh-reh-sah lah roh-dee-yah)*
Move your leg.	**Mueve tu pierna.** *(Moo-eh-beh too pee-ehr-nah)*
Forward.	**Adelante.** *(Ah-deh-lahn-teh)*
Backward.	**Atrás.** *(Ah-trahs)*
I am going to examine your foot.	**Voy a examinar tu pie.** *(Boy ah ehx-ah-mee-nahr too pee-eh)*
Turn it to the left.	**Voltéalo hacia la izquierda.** *(Bohl-teh-ah-loh ah-see-ah lah ees-kee-ehr-dah)*
Turn it to the right.	**Voltéalo hacia la derecha.** *(Bohl-teh-ah-loh ah-see-ah lah deh-reh-chah)*

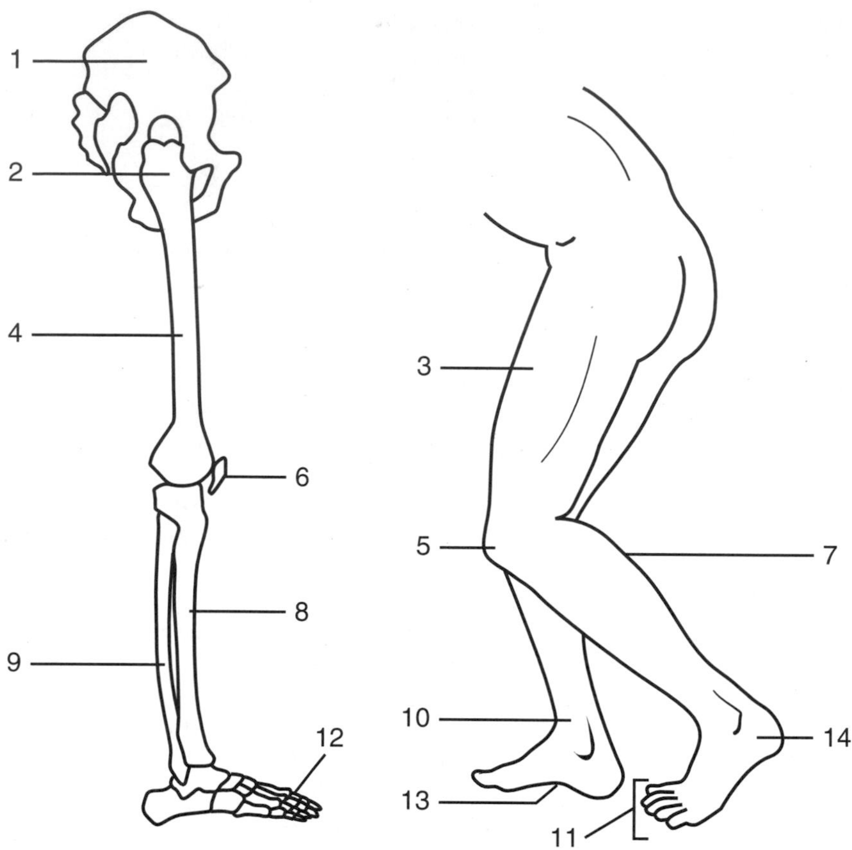

Figure 22–4 The leg and foot. (1) La pelvis (*pelvis*), (2) la cabeza del fémur (*head of the femur*), (3) el muslo (*thigh*), (4) el fémur (*femur*), (5) la rodilla (*knee*), (6) la rótula (*knee cap*), (7) la pantorrilla (*calf*), (8) la tibia (*tibia*), (9) el peroné (*fibula*), (10) el tobillo (*ankle*), (11) los dedos (*toes*), (12) las falanges (*phalanges*), (13) la planta (*plantar area*), (14) el talón (*heel*).

Push.	**Haz fuerza, empuja.** ***(Ahs foo-ehr-sah, ehm-poo-hah)***
Lift your foot.	**Levanta tu pie.** ***(Leh-bahn-tah too pee-eh)***
Bend your toes.	**Dobla tus dedos (del pie).** ***(Doh-blah toos deh-dohs [dehl pee-eh])***
Lower your foot.	**Baja el pie.** ***(Bah-hah ehl pee-eh)***

I am going to palpate your feet and ankles.	**Voy a palpar tus pies y tobillos.** *(Boy ah pahl-pahr toos pee-ehs ee toh-bee-yohs)*
Flex the foot upward.	**Dobla el pie hacia arriba.** *(Doh-blah ehl pee-eh ah-see-ah ah-ree-bah)*
Hold it like this.	**Manténlo así.** *(Mahn-tehn-loh ah-see)*
I am going to press on your big toe.	**Voy a apretar tu dedo grueso.** *(Boy ah ah-preh-tahr too deh-doh groo-eh-soh)*
I am going to palpate your knees.	**Voy a palpar tus rodillas.** *(Boy ah pahl-pahr toos roh-dee-yahs)*
Pull your knee to your chest.	**Estira la rodilla hacia el pecho.** *(Ehs-tee-rah lah roh-dee-yah ah-see-ah ehl peh-choh)*
Place your foot on the opposite knee.	**Pon tu pie sobre la rodilla opuesta.** *(Pohn too pee-eh soh-breh lah roh-dee-yah oh-poo-ehs-tah)*
Flex your knee and turn it to the middle.	**Dobla tu rodilla y voltéala hacia adentro.** *(Doh-blah too roh-dee-yah ee bohl-teh-ah-lah ah-see-ah ah-dehn-troh)*
Cross your legs.	**Cruza tus piernas.** *(Kroo-sah toos pee-ehr-nahs)*
Straighten your leg.	**Endereza tu pierna.** *(Ehn-deh-reh-sah too pee-ehr-nah)*
Don't let me bend it.	**No me dejes que la doble.** *(Noh meh deh-hehs keh lah doh-bleh)*
Relax your muscle.	**Relaja tu músculo.** *(Reh-lah-hah too moos-koo-loh)*
Stand up!	**¡Levántate!** *(Leh-bahn-tah-teh!)*
Please walk.	**Camina, por favor.** *(Kah-mee-nah, pohr fah-bohr)*
Stop!	**¡Para!/¡Deténte!** *(Pah-rah/Deh-tehn-teh)*
Jump on one foot.	**Brinca con un pie.** *(Breen-kah kohn oon pee-eh)*
Take your shoes off.	**Quítate los zapatos.** *(Kee-tah-teh lohs sah-pah-tohs)*

Take your socks off.	**Quítate los calcetines.** *(Kee-tah-teh lohs kahl-seh-tee-nehs)*
Now, I am going to examine your skin.	**Ahora, voy a revisar tu piel.** *(Ah-oh-rah boy ah reh-bee-sahr too pee-ehl)*
You have bruises and white spots.	**Tiene moretones y manchas blancas.** *(Tee-eh-neh moh-reh-toh-nehs ee mahn-chahs blahn-kahs)*
Now, I am going to examine your chest.	**Ahora, voy a revisar tu pecho.** *(Ah-oh-rah boy ah reh-bee-sahr too peh-choh)*
I am going to listen to your heart.	**Voy a escuchar el corazón.** *(Boy ah ehs-koo-chahr ehl koh-rah-sohn)*
Don't talk.	**No hables.** *(Noh ah-blehs)*
Breathe!	**¡Respira!** *(Rehs-pee-rah)*
Breathe regularly.	**Respira regularmente.** *(Rehs-pee-rah reh-goo-lahr-mehn-teh)*
Now, take a deep breath.	**Ahora, respira hondo.** *(Ah-oh-rah, rehs-pee-rah ohn-doh)*
Hold it!	**¡Deténlo!** *(Deh-tehn-loh)*
Does it hurt to breathe?	**¿Te duele al respirar?** *(Teh doo-eh-leh ahl rehs-pee-rahr)*
Cough!	**¡Tose!** *(Toh-seh)*
Cough harder!	**¡Tose más fuerte!** *(Toh-seh mahs foo-ehr-teh)*
I am going to palpate your chest.	**Voy a palpar el pecho.** *(Boy ah pahl-pahr ehl peh-choh)*
Relax.	**Descansa.** *(Dehs-kahn-sah)*
Sit upright!	**¡Siéntate derecho!** *(See-ehn-tah-teh deh-reh-choh)*
Please lie down.	**Acuéstate, por favor.** *(Ah-koo-ehs-tah-teh pohr fah-bohr)*
I am going to palpate the breast.	**Voy a palpar el seno.** *(Boy ah pahl-pahr ehl seh-noh)*
I am going to palpate the axillary nodes.	**Voy a palpar los nodos de la axila.** *(Boy ah pahl-pahr lohs noh-dohs deh lah ahx-ee-lah)*

TABLE 22–2
Skin-Related Terms

TABLA 22–2
Términos relacionados con la piel

English	Spanish	Pronunciation
acne	**acné**	*(ahk-neh)*
birthmark	**lunar**	*(loo-nahr)*
bruises/echymosis	**moretones/equimosis**	*(moh-reh-toh-nehs/eh-kee-moh-sees)*
burns	**quemaduras**	*(keh-mah-doo-rahs)*
dry	**seca**	**(seh-kah)**
eczema	**eczema**	*(ehk-seh-mah)*
freckles	**pecas**	*(peh-kahs)*
fungus	**hongos**	*(ohn-gohs)*
hematoma	**hematoma**	*(eh-mah-toh-mah)*
infection	**infección**	*(een-fehk-see-ohn)*
inflammation	**inflamación**	*(een-flah-mah-see-ohn)*
mole	**verruga**	*(beh-roo-gah)*
psoriasis	**soriasis**	*(soh-ree-ah-sees)*
red spots/white spots	**manchas rojas/ manchas blancas**	*(mahn-chahs roh-hahs/ mahn-chahs blahn-kahs)*
scratch	**raspón**	*(rahs-pohn)*
ulcers	**úlceras**	*(ool-seh-rahs)*
wound	**herida**	*(eh-ree-dah)*

I am going to tap.
Voy a percutir/golpear.
(Boy ah pehr-koo-teer/gohl-peh-ahr)

I am going to auscultate.
Voy a auscultar/escuchar.
(Boy ah ah-oos-kool-tahr/ehs-koo-chahr)

I am going to listen to your apical pulse/your heartbeat.
Voy a oír tu pulso apical/los latidos del corazón.
(Boy ah oh-eer too pool-soh ah-pee-kahl/lohs lah-tee-dohs dehl koh-rah-sohn)

I am going to palpate your carotid pulse.
Voy a palpar tu pulso en la carótida/ en el cuello.
(Boy ah pahl-pahr too pool-soh ehn lah kah-roh-tee-dah/ehn ehl koo-eh-yoh)

I am going to take the radial pulse.
Voy a tomar tu pulso radial.
(Boy ah toh-mahr too pool-soh rah-dee-ahl)

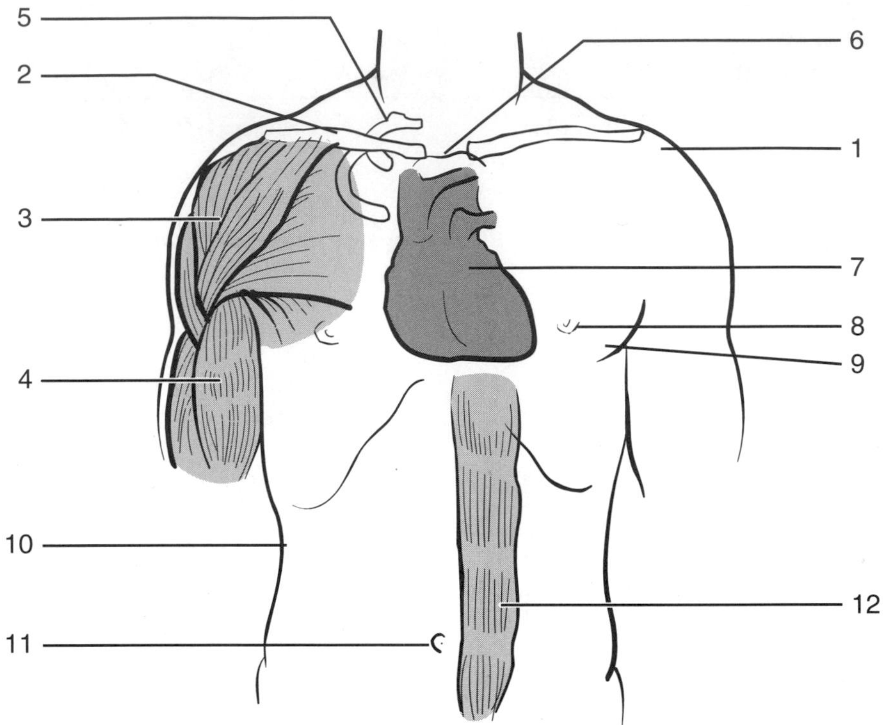

Figure 22–5 The chest. (1) El hombro (*shoulder*), (2) la clavícula (*clavicle*), (3) los deltoides (*deltoids*), (4) el bíceps (*biceps*), (5) la costilla (*rib*), (6) el esternón (*sternum*), (7) el corazón (*heart*), (8) la aréola/el pezón (*areola/nipple*), (9) el pecho/seno (*chest/breast*), (10) la cintura (*waist*), (11) el ombligo (*umbilicus*), (12) el músculo abdominal (*abdominal muscle*).

I am going to observe the jugular vein.	**Voy a observar tu vena yugular.** ***(Boy ah ohb-sehr-bahr too beh-nah yoo-goo-lahr)***
Now, I am going to examine your abdomen.	**Ahora, voy a revisar tu abdomen/vientre.** ***(Ah-oh-rah boy ah reh-bee-sahr too ahb-doh-mehn/bee-ehn-treh)***
I am going to check your liver.	**Voy a revisar tu hígado.** ***(Boy ah reh-bee-sahr too ee-gah-doh)***
I am going to palpate lightly.	**Voy a palpar/tocar ligero.** ***(Boy ah pahl-pahr/toh-kahr lee-heh-roh)***

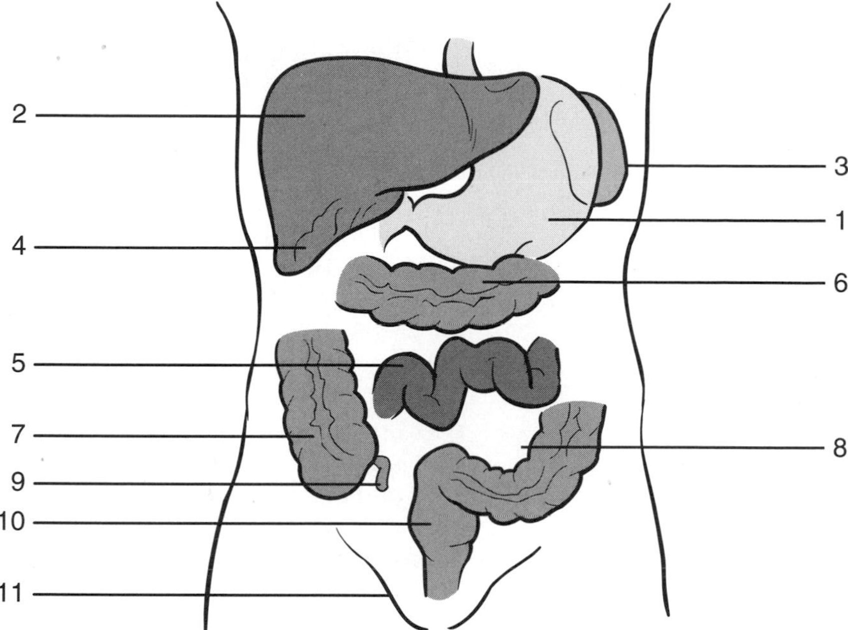

Figure 22–6 The abdomen. (1) El estómago (*stomach*), (2) el hígado (*liver*), (3) el bazo (*spleen*), (4) la vesícula biliar (*gallbladder*), (5) el intestino delgado (*small intestine*), (6) el intestino transverso (*transverse intestine*), (7) el colon ascendente (*ascending colon*), (8) el área pélvica (*lower pelvic area*), (9) el apéndice (*appendix*), (10) el recto (*rectum*), (11) la ingle (*groin*).

I am going to palpate deeply.	**Voy a palpar hondo.** ***(Boy ah pahl-pahr ohn-doh)***
Tell me if it hurts.	**Dime si duele.** ***(Dee-meh see doo-eh-leh)***
Does it hurts when I press?	**¿Duele cuando presiono?** ***(Doo-eh-leh koo-ahn-doh preh-see oh-noh)***
Does it hurts when I let go?	**¿Duele cuando retiro la mano?** ***(Doo-eh-leh koo-ahn-doh reh-tee-roh lah mah-noh)***
I am going to palpate with both hands.	**Voy a palpar/tocar con las dos manos.** ***(Boy ah pahl-pahr/toh-kahr kohn lahs dohs mah-nohs)***
Raise your head.	**Levanta tu cabeza.** ***(Leh-bahn-tah too kah-beh-sah)***

I am going to check how strong your abdominal muscle is.	**Voy a ver la fuerza del músculo abdominal.** *(Boy ah behr lah foo-ehr-sah dehl moos-koo-loh ahb-doh-mee-nahl)*
Turn onto your side:	**Voltéate de lado:** *(Bohl-teh-ah-teh deh lah-doh)*
left . . .	**izquierdo...** *(ees-kee-ehr-doh)*
right . . .	**derecho...** *(deh-reh-choh)*
Take a deep breath.	**Respira hondo.** *(Rehs-pee-rah ohn-doh)*
Let it out.	**Exhala.** *(Ehx-ah-lah)*
I am going to palpate the groin.	**Voy a palpar la ingle.** *(Boy ah pahl-pahr lah een-gleh)*
Push down.	**Empuja.** *(Ehm-poo-hah)*
I am going to examine the rectum.	**Voy a examinar el recto.** *(Boy ah ehx-ah-mee-nahr ehl rehk-toh)*
I am going to collect a stool sample.	**Voy a recoger una muestra de excremento.** *(Boy ah reh-koh-hehr oo-nah moo-ehs-trah deh ehx-kreh-mehn-toh)*
I am going to examine the genitalia.	**Voy a examinar los genitales.** *(Boy ah ehx-ah-mee-nahr lohs heh-nee-tah-lehs)*
I am going to examine your back.	**Voy a examinar tu espalda.** *(Boy ah ehx-ah-mee-nahr too ehs-pahl-dah)*
I am going to listen to the lungs.	**Voy a oír los pulmones.** *(Boy ah oh-eer lohs pool-moh-nehs)*
Breathe through the mouth.	**Respira con la boca abierta.** *(Rehs-pee-rah kohn lah boh-kah ah-bee-ehr-tah)*
Again.	**Otra vez.** *(Oh-trah behs)*
Repeat one, two, three.	**Repite uno, dos, tres.** *(Reh-pee-teh oo-noh, dohs, trehs)*
Now, stand up.	**Ahora, levántate.** *(Ah-oh-rah, leh-bahn-tah-teh)*

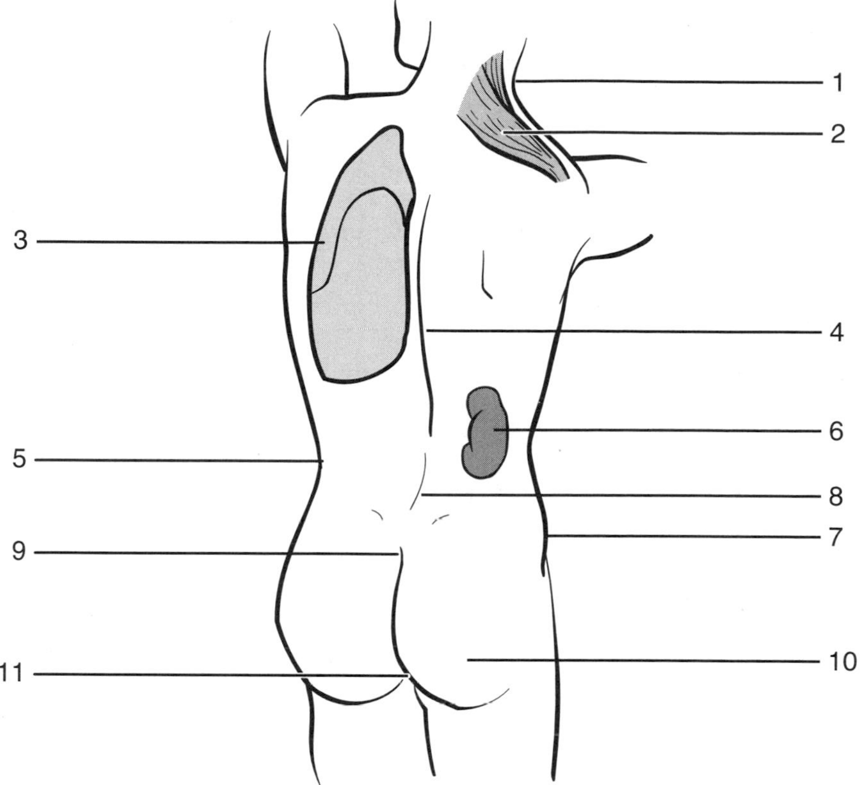

Figure 22–7 The back. (1) La nuca (*nape*), (2) el trapezoide (*trapezius*), (3) el pulmón (*lung*), (4) la vertebra (*spine*), (5) la cintura (*waist*), (6) el riñón (*kidney*), (7) la cadera (*hip*), (8) el lumbar (*lumbar*), (9) el sacro (*sacrum*), (10) la nalga (*buttock*), (11) el ano/la cola (*anus*).

Now, bend over.	**Ahora, agáchate.** ***(Ah-oh-rah, ah-gah-chah-teh)***
Cross your arms.	**Cruza tus brazos.** ***(Kroo-sah toos brah-sohs)***
Twist your waist.	**Tuerce la cintura.** ***(Too-ehr-seh lah seen-too-rah)***
Repeat the word "99."	**Repite las palabras "noventa y nueve."** ***(Reh-pee-teh lahs pah-lah-brahs "noh-behn-tah ee noo-eh-beh")***

Say your name.	**Dí tu nombre.** *(Dee too nohm-breh)*
Bend your shoulder.	**Dobla tu hombro.** *(Doh-blah too ohm-broh)*
I have finished the exam.	**Terminé de revisarte.** *(Tehr-mee-neh deh reh-bee-sahr-teh)*
[Do you have] Any questions?	**¿Alguna pregunta?** *(Ahl-goo-nah preh-goon-tah)*

Chapter Twenty-three | Capítulo veintitrés

Greetings and Common Expressions | Saludos y expresiones comunes

Greetings and expressions are used specially to address a person or get someone's attention. Hispanics are generally very friendly and will greet you even when they do not know you. In this chapter we will only provide those greetings that are used most frequently.

Los saludos y expresiones se hacen en forma particular para llamar la atención de la persona. Los hispanos son generalmente muy amigables y saludan aún sin conocer a la persona. En este capítulo sólo hablamos de los saludos que usamos con más frecuencia.

Hi!	**¡Hola!** *(Oh-lah)*
Good morning.	**Buenos días.** *(Boo-eh-nohs dee-ahs)*
Good afternoon.	**Buenas tardes.** *(Boo-eh-nahs tahr-dehs)*
Good evening.	**Buenas noches.** *(Boo-eh-nahs noh-chehs)*
Good night.	**Buenas noches.** *(Boo-eh-nahs noh-chehs)*
Do you speak English?	**¿Habla inglés?** *(Ah-blah een-glehs)*
Yes, I speak English.	**Sí, yo hablo inglés.** *(See, yoh ah-bloh een-glehs)*
No, I do not speak English.	**No, no hablo inglés.** *(Noh, noh ah-bloh een-glehs)*
Do you speak Spanish?	**¿Habla español?** *(Ah-blah ehs-pah-nyohl)*
Yes, I speak Spanish.	**Sí, hablo español.** *(See, ah-bloh ehs-pah-nyohl)*

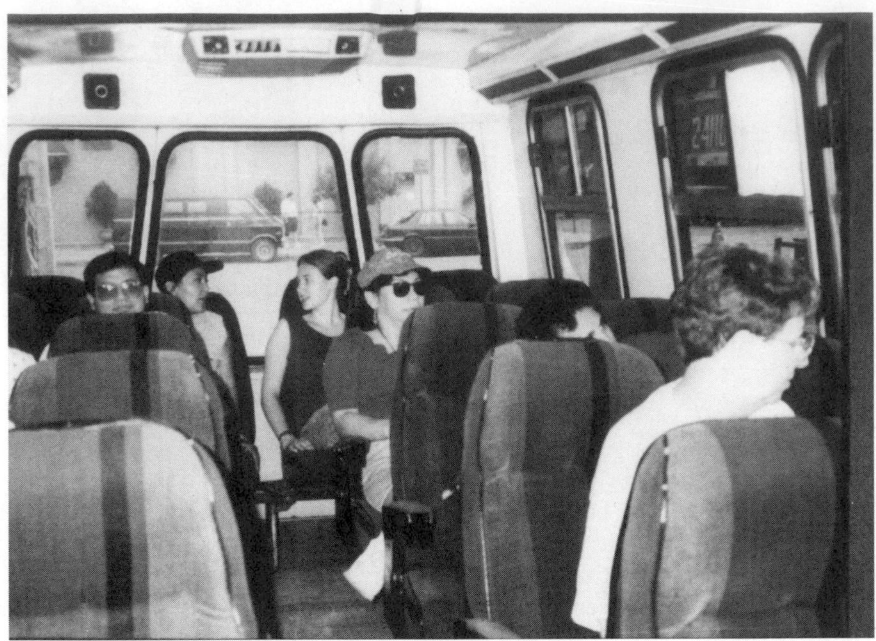

Figure 23–1 Hispanics are generally very friendly.

No, I do not speak Spanish.	**No, no hablo español.** *(Noh, noh ah-bloh ehs-pah-nyohl)*
Yes, a little.	**Sí, un poco.** *(See, oon poh-koh)*
No, I don't understand.	**No, no comprendo/no entiendo.** *(Noh, noh kohm-prehn-doh/noh ehn-tee-ehn-doh)*
Speak slowly, please.	**Hable despacio, por favor.** *(Ah-bleh dehs-pah-see-oh, pohr fah-bohr)*
Slowly, please.	**Despacio, por favor.** *(Dehs-pah-see-oh, pohr fah-bohr)*
Thank you!	**¡Gracias!** *(Grah-see-ahs)*
Thank you very much!	**¡Muchas gracias!** *(Moo-chahs grah-see-ahs)*
It's nothing./You are welcome.	**De nada.** *(Deh nah-dah)*
I am . . .	**Yo soy...** *(Yoh soh-ee)*

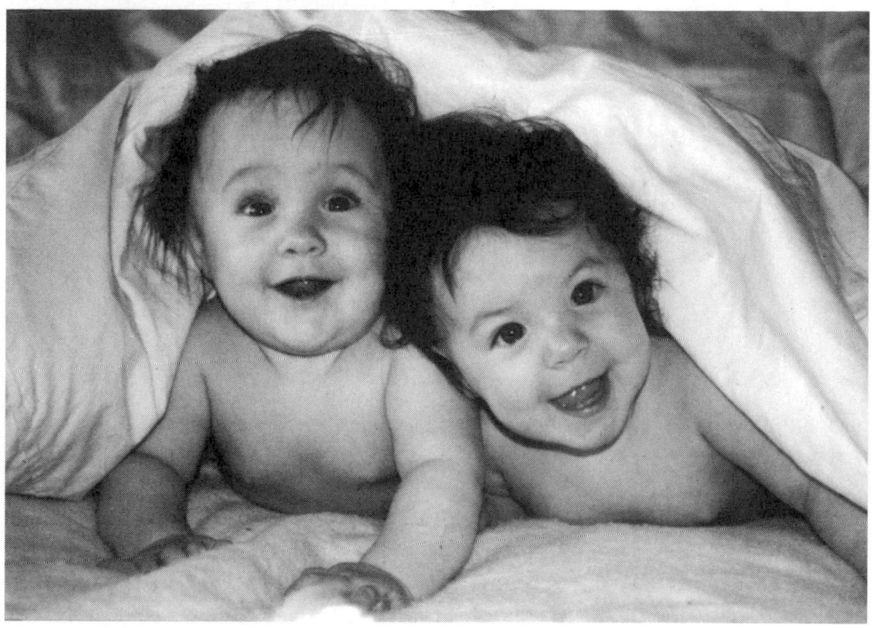

Figure 23–2 Friendliness is a trait that is acquired while very young.

I am the doctor (*male*).	**Yo soy el doctor.** *(Yoh soh-ee ehl dohk-tohr)*
I am the doctor (*female*).	**Yo soy la doctora.** *(Yoh soh-ee lah dohk-tohr-ah)*
I am the nurse (*female*).	**Yo soy la enfermera.** *(Yoh soh-ee lah ehn-fehr-meh-rah)*
I am the nurse (*male*).	**Yo soy el enfermero.** *(Yoh soh-ee ehl ehn-fehr-meh-roh)*
What is your name (formal)?	**¿Cómo se llama usted?** *(Koh-moh seh yah-mah oos-tehd)*
What is your name (informal)?	**¿Cómo te llamas?** *(Koh-moh teh yah-mahs)*
My name is . . .	**Me llamo...** *(Meh yah-moh)*
May I join you?	**¿Lo/La puedo acompañar?** *(Loh/Lah poo-eh-doh ah-kohm-pah-nyahr)*

Chapter Twenty-four | Capítulo veinticuatro

Commands | Órdenes o mandatos

Commands or orders are used in hospitals, private offices, and health care centers. This gives responsibility to patients related to their well-being and state of health. These commands should be given firmly and with confidence. In this manner, the patient is able to understand the outcome of such commands.

Las órdenes o mandatos se usan en los hospitales, las consultas privadas y los centros de salud. Esto crea en los pacientes una responsabili-

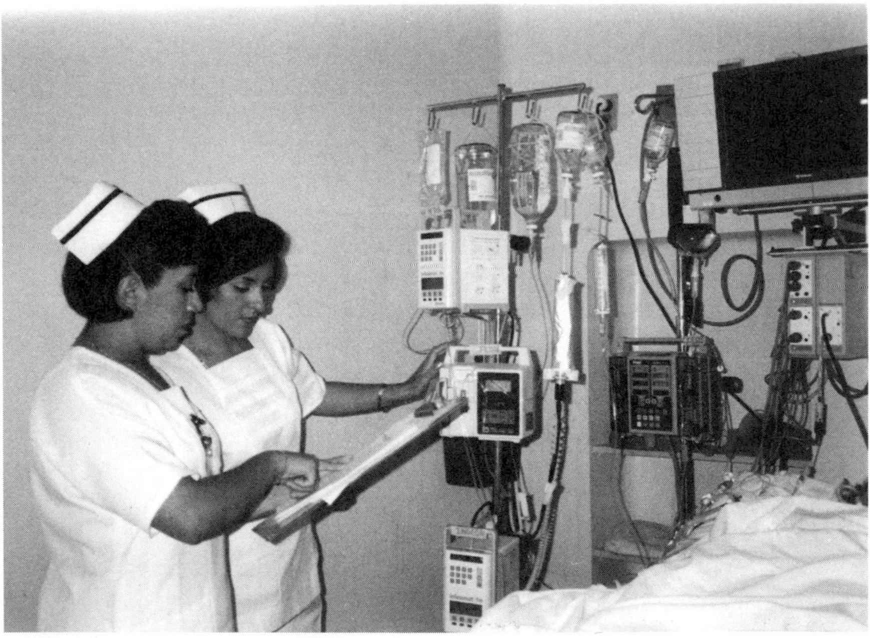

Figure 24–1 Knowledge of commands is useful in the clinical setting to make sure that instructions are clear.

dad acerca de su bienestar y curación total. Estas órdenes deben darse con mucha firmeza y seguridad. De esta manera el paciente capta en su totalidad la finalidad que se persigue al indicárselas.

Wake up!	**¡Despierte!** *(Dehs-pee-ehr-teh)*
Get up.	**Levántese.** *(Leh-bahn-teh-seh)*
Do not get up!	**¡No se levante!** *(Noh seh leh-bahn-teh)*
Sit up!	**¡Siéntese!** *(See-ehn-teh-seh)*
Walk.	**Camine.** *(Kah-mee-neh)*
Sit (on the chair)!	**¡Siéntese (en la silla)!** *(See-ehn-teh-seh [ehn lah see-yah])*
Stop!	**¡Párese!** *(Pah-reh-seh)*

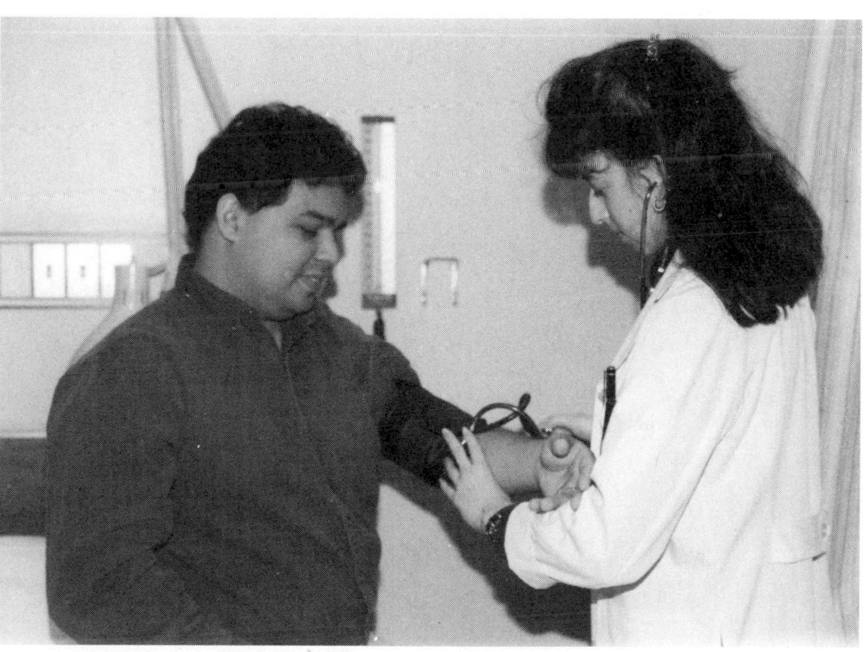

Figure 24–2 The patient will follow your instructions when you give the appropriate commands.

Look up/down.	**Vea arriba/abajo.** *(Beh-ah ah-ree-bah/ah-bah-hoh)*
Move!	**¡Muévase!** *(Moo-eh-bah-seh)*
Listen!	**¡Oiga!/¡Escuche!** *(Oh-ee-gah/Ehs-koo-cheh)*
Don't talk!	**¡No hable!** *(Noh ah-bleh)*
Open your mouth.	**Abra la boca.** *(Ah-brah lah boh-kah)*
Show me your tongue.	**Muéstreme la lengua.** *(Moo-ehs-treh-meh lah lehn-goo-ah)*
Close your mouth.	**Cierre la boca.** *(See-eh-reh lah boh-kah)*
Bite!	**¡Muerda!** *(Moo-ehr-dah)*
Talk.	**Hable.** *(Ah-bleh)*
Breathe deeply!	**¡Respire hondo/profundo!** *(Rehs-pee-reh ohn-doh/proh-foon-doh)*
Don't breathe!	**¡No respire!** *(Noh rehs-pee-reh)*
Turn!	**¡Voltee!** *(Bohl-teh-eh)*
Take a bath.	**Báñese.** *(Bah-nyeh-seh)*
Wash your face!	**¡Lávese la cara!** *(Lah-beh-seh lah kah-rah)*
Brush your teeth!	**¡Cepíllese los dientes!** *(Seh-pee-yeh-seh lohs dee-ehn-tehs)*
Bend over.	**Agáchese.** *(Ah-gah-cheh-seh)*
Kneel down.	**Póngase de rodillas.** *(Pohn-gah-seh deh roh-dee-yahs)*
Open your eyes!	**¡Abra los ojos!** *(Ah-brah lohs oh-hohs)*
Close your eyes!	**¡Cierre los ojos!** *(See-eh-reh lohs oh-hohs)*
Lie down!	**¡Acuéstese!** *(Ah-koo-ehs-teh-seh)*
Eat!	**¡Coma!** *(Koh-mah)*

Swallow!	**¡Trague!** *(Trah-gheh)*
Drink.	**Beba./Tome.** *(Beh-bah/Toh-meh)*
Relax!	**¡Relaje!/¡Descanse!** *(Reh-lah-heh/Dehs-kahn-seh)*
Run!	**¡Corra!** *(Koh-rah)*
Wait!	**¡Espere!** *(Ehs-peh-reh)*
Don't sit.	**No se siente.** *(Noh seh see-ehn-teh)*
Bend your knee!	**¡Doble su rodilla!** *(Doh-bleh soo roh-dee-yah)*
Move your eyes.	**Mueva sus ojos.** *(Moo-eh-bah soos oh-hohs)*
Squeeze my hand.	**Apriete mi mano.** *(Ah-pree-eh-teh mee mah-noh)*
Cough!	**¡Tosa!** *(Toh-sah)*
Don't push!	**¡No haga esfuerzo!** *(Noh ah-gah ehs-foo-ehr-soh)*
Watch your bleeding!	**¡Vigile su sangrado!** *(Bee-hee-leh soo sahn-grah-doh)*
Take care of yourself!	**¡Cuídese mucho!** *(Koo-ee-deh-seh moo-choh)*

Chapter Twenty-five / Capítulo veinticinco

Phrases / Frases

Phrases consist of a series of words that add "feeling" to a short conversation. They can also mean more than what is expressed. For example, if you ask a person, "How are you?" and he/she replies, "Marvelous," we should understand that this individual feels well and is happy.

Las frases son una serie de palabras que le dan sentido a una conversación corta. Significan más de lo que se expresa en ellas. Por ejemplo, al preguntarle a una persona *¿Cómo se siente?* y nos contesta *"Maravilloso(a)"* debemos entender que este individuo se siente muy bien y está contento.

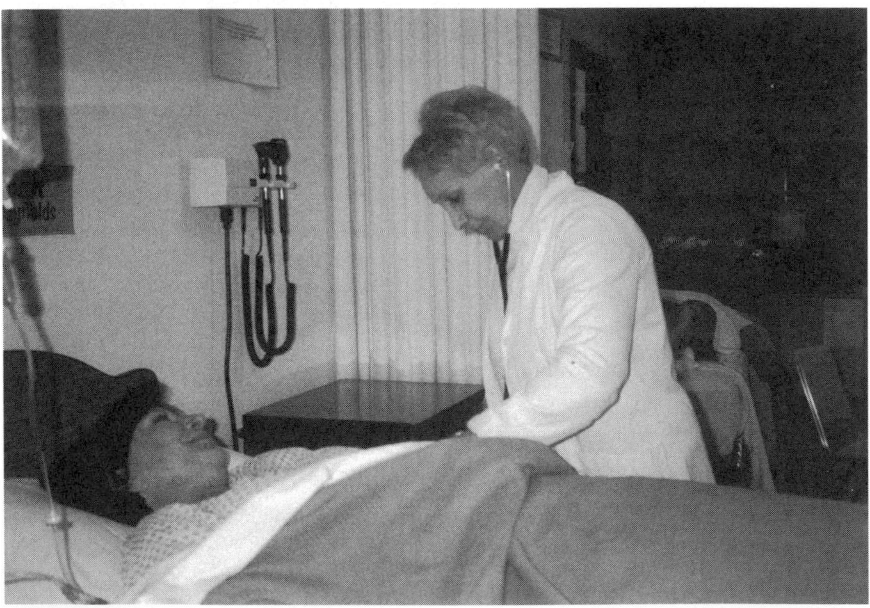

Figure 25–1 Specific phrases make conversation interesting and meaningful.

to find out	**descubrir** *(dehs-koo-breehr)*
from time to time	**de vez en cuando** *(deh behs ehn koo-ahn-doh)*
for the most part	**por la mayor parte** *(pohr lah mah-yohr pahr-teh)*
to deal with	**tratar** *(trah-tahr)*
Don't be afraid!	**¡No tenga miedo!** *(Noh tehn-gah mee-eh-doh)*
to call for	**llamar** *(yah-mahr)*
as a whole	**en conjunto/en todo** *(ehn kohn-hoon-toh/ehn toh-doh)*
according to	**de acuerdo con** *(deh ah-koo-ehr-doh kohn)*
to go through	**atravesar/cruzar** *(ah-trah-beh-sahr/kroo-sahr)*
to go by	**pasar** *(pah-sahr)*
to gain by	**ganar con** *(gah-nahr kohn)*
helpful	**útil** *(oo-teel)*
in addition	**además** *(ah-deh-mahs)*
in large part	**en gran parte** *(ehn grahn pahr-teh)*
in the middle of . . .	**a mediados de...** *(ah meh-dee-ah-dohs deh)*
all of a sudden . . .	**de golpe...** *(Deh gohl-peh)*
to keep up	**continuar** *(kohn-tee-noo-ahr)*
to leave behind	**abandonar** *(ah-bahn-doh-nahr)*
to meet with	**encontrarse con** *(ehn-kohn-trahr-seh kohn)*
Never mind.	**No importa.** *(Noh eem-pohr-tah)*
nonetheless	**sin embargo** *(seen ehm-bahr-goh)*

not at all	**de ningún modo** *(deh neen-goon moh-doh)*
Of course.	**Desde luego.** *(Dehs-deh loo-eh-goh)*
registered/on record	**registrado** *(reh-hees-trah-doh)*
over a period	**durante un período** *(doo-rahn-teh oon peh-ree-oh-doh)*
on the one hand	**por un lado** *(pohr oon lah-doh)*
to point out	**señalar/apuntar** *(seh-nyah-lahr/ah poon-tahr)*
modern/present day	**moderno** *(moh-dehr-noh)*
each hour	**cada hora** *(kah-dah oh-rah)*
every 2 hours	**cada dos horas** *(kah-dah dohs oh-rahs)*
four times	**cuatro veces** *(koo-ah-troh beh-sehs)*
to recall	**recordar** *(reh-kohr-dahr)*
rather than	**más bien que** *(mahs bee-ehn keh)*
to rely on	**confiar** *(kohn-fee-ahr)*
Say it again.	**Dígalo otra vez./Repita.** *(Dee-gah-loh oh-trah behs/Reh-pee-tah)*
so far/until now	**hasta ahora** *(ahs-tah ah-oh-rah)*
to select	**seleccionar** *(seh-lehk-see-oh-nahr)*
to sort out	**escoger** *(ehs-koh-hehr)*
such as	**tal como** *(tahl koh-moh)*
thought to be/considering	**considerando** *(kohn-see-deh-rahn-doh)*
to some extent	**hasta cierto punto** *(ahs-tah see-ehr-toh poon-toh)*
Try again!	**¡Pruebe otra vez!** *(Proo-eh-beh oh-trah behs)*

buzzing in the/one's ears	**zumbido en los oídos** *(soom-bee-doh ehn lohs oh-ee-dohs)*
sore throat	**dolor de garganta** *(doh-lohr deh gahr-gahn-tah)*
toothache	**dolor de muelas** *(doh-lohr deh moo-eh-lahs)*
difficulty in swallowing	**dificultad al tragar** *(dee-fee-kool-tahd ahl trah-gahr)*
I am continuously . . .	**Continuamente estoy...** *(Kohn-tee-noo-ah-mehn-teh ehs-toh-ee)*
Have you had this happen before?	**¿Le ha pasado esto antes?** *(Leh ha pah-sah-doh ehs-toh ahn-tehs)*
Don't worry.	**No se preocupe.** *(Noh seh preh-oh-koo-peh)*
See you later!	**¡Hasta luego!** *(Ahs-tah loo-eh-goh)*

Unit 5

Unidad 5

Chapter Twenty-six | Capítulo veintiséis

Useful Vocabulary at Home

Vocabulario útil sobre la vivienda

Vocabulary is a group of words from a language. Here we will introduce the most common or useful words used during an interview or conversation with a patient. This will give us an idea how the patient lives at home or what is available to him.

El vocabulario es un conjunto de palabras de un idioma. En esta ocasión presentaremos las palabras más usuales o útiles en una entrevista o una conversación con el paciente. Esto nos indicará la forma de vivir del paciente.

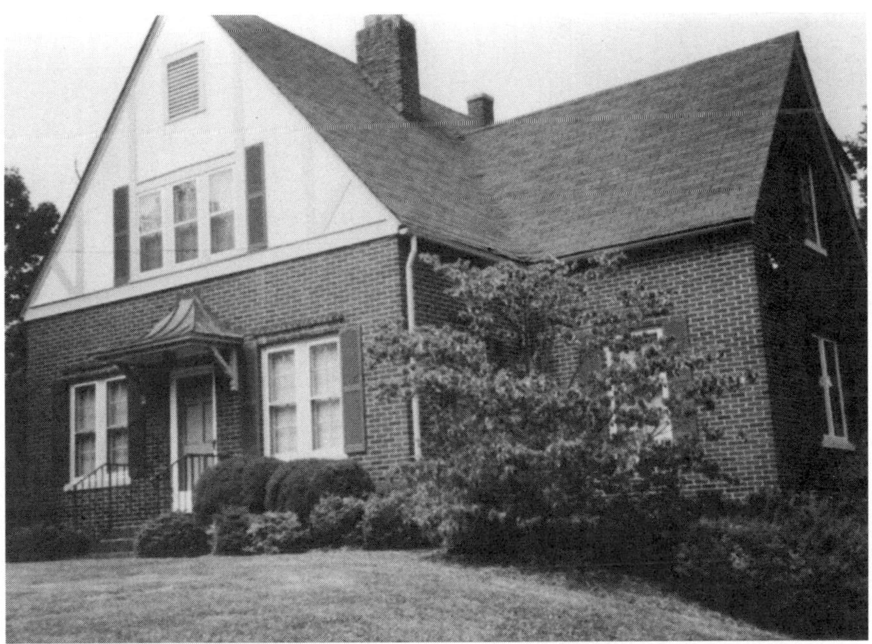

Figure 26–1 The home lets us know how the patient lives.

BATHROOM	**BAÑO**	**(BAH-NYOH)**
basin	**lavabo**	*(lah-bah-boh)*
shower	**regadera/ ducha**	*(reh-gah-deh-rah/doo-chah)*
toilet	**excusado**	*(ehx-koo-sah-doh)*
toothbrush	**cepillo de dientes**	*(seh-pee-yoh deh dee-ehn-tehs)*
toothpaste	**pasta de dientes**	*(pahs-tah deh dee-ehn-tehs)*
towel	**toalla**	*(too-ah-yah)*

BEDROOM	**RECÁMARA**	**(REH-KAH-MAH-RAH)**
bed	**cama**	*(kah-mah)*
bed cover	**colcha**	*(kohl-chah)*
clock	**reloj**	*(reh-lohj)*
comb	**peine**	*(peh-ee-neh)*
dresser	**aparador**	*(ah-pah-rah-dohr)*
hairbrush	**cepillo de pelo**	*(seh-pee-yoh deh peh-loh)*
mattress	**colchón**	*(kohl-chohn)*
phone	**teléfono**	*(teh-leh-foh-noh)*
pillow	**almohada**	*(ahl-moh-ah-dah)*
radio	**radio**	*(rah-dee-oh)*
sheet	**sábana**	*(sah-bah-nah)*

DINING ROOM	**COMEDOR**	**(KOH-MEH-DOHR)**
cabinet	**gabinete**	*(gah-bee-neh-teh)*
chairs	**sillas**	*(see-yahs)*
drapes	**cortinas**	*(kohr-tee-nahs)*
table	**mesa**	*(meh-sah)*

INSIDE THE HOME	**DENTRO DE LA CASA**	**(DEHN-TROH DEH LAH KAH-SAH)**
air conditioning	**aire acondici-onado**	*(ah-ee-reh ah-kohn-dee-see-oh-nah-doh)*
carpet	**alfombra**	*(ahl-fohm-brah)*
heater	**calentador**	*(kah-lehn-tah-dohr)*
mirror	**espejo**	*(ehs-peh-hoh)*
picture	**retrato**	*(reh-trah-toh)*
room	**cuarto**	*(koo-ahr-toh)*
water heater	**calentador de agua**	*kah-lehn-tah-dohr deh ah-goo-ah)*

KITCHEN	COCINA	(KOH-SEE-NAH)
can opener	**abrelatas**	*(ah-breh-lah-tahs)*
coffee pot	**cafetera**	*(kah-feh-teh-rah)*
cold water	**agua fría**	*(ah-goo-ah free-ah)*
cup	**tasa**	*(tah-sah)*
dish	**plato**	*(plah-toh)*
dishwasher	**lavaplatos**	*(lah-bah-plah-tohs)*
glass	**vaso**	*(bah-soh)*
hot water	**agua caliente**	*(ah-goo-ah kah-lee-ehn-teh)*
microwave	**microondas**	*(mee-kroh-ohn-dahs)*
plate	**platón**	*(plah-tohn)*
pot/pan	**traste/vasija**	*(trahs-teh/bah-see-hah)*
refrigerator	**refrigerador**	*(reh-free-heh-rah-dohr)*
stove	**estufa**	*(ehs-too-fah)*
table	**mesa**	*(meh-sah)*

LIVING ROOM	SALA/ESTANCIA	(SAH-LAH/EHS-TAHN-SEE-AH)
armchair	**sillón**	*(see-yohn)*
lamp	**lámpara**	*(lahm-pah-rah)*
sofa	**sofá**	*(soh-fah)*
stereo	**estereo**	*(ehs-teh-reh-oh)*
television	**televisor**	*(teh-leh-bee-sohr)*
VCR	**VCR**	*(beh-seh-eh-reh)*

OUTSIDE THE HOME	EXTERIOR DE LA CASA	(EHX-TEH-REE-OHR DEH LAH KAH-SAH)
address	**dirección**	*(dee-rehk-see-ohn)*
door	**puerta**	*(poo-ehr-tah)*
driveway	**entrada para vehículos**	*(ehn-trah-dah pah-rah beh-ee-koo-lohs)*
garage	**garaje**	*(gah-rah-heh)*
home	**hogar**	*(oh-gahr)*
house	**casa**	*(kah-sah)*
number	**número**	*(noo-meh-roh)*
porch/patio	**pórtico/patio**	*(pohr-tee-koh/pah-tee-oh)*
street/avenue	**calle/avenida**	*(kah-yeh/ah-beh-nee-dah)*
window	**ventana**	*(behn-tah-nah)*

OFFICE	OFICINA	(OH-FEE-SEE-NAH)
computer	**computadora**	*(kohm-poo-tah-doh-rah)*
desk	**escritorio**	*(ehs-kree-toh-ree-oh)*

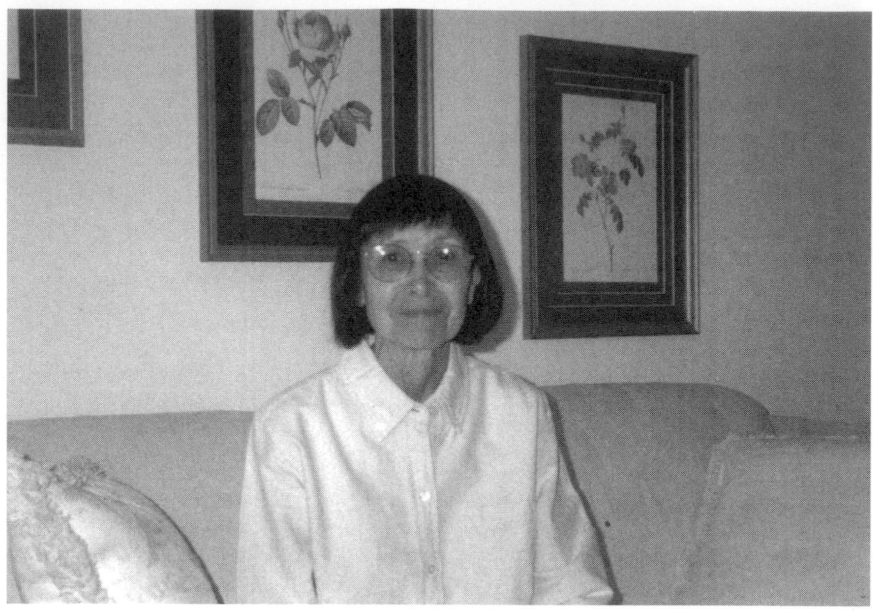

Figure 26–2 The home environment tells us about a patient's disposition.

monitor	**monitor**	*(moh-nee-tohr)*
paper	**papel**	*(pah-pehl)*
pencil	**lápiz**	*(lah-pee-seh)*
book	**libro**	*(lee-broh)*
bookcase	**armario/ estante**	*(ahr-mah-ree-oh/ehs-tahn-teh)*
magazine	**revista**	*(reh-bees-tah)*
typewriter	**máquina de escribir**	*(mah-kee-nah deh ehs-kree-beer)*

Chapter Twenty-seven — Capítulo veintisiete

Cognates — Cognados

Similar terms are those in which words are written and/or pronounced almost like others in a different language. These similar terms have very small variations in their spelling. In this chapter, we will mention only those terms useful to the medical practice.

Los términos similares son aquéllos en los cuales las palabras se escriben y se pronuncian casi igual en ambos idiomas. Estos términos tienen variaciones muy pequeñas en ortografía. En este capítulo mencionaremos términos útiles en la práctica de la medicina.

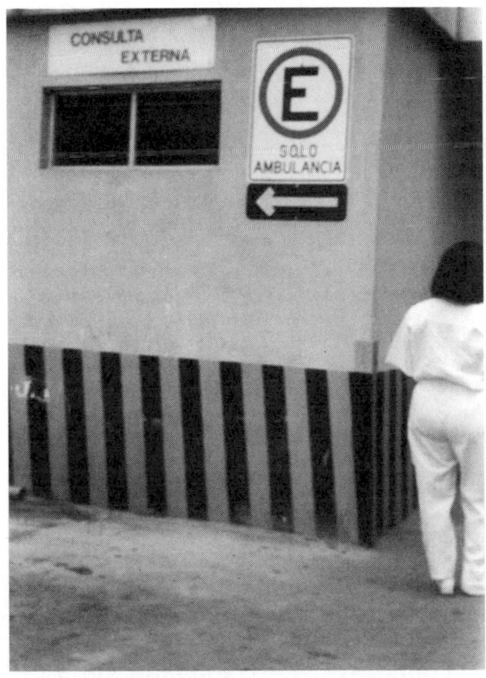

Figure 27–1 Similarities in written words make communication easier.

abdomen	**abdomen**	*(ahb-doh-mehn)*
accident	**accidente**	*(ahk-see-dehn-teh)*
acetic	**acético**	*(ah-seh-tee-koh)*
acid	**ácido**	*(ah-see-doh)*
acne	**acné**	*(ahk-neh)*
acoustic	**acústico**	*(ah-koos-tee-koh)*
adenoid	**adenoide**	*(ah-deh-noh-ee-deh)*
adrenalism	**adrenalismo**	*(ah-dreh-nah-lees-moh)*
air	**aire**	*(ah-ee-reh)*
alcohol	**alcohol**	*(ahl-kohl)*
alcoholic	**alcohólico**	*(ahl-koh-lee-koh)*
allergy	**alergia**	*(ah-lehr-hee-ah)*
amebic	**amébico**	*(ah-meh-bee-koh)*
amygdala	**amígdala**	*(ah-meeg-dah-lah)*
analyze	**analizar**	*(ah-nah-lee-sahr)*
anemia	**anemia**	*(ah-neh-mee-ah)*
anesthesia	**anestesia**	*(ah-nehs-teh-see-ah)*
angioma	**angioma**	*(ahn-hee-oh-mah)*
angle	**ángulo**	*(ahn-goo-loh)*
antibiotic	**antibiótico**	*(ahn-tee-bee-oh-tee-koh)*
anticoagulant	**anticoagulante**	*(ahn-tee-koo-ah-goo-lahn-teh)*
asthma	**asma**	*(ahs-mah)*
bacteria	**bacteria**	*(bahk-teh-ree-ah)*
barbaric	**bárbaro**	*(bahr-bah-roh)*
bradycardia	**bradicardia**	*(brah-dee-kahr-dee-ah)*
cafe (coffee)	**café**	*(kah-feh)*
caffeine	**cafeína**	*(kah-feh-ee-nah)*
callus	**callo**	*(kah-yoh)*
calm	**calma**	*(kahl-mah)*
cancer	**cáncer**	*(kahn-sehr)*
cardiac	**cardíaco**	*(kahr-dee-ah-koh)*
caries	**caries**	*(kah-ree-ehs)*
carothid	**carótida**	*(kah-roh-tee-dah)*
cause	**causa**	*(kah-oo-sah)*
cavity	**cavidad**	*(kah-bee-dahd)*
chancre	**chancro**	*(chahn-kroh)*
chemotherapy	**quimioterapia**	*(kee-mee-oh-teh-rah-pee-ah)*
chocolate	**chocolate**	*(choh-koh-lah-teh)*
claustrophobia	**claustrofobia**	*(klah-oos-troh-foh-bee-ah)*
coagulation	**coagulación**	*(koh-ah-goo-lah-see-ohn)*
coma	**coma**	*(koh-mah)*
comatose	**comatoso**	*(koh-mah-toh-soh)*
common	**común**	*(koh-moon)*

communication	**comunicación**	*(koh-moo-nee-kah-see-ohn)*
compromise	**compromiso**	*(kohm-proh-mee-soh)*
consultant	**consultante**	*(kohn-sool-tahn-teh)*
continued	**continuado**	*(kohn-tee-noo-ah-doh)*
control	**control**	*(kohn-trohl)*
cortisone	**cortisona**	*(kohr-tee-soh-nah)*
deficiency	**deficiencia**	*(deh-fee-see-ehn-see-ah)*
dehydration	**deshidratación**	*(deh-see-drah-tah-see-ohn)*
delirious	**delirio**	*(deh-lee-ree-oh)*
demented	**demente**	*(deh-mehn-teh)*
dental	**dental**	*(dehn-tahl)*
dentifrice	**dentífrico**	*(dehn-tree-fee-koh)*
echymosis	**equimosis**	*(eh-kee-moh-sees)*
eczema	**eczema**	*(ehk-seh-mah)*
embolism	**embolismo**	*(ehm-boh-lees-moh)*
emetic	**emético**	*(ehm-eh-tee-koh)*
employ	**emplear**	*(ehm-pleh-ahr)*
English	**inglés**	*(een-glehs)*
epilepsy	**epilepsia**	*(eh-peel-ehp-see-ah)*
error	**error**	*(eh-rohr)*
exercise	**ejercicio**	*(eh-hehr-see-see-oh)*
explain	**explicar**	*(ehx-plee-kahr)*
extraction	**extracción**	*(ehx-trahk-see-ohn)*
exudate	**exudado**	*(ehx-oo-dah-doh)*
facial	**facial**	*(fah-see-ahl)*
fail	**fallar**	*(fah-yahr)*
false	**falso**	*(fahl-soh)*
family	**familia**	*(fah-mee-lee-ah)*
fatal	**fatal**	*(fah-tahl)*
fever	**fiebre**	*(fee-eh-breh)*
fibroid	**fibroide**	*(fee-broh-ee-deh)*
fistula	**fístula**	*(fees-too-lah)*
form	**forma**	*(fohr-mah)*
fremitus	**frémito**	*(freh-mee-toh)*
fresh	**fresco**	*(frehs-koh)*
frontal	**frontal**	*(frohn-tahl)*
function	**función**	*(foon-see-ohn)*
fundamental	**fundamental**	*(foon-dah-mehn-tahl)*
gastroenteritis	**gastroenteritis**	*(gahs-troh-ehn-teh-ree-tees)*
generic	**genérico**	*(heh-neh-ree-koh)*
genial	**genial**	*(heh-nee-ahl)*
glaucoma	**glaucoma**	*(glah-oo-koh-mah)*
globule	**glóbulo**	*(gloh-boo-loh)*

grave	**grave**	*(grah-beh)*
gynecologist	**ginecólogo**	*(hee-neh-koh-loh-goh)*
hematoma	**hematoma**	*(eh-mah-toh-mah)*
hemolysis	**hemólisis**	*(eh-moh-lee-sees)*
hepatitis	**hepatitis**	*(eh-pah-tee-tees)*
history	**historia**	*(ees-toh-ree-ah)*
hygienist	**higienista**	*(ee-hee-eh-nees-tah)*
ignore	**ignorar**	*(eeg-noh-rahr)*
impression	**impresión**	*(eem-preh-see-ohn)*
independence	**independencia**	*(een-deh-pehn-dehn-see-ah)*
indigestion	**indigestión**	*(een-dee-hehs-tee-ohn)*
infancy	**infancia**	*(een-fahn-see-ah)*
infection	**infección**	*(een-fehk-see-ohn)*
inflammation	**inflamación**	*(een-flah-mah-see-ohn)*
injection	**inyección**	*(een-yehk-see-ohn)*
insect	**insecto**	*(een-sehk-toh)*
instrument	**instrumento**	*(een-stroo-mehn-toh)*
insulin	**insulina**	*(een-soo-lee-nah)*
intimate	**íntimo**	*(een-tee-moh)*
jugular	**yugular**	*(yoo-goo-lahr)*
just	**justo**	*(hoos-toh)*
juvenile	**juvenil**	*(hoo-beh-neel)*
kleptomania	**cleptomanía**	*(klehp-toh-mah-nee-ah)*
laboratory	**laboratorio**	*(lah-boh-rah-toh-ree-oh)*
lancet	**lanceta**	*(lahn-seh-tah)*
laparoscopy	**laparoscopia**	*(lah-pah-rohs-koh-pee-ah)*
ligament	**ligamento**	*(lee-gah-mehn-toh)*
linen	**lino**	*(lee-noh)*
lingual	**lingual**	*(leen-goo-ahl)*
lithium	**litio**	*(lee-tee-oh)*
lupus	**lupus**	*(loo-poos)*
manual	**manual**	*(mah-noo-ahl)*
material	**material**	*(mah-teh-ree-ahl)*
maternal	**maternal**	*(mah-tehr-nahl)*
mathematics	**matemáticas**	*(mah-teh-mah-tee-kahs)*
medication	**medicamento**	*(meh-dee-kah-mehn-toh)*
medicine	**medicina**	*(meh-dee-see-nah)*
medulla	**médula**	*(meh-doo-lah)*
memory	**memoria**	*(meh-moh-ree-ah)*
meningitis	**meningitis**	*(meh-neen-hee-tees)*
minimum	**mínimo**	*(mee-nee-moh)*
model	**modelo**	*(moh-deh-loh)*

modern	**moderno**	*(moh-dehr-noh)*
molar	**muela**	*(moo-eh-lah)*
moral	**moral**	*(moh-rahl)*
nasal	**nasal**	*(nah-sahl)*
nausea	**náusea**	*(nah-oo-seh-ah)*
neonatal	**neonatal**	*(neh-oh-nah-tahl)*
nervous	**nervioso**	*(nehr-bee-oh-soh)*
neurotic	**neurótico**	*(neh-oo-roh-tee-koh)*
neutral	**neutral**	*(neh-oo-trahl)*
normal	**normal**	*(nohr-mahl)*
note	**nota**	*(noh-tah)*
Novocaine	**Novocaína**	*(Noh-boh-kah-ee-nah)*
nutrition	**nutrición**	*(noo-tree-see-ohn)*
obsession	**obsesión**	*(ohb-seh-see-ohn)*
obstruction	**obstrucción**	*(ohb-strook-see-ohn)*
occipital	**occipital**	*(ohk-see-pee-tahl)*
occur	**ocurrir**	*(oh-koo-reer)*
office	**oficina**	*(oh-fee-see-nah)*
opinion	**opinión**	*(oh-pee-nee-ohn)*
optic	**óptico**	*(ohp-tee-koh)*
organ	**órgano**	*(ohr-gah-noh)*
ovary	**ovario**	*(oh-bah-ree-oh)*
oxygen	**oxígeno**	*(ohx-ee-heh-noh)*
palate	**paladar**	*(pahl-ah-dahr)*
palmar	**palmar**	*(pahl-mahr)*
palpation	**palpación**	*(pahl-pah-see-ohn)*
pancreas	**páncreas**	*(pahn-kreh-ahs)*
panic	**pánico**	*(pah-nee-koh)*
paralytic	**paralítico**	*(pah-rah-lee-tee-koh)*
pathogen	**patogénico**	*(pah-toh-heh-nee-koh)*
pathological	**patológico**	*(pah-toh-loh-hee-koh)*
pelvis	**pelvis**	*(pehl-bees)*
pharmacy	**farmacia**	*(fahr-mah-see-ah)*
philosophy	**filosofía**	*(fee-loh-soh-fee-ah)*
physique	**físico**	*(fee-see-koh)*
piece	**pieza**	*(pee-eh-sah)*
plan	**plan**	*(plahn)*
porcelain	**porcelana**	*(pohr-seh-lah-nah)*
practice	**práctica**	*(prahk-tee-kah)*
prepare	**preparar**	*(preh-pah-rahr)*
preventive	**preventivo**	*(preh-behn-tee-boh)*
probable	**probable**	*(proh-bah-bleh)*

problem	**problema**	*(proh-bleh-mah)*
pruritic	**prurítico**	*(proo-ree-tee-koh)*
pubic	**púbico**	*(poo-bee-koh)*
pulse	**pulso**	*(pool-soh)*
pure	**puro**	*(poo-roh)*
pyorrhea	**piorrea**	*(pee-oh-reh-ah)*
racial	**racial**	*(rah-see-ahl)*
radical	**radical**	*(rah-dee-kahl)*
radioactive	**radioactivo**	*(rah-dee-oh-ahk-tee-boh)*
rare	**raro**	*(rah-roh)*
rectal	**rectal**	*(rehk-tahl)*
repell	**repeler**	*(reh-peh-lehr)*
residue	**residuo**	*(reh-see-doo-oh)*
resin	**resina**	*(reh-see-nah)*
respect	**respeto**	*(rehs-peh-toh)*
rheumatic	**reumático**	*(reh-oo-mah-tee-koh)*
roseola	**roseola**	*(roh-seh-oh-lah)*
rubella	**rubella**	*(roo-beh-lah)*
rubeola	**rubéola**	*(roo-beh-oh-lah)*
saliva	**saliva**	*(sah-lee-bah)*
salt	**sal**	*(sahl)*
sanitary	**sanitario**	*(sah-nee-tah-ree-oh)*
science	**ciencia**	*(see-ehn-see-ah)*
scleral	**escleral**	*(ehs-kleh-rahl)*
sebaceous	**sebásceo**	*(seh-bah-seh-oh)*
secrete	**secretar**	*(seh-kreh-tahr)*
selection	**selección**	*(seh-lehk-see-ohn)*
serology	**serología**	*(seh-roh-loh-hee-ah)*
sex	**sexo**	*(sehx-oh)*
sexual	**sexual**	*(sehx-oo-ahl)*
situation	**situación**	*(see-too-ah-see-ohn)*
social	**social**	*(soh-see-ahl)*
solution	**solución**	*(soh-loo-see-ohn)*
solvent	**solvente**	*(sohl-behn-teh)*
somatic	**somático**	*(soh-mah-tee-koh)*
Spanish	**español**	*(ehs-pah-nyohl)*
spectrum	**espectro**	*(ehs-pehk-troh)*
spinal	**espinal**	*(ehs-pee-nahl)*
spirit	**espíritu**	*(ehs-pee-ree-too)*
stethoscope	**estetoscopio**	*(ehs-teh-tohs-koh-pee-oh)*
stupor	**estupor**	*(ehs-too-pohr)*
subaxillary	**subaxilar**	*(soob-ahx-ee-lahr)*

subnormal	**subnormal**	*(soob-nohr-mahl)*
substernal	**subesternal**	*(soob-ehs-tehr-nahl)*
suffer	**sufrir**	*(soo-freer)*
syncope	**síncope**	*(seen-koh-peh)*
systole	**sístole**	*(sees-toh-leh)*
tea	**té**	*(teh)*
technician	**técnico**	*(tehk-nee-koh)*
temporal	**temporal**	*(tehm-poh-rahl)*
tension	**tensión**	*(tehn-see-ohn)*
tetanus	**tétanos**	*(teh-tah-nohs)*
thermometer	**termómetro**	*(tehr-moh-meh-troh)*
tolerant	**tolerante**	*(toh-leh-rahn-teh)*
torso	**torso**	*(tohr-soh)*
treatment	**tratamiento**	*(trah-tah-mee-ehn-toh)*
tube	**tubo**	*(too-boh)*
tumor	**tumor**	*(too-mohr)*
ulcer	**úlcera**	*(ool-seh-rah)*
union	**unión**	*(oo-nee-ohn)*
universal	**universal**	*(oo-nee-behr-sahl)*
urea	**urea**	*(oo-reh-ah)*
uremia	**uremia**	*(oo-reh-mee-ah)*
ureteritis	**uretritis**	*(oo-reh-tree-tees)*
urticaria	**urticaria**	*(oor-tee-kah-ree-ah)*
use	**usar**	*(oo-sahr)*
uterus	**útero**	*(oo-teh-roh)*
uvula	**úvula**	*(oo-boo-lah)*
vaginal	**vaginal**	*(bah-hee-nahl)*
vagus	**vago**	*(bah-goh)*
valve	**válvula**	*(bahl-boo-lah)*
vapor	**vapor**	*(bah-pohr)*
varicocele	**varicocele**	*(bah-ree-koh-seh-leh)*
vein	**vena**	*(beh-nah)*
venereal	**venéreo**	*(beh-neh-reh-oh)*
vertebrate	**vertebrado**	*(behr-teh-brah-doh)*
vertigo	**vértigo**	*(behr-tee-goh)*
vestibule	**vestíbulo**	*(behs-tee-boo-loh)*
veterinary	**veterinaria**	*(beh-teh-ree-nah-ree-ah)*
vinegar	**vinagre**	*(bee-nah-greh)*
visible	**visible**	*(bee-see-bleh)*
vision	**visión**	*(bee-see-ohn)*
vital	**vital**	*(bee-tahl)*
volume	**volumen**	*(boh-loo-mehn)*

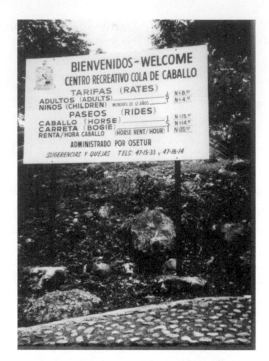

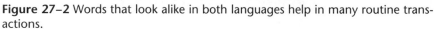

Figure 27–2 Words that look alike in both languages help in many routine transactions.

vomit **vómito** ***(boh-mee-toh)***
X-rays **rayos X** ***(rah-yohs eh-kees)***
xiphoid **xifoide** ***(see-foh-ee-deh)***
yogurt **yogurt** ***(yoh-goohrt)***
zone **zona** ***(soh-nah)***
zoology **zoología** ***(soh-oh-loh-hee-ah)***
zygomatic **cigomático** ***(see-goh-mah-tee-koh)***

Chapter Twenty-eight | Capítulo veintiocho

Numbers | Números

Numbers are as important as nouns and verbs. Everybody needs numbers to buy, sell, mention dates, indicate hours of the day, determine temperature, and state measurements and quantities. Numbers are also needed to make phone calls, to use in all the sciences and thousands of other things. There is a difference between knowing the numbers and how to use them. In medicine, especially, errors can be made if we do not take numbers seriously.

Los números son tan importantes como los nombres y los verbos. Todas las personas necesitamos números para comprar, vender, mencionar fechas, indicar la hora del día, determinar la temperatura y expresar medidas y cantidades. También los números son necesarios para telefonear, para todas las ciencias y para miles de cosas más. Hay diferencia entre saber los números y el saber usarlos. Especialmente en la medicina, se pueden cometer muchos errores si no tomamos en serio a los números.

1	one	**uno**	*(oo-noh)*
2	two	**dos**	*(dohs)*
3	three	**tres**	*(trehs)*
4	four	**cuatro**	*(koo-ah-troh)*
5	five	**cinco**	*(seen-koh)*
6	six	**seis**	*(seh-ees)*
7	seven	**siete**	*(see-eh-teh)*
8	eight	**ocho**	*(oh-choh)*
9	nine	**nueve**	*(noo-eh-beh)*
10	ten	**diez**	*(dee-ehs)*
11	eleven	**once**	*(ohn-seh)*
12	twelve	**doce**	*(doh-seh)*
13	thirteen	**trece**	*(treh-seh)*
14	fourteen	**catorce**	*(kah-tohr-seh)*
15	fifteen	**quince**	*(keen-seh)*
16	sixteen	**dieciséis**	*(dee-ehs-ee-seh-ees)*

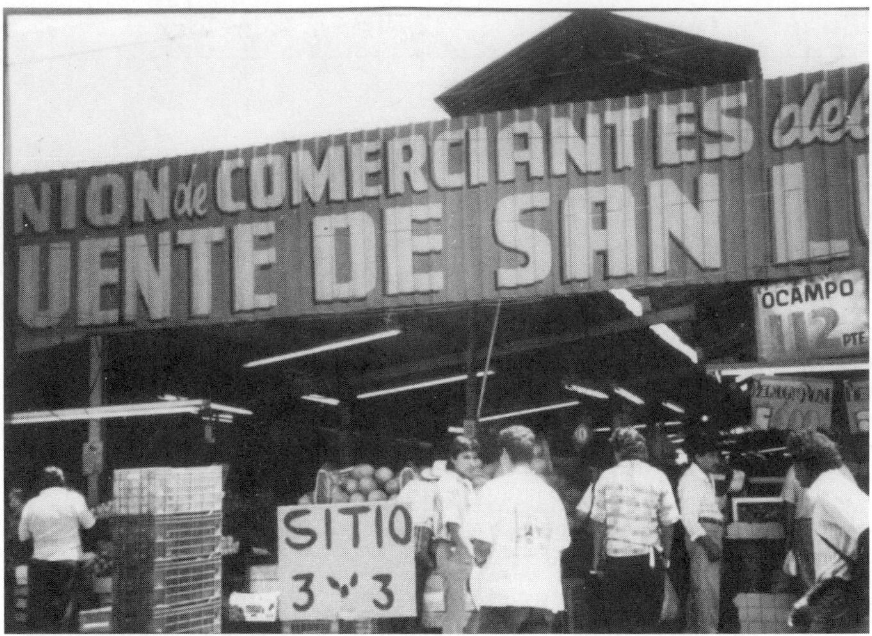

Figure 28–1 Numbers are used in a variety of verbal and written transactions.

17	seventeen	**diecisiete**	*(dee-ehs-ee-see-eh-teh)*
18	eighteen	**dieciocho**	*(dee-ehs-ee-oh-choh)*
19	nineteen	**diecinueve**	*(dee-ehs-ee-noo-eh-beh)*
20	twenty	**veinte**	*(beh-een-teh)*

After number 20, use the root of the number (20) and add the first nine numbers in order. See Table 28–1.

Después del número veinte, use la raíz del número (veinte) y agregue los primeros nueve números en orden. Vea la Tabla 28–1.

30	thirty	**treinta**	*(treh-een-tah)*
40	forty	**cuarenta**	*(koo-ah-rehn-tah)*
50	fifty	**cincuenta**	*(seen-koo-ehn-tah)*
60	sixty	**sesenta**	*(seh-sehn-tah)*
70	seventy	**setenta**	*(seh-tehn-tah)*
80	eighty	**ochenta**	*(oh-chehn-tah)*
90	ninety	**noventa**	*(noh-behn-tah)*
100	one hundred	**cien**	*(see-ehn)*

TABLE 28–1
Add the Roots

TABLA 28–1
Agregue la raíz

English	Spanish	Pronunciation
twenty-one	**veintiuno**	*(beh-een-tee-oo-noh)*
twenty-two	**veintidós**	*(beh-een-tee-dohs)*
twenty-three	**veintitrés**	*(beh-een-tee-trehs)*
twenty-four	**veinticuatro**	*(beh-een-tee-koo-ah-troh)*
twenty-five	**veinticinco**	*(beh-een-tee-seen-koh)*
twenty-six	**veintiseis**	*(beh-een-tee-seh-ees)*
twenty-seven	**veintisiete**	*(beh-een-tee-see-eh-teh)*
twenty-eight	**veintiocho**	*(beh-een-tee-oh-choh)*
twenty-nine	**veintinueve**	*(beh-een-tee-noo-eh-beh)*

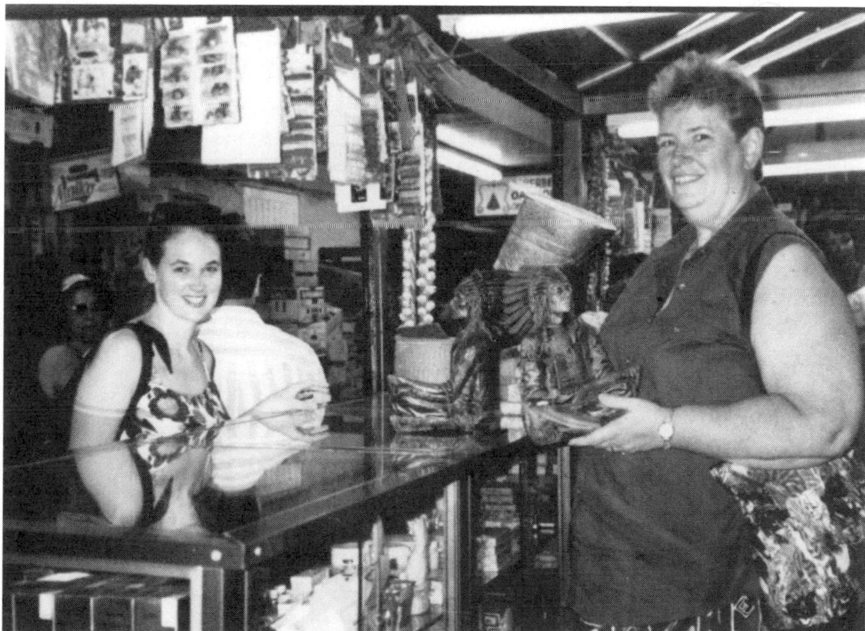

Figure 28–2 Numbers are helpful when inquiring about prices, buying merchandise, or working on a budget.

TABLE 28–2 **In the Hundreds**	**TABLA 28–2** **En los cientos**	
English	**Spanish**	**Pronunciation**
two hundred	**doscientos**	*(doh-see-ehn-tohs)*
three hundred	**trescientos**	*(treh-see-ehn-tohs)*
four hundred	**cuatrocientos**	*(koo-ah-troh-see-ehn-tohs)*
five hundred	**quinientos**	*(kee-nee-ehn-tohs)*
six hundred	**seiscientos**	*(seh-ee-see-ehn-tohs)*
seven hundred	**setecientos**	*(seh-teh-see-ehn-tohs)*
eight hundred	**ochocientos**	*(oh-choh-see-ehn-tohs)*
nine hundred	**novecientos**	*(noh-beh-see-ehn-tohs)*

When forming hundreds, you will use numbers 2, 3, 4, 6, 8 and add the word **cientos.** See Table 28–2.

Cuando se forman números en los cientos, usará los números 2, 3, 4, 6, 8 y agregue la palabra "cientos". Vea la Tabla 28–2.

Larger numbers are easier to deal with. You add the first nine numbers before or after. See below.

Los números mayores ofrecen menos problemas. A la raíz se le agregan los primeros números antes o después. Vea abajo.

1,000	one thousand	**mil**	*(meel)*
1,001	one thousand one	**mil uno**	*(meel-oo-noh)*
2,000	two thousand	**dos mil**	*(dohs meel)*
2,002	two thousand two	**dos mil dos**	*(dohs meel dohs)*

In medicine we use fractions. It is necessary to know exact quantities since dosages vary, especially for children. See below.

En medicina usamos números fraccionados. Es necesario saber las cantidades exactas ya que las dosis varían mucho, especialmente para niños. Vea abajo.

1/4	one fourth	**un cuarto**	*(oon koo-ahr-toh)*
1/3	one third	**un tercio**	*(oon tehr-see-oh)*
1/2	one half	**un medio**	*(oon meh-dee-oh)*
3/4	three fourths	**tres cuartos**	*(trehs koo-ahr-tohs)*

When there is a need to emphasize degree or a category of items or persons, you must use ordinal numbers as listed below.

Cuando hay necesidad de enfatizar ciertos grados o categorías se deben usar los números ordinales como se enlistan abajo.

1st	first	**primero(a)**	*(pree-meh-roh[rah])*
2nd	second	**segundo(a)**	*(seh-goon-doh[dah])*
3rd	third	**tercero(a)**	*(tehr-seh-roh[rah])*
4th	fourth	**cuarto(a)**	*(koo-ahr-toh[tah])*
5th	fifth	**quinto(a)**	*(keen-toh[tah])*
6th	sixth	**sexto(a)**	*(sehx-toh[tah])*
7th	seventh	**séptimo(a)**	*(sehp-tee-moh[mah])*
8th	eighth	**octavo(a)**	*(ohk-tah-boh[bah])*
9th	ninth	**noveno(a)**	*(noh-beh-noh[nah])*
10th	tenth	**décimo(a)**	*(deh-see-moh[mah])*

Chapter Twenty-nine	Capítulo veintinueve

Time — La hora

Time is so important throughout the world that all of us want to know—What time is it? At what time do we eat? At what time do we go to the movies?—and millions of other questions. Time varies depending on the country where you reside. There are places where time schedules are very different. So, if we wish to travel to faraway places, we must consult our travel agent or a time chart that shows the standard times in various parts of the world with reference to a specified place. In hospitals, time is of the essence, since we can save or lose a life in seconds.

El tiempo es tan importante en el mundo entero que todos queremos saber—¿Qué hora es? ¿A qué hora comemos? ¿A qué hora nos vamos al cine?—y un millón de otras preguntas. El tiempo varía de acuerdo al país donde nos encontremos. Hay lugares en los que el horario es muy diferente. Por lo tanto, debemos consultar con nuestro agente de viajes o un esquema que muestre la hora estándar (oficial) en varias partes del mundo con referencia a un lugar específico. En los hospitales, el tiempo es la esencia, ya que una vida se puede salvar o perder en segundos.

In many hospitals standard time is used. In others, military time is used after noon. See below to compare.

En muchos hospitales se usa la hora estándar. En otros se usa el horario militar después del mediodía. Vea abajo para comparar.

TIME	STANDARD	MILITARY (HOURS P.M.)
one o'clock	**la una** *(la oo-nah)*	**las trece horas** *(lahs treh-seh oh-rahs)*
two o'clock	**las dos** *(lahs dohs)*	**las catorce horas** *(lahs kah-tohr-seh oh-rahs)*
three o'clock	**las tres** *(lahs trehs)*	**las quince horas** *(lahs keen-seh oh-rahs)*

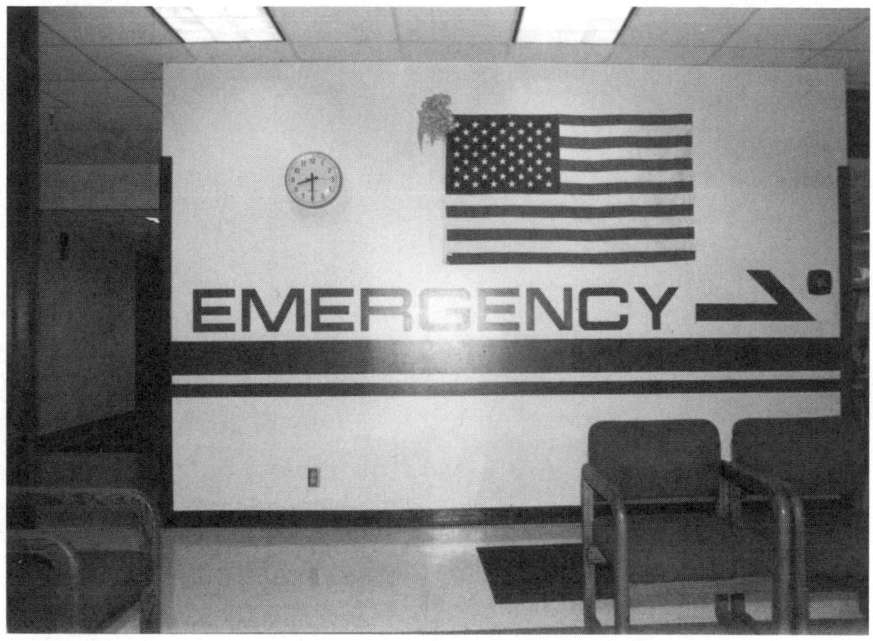

Figure 29–1 Clocks are hung throughout the hospital because knowing the time can be essential.

four o'clock	**las cuatro** *(lahs koo-ah-troh)*	**las dieciséis horas** *(lahs dee-ehs-ee-seh-ees oh-rahs)*
five o'clock	**las cinco** *(lahs seen-koh)*	**las diecisiete horas** *(lahs dee-ehs-ee-see-eh-teh oh-rahs)*
six o'clock	**las seis** *(lahs seh-ees)*	**las dieciocho horas** *(lahs dee-ehs-ee-oh-choh oh-rahs)*
seven o'clock	**las siete** *(lahs see-eh-teh)*	**las diecinueve horas** *(lahs dee-ehs-ee-noo-eh-beh oh-rahs)*
eight o'clock	**las ocho** *(lahs oh-choh)*	**las veinte horas** *(lahs beh-een-teh oh-rahs)*
nine o'clock	**las nueve** *(lahs noo-eh-beh)*	**las veintiuna horas** *(lahs beh-een-tee-oo-nah oh-rahs)*
ten o'clock	**las diez** *(lahs dee-ehs)*	**las veintidós horas** *(lahs beh-een-tee-dohs oh-rahs)*

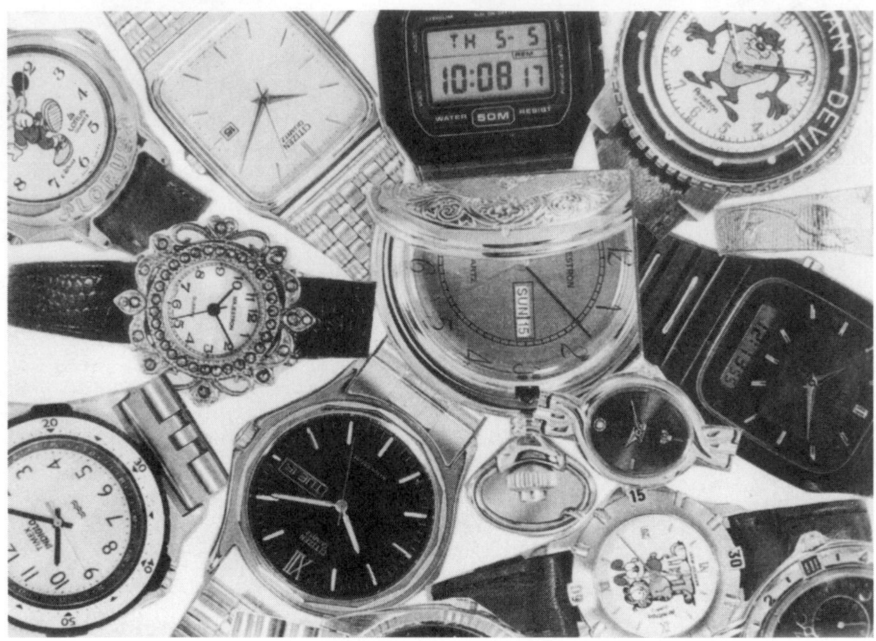

Figure 29–2 Time changes continuously.

eleven o'clock	**las once** *(lahs ohn-seh)*	**las veintitrés horas** *(lahs beh-een-tee-trehs oh-rahs)*
twelve o'clock/ midnight	**las doce/la media noche** *(lahs doh-seh/ lah meh-dee-ah non-cheh)*	**las cero horas** *(lahs-seh-roh-oh-rahs)* *(lahs beh-een-tee-koo-ah-troh oh-rahs)*

Chapter Thirty | Capítulo treinta

The Colors, the Seasons, the Months, the Days

Los colores, las estaciones del año, los meses, los días

The Colors — *Los colores*

Colors are used frequently in medicine. In daily care, the physician notes the condition of the patient through observation of the color of the skin, hair, eyes, tongue, lips, etc. Colors also assist in making a medical diagnosis. For example, when one notices a reddish tint in the urine, one thinks that it may be caused by kidney problems.

Los colores se utilizan a menudo en el área médica. En el cuidado diario, el médico observa la condición del paciente y vigila el color de la piel, pelo, ojos, lengua, labios, etc. Los colores también apoyan el diagnóstico médico. Por ejemplo, al notar una orina color rojizo, esto indica que hay problemas de riñón.

albino	**albino**	*(ahl-bee-noh)*
amber	**ámbar**	*(ahm-bahr)*
black	**negro**	*(neh-groh)*
blonde	**rubio**	*(roo-bee-oh)*
blue	**azul**	*(ah-sool)*
brown	**café**	*(kah-feh)*
brown (*skin tone*)	**moreno**	*(moh-reh-noh)*
clear	**claro**	*(klah-roh)*
emerald	**esmeralda**	*(ehs-meh-rahl-dah)*
gold	**dorado**	*(doh-rah-doh)*
gray	**gris**	*(grees)*
grayish-white	**canoso**	*(kah-noh-soh)*

green	**verde**	*(behr-deh)*
hazel	**castaño**	*(kahs-tah-nyoh)*
orange	**naranja**	*(nah-rahn-hah)*
pink	**rosa**	*(roh-sah)*
red	**rojo**	*(roh-hoh)*
violet	**violeta**	*(bee-oh-leh-tah)*
yellow	**amarillo**	*(ah-mah-ree-yoh)*
white	**blanco**	*(blahn-koh)*

The Seasons *Las estaciones del año*

We also use the seasons of the year to guide us during our practice. The human body reacts differently when exposed to temperature variations: cold, warm, hot. These variations cause the skin to be sweaty, dry, or warm. One can detect potential dangers such as dehydration or burns caused by very low temperatures.

También usamos las estaciones del año para guiar nuestra práctica. El cuerpo humano reacciona de manera diferente cuando se expone a variaciones en la temperatura, tales como el frío, la humedad o el calor. Estas variaciones causan que la piel se sienta caliente, húmeda, fría o seca. Uno puede detectar posibles peligros tales como la deshidratación por el calor durante el verano, o las quemaduras causadas por una temperatura muy baja en el invierno.

season	**estación**	*(ehs-tah-see-ohn)*
spring	**primavera**	*(pree-mah-beh-rah)*
summer	**verano**	*(beh-rah-noh)*
fall	**otoño**	*(oh-toh-nyoh)*
winter	**invierno**	*(een-bee-ehr-noh)*

The Months *Los meses*

Months become important during a pregnancy, since one can calculate a tentative delivery date. One can program the instruction for the mother and prepare her for the birth date. Also, months help us watch the growth and development of babies since they require scheduled vaccinations at specific times in their lives. In our personal lives, the months indicate all the dates that are important to us when we plan vacations, celebrations, and anniversaries.

Los meses son importantes durante el embarazo, ya que se puede calcular una fecha probable de parto. Se puede entonces programar la educación de la madre y prepararla para el evento del parto. También los meses nos ayudan a vigilar el desarrollo de los bebés ya que ellos requieren de vacunación en cierto tiempo de su vida. Los meses indican, en la vida personal, todas las fechas y eventos que tienen importancia y por los cuales disfrutamos de vacaciones, festejos y aniversarios.

month	**mes**	*(mehs)*
January	**enero***	*(eh-neh-roh)*
February	**febrero**	*(feh-breh-roh)*
March	**marzo**	*(mahr-soh)*
April	**abril**	*(ah-breel)*
May	**mayo**	*(mah-yoh)*
June	**junio**	*(hoo-nee-oh)*
July	**julio**	*(hoo-lee-oh)*
August	**agosto**	*(ah-gohs-toh)*
September	**septiembre**	*(sehp-tee-ehm-breh)*
October	**octubre**	*(ohk-too-breh)*
November	**noviembre**	*(noh-bee-ehm-breh)*
December	**diciembre**	*(dee-see-ehm-breh)*

TABLE 30–1
Descriptive Words

TABLA 30–1
Palabras descriptivas

English	**Spanish**	**Pronunciation**
amber	ambarino	(ahm-bah-ree-noh)
bluish	azuloso	(ah-soo-loh-soh)
cianotic	cianótico/ violáceo	(see-ah-noh-tee-koh/ bee-oh-lah-se-oh)
grayish	grisáseo	(gree-sah-seh-oh)
icteric	ictérico	(eek-teh-ree-koh)
opaque	opaco	(oh-pah-koh)
orangy	anaranjado	(ah-nah-rahn-hah-doh)
pale	pálido	(pah-lee-doh)
pinkish	rosado	(roh-sah-doh)
transparent	transparente	(trahns-pah-rehn-teh)

*The names of months and days of the week are not capitalized in Spanish.

The Days of the Week — *Los días de la semana*

The use of days is indispensable in a hospital. We use them in all the medical records, appointments, visits to the laboratory, X-ray department, rehabilitation, or home visits. The days serve as a control. We use the number of hospital days to determine the cost of a hospitalization.

El uso de los días es indispensable en un hospital. Se usan en todas las notas de evolución de los pacientes, citas en el laboratorio, departamento de rayos X, rehabilitación o visitas comunitarias. Los días sirven para controlar la estancia del paciente en el hospital. Se usa el número de días de estancia para determinar el costo de la hospitalización.

Monday	**lunes***	*(loo-nehs)*
Tuesday	**martes**	*(mahr-tehs)*
Wednesday	**miércoles**	*(mee-ehr-koh-lehs)*
Thursday	**jueves**	*(hoo-eh-behs)*
Friday	**viernes**	*(bee-ehr-nehs)*
Saturday	**sábado**	*(sah-bah-doh)*
Sunday	**domingo**	*(doh-meen-goh)*

Cardinal Points — *Los puntos cardinales*

Cardinal points serve as orientation, especially when one asks for directions.

Los puntos cardinales sirven de orientación, especialmente cuando uno requiere direcciones.

north	**norte**	*(nohr-teh)*
south	**sur**	*(soor)*
east	**este**	*(ehs-teh)*
west	**oeste**	*(oh-ehs-teh)*

*The names of months and days of the week are not capitalized in Spanish.

Chapter Thirty-one | Capítulo treinta y uno

The Members of the Family | Los miembros de la familia

In the past, it was difficult to mention or count all the members of a family. This happened because they were numerous and they lived a long time. One could easily confuse the relationships between members. Today, because families are smaller, one knows who makes up the nuclear family and where we find the best relationships.

En épocas pasadas era tan difícil enumerar o contar a todos los miembros que integraban una familia. Esto sucedía por lo numeroso y por los muchos años que vivían. Fácilmente se podía confundir el parentesco. Ahora, gracias a que las familias son más pequeñas, se pueden conocer mejor los integrantes del núcleo familiar y en donde encontramos las mejores convivencias.

the family	**la familia**	*(lah fah-mee-lee-ah)*
father	**padre**	*(pah-dreh)*
dad	**papá**	*(pah-pah)*
mother	**madre**	*(mah-dreh)*
mom	**mamá**	*(mah-mah)*
husband	**esposo**	*(ehs-poh-soh)*
wife	**esposa**	*(ehs-poh-sah)*
sister	**hermana**	*(ehr-mah-nah)*
brother	**hermano**	*(ehr-mah-noh)*
son	**hijo**	*(ee-hoh)*
daughter	**hija**	*(ee-hah)*
niece	**sobrina**	*(soh-bree-nah)*
nephew	**sobrino**	*(soh-bree-noh)*
grandmother	**abuela**	*(ah-boo-eh-lah)*
grandfather	**abuelo**	*(ah-boo-eh-loh)*
grandparents	**abuelos**	*(ah-boo-eh-lohs)*
aunt	**tía**	*(tee-ah)*
uncle	**tío**	*(tee-oh)*
stepfather	**padrastro**	*(pah-drahs-troh)*

stepmother	**madrastra**	*(mah-drahs-trah)*
stepson	**hijastro**	*(ee-hahs-troh)*
stepdaughter	**hijastra**	*(ee-hahs-trah)*
children	**hijos**	*(eeh-hohs)*
great-grandparents	**bisabuelos**	*(bee-sah-boo-eh-lohs)*
mother-in-law	**suegra**	*(soo-eh-grah)*
father-in-law	**suegro**	*(soo-eh-groh)*
sister-in-law	**cuñada**	*(koo-nyah-dah)*
brother-in-law	**cuñado**	*(koo-nyah-doh)*
concubine/ common law	**concubina**	*(kohn-koo-bee-nah)*
cousins	**primos**	*(pree-mohs)*
cousin (female)	**prima**	*(pree-mah)*
cousin (male)	**primo**	*(pree-moh)*
grandchildren	**nietos**	*(nee-eh-tohs)*
godparents	**padrinos**	*(pah-dree-nohs)*
godfather	**padrino**	*(pah-dree-noh)*
godmother	**madrina**	*(mah-dree-nah)*

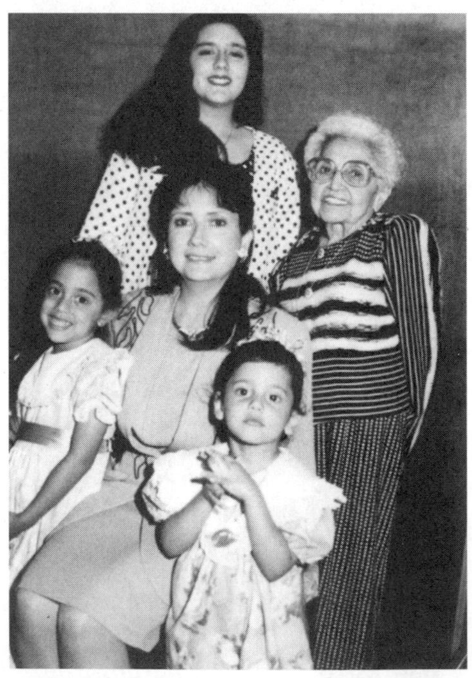

Figure 31–1 Sometimes we find several generations in a group.

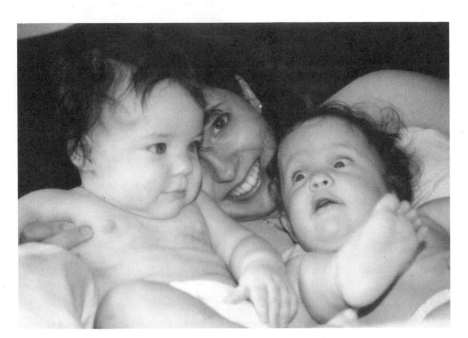

Figure 31–2 Potential health problems may be prevented if you know the family background.

It is important to determine the family composition soon after you interview the patient. This will give you an idea of the family support for the patient. It may also show potential familial problems. Many problems may be prevented if we know which members of the family have chronic illnesses.

Es muy importante determinar la composición de la familia inmediatamente después de la entrevista. Esto le dará una idea del apoyo de la familia para el paciente. También puede demostrar posibles problemas hereditarios. Muchos problemas se pueden prevenir si sabemos cuales de los miembros de la familia tienen enfermedades crónico-degenerativas.

We must keep in mind that the family composition is changing. A parent may be missing due to death, divorce, or abandonment. This means that we must be alert to potential problems, especially when the family has few economic resources, is educationally deprived, or is new to your area.

Debemos considerar que la composición de la familia está evolucionando. El padre o la madre pueden faltar en la familia debido a muerte, divorcio o abandono. Esto nos debe alertar a posibles problemas, especialmente cuando la familia posee escasos recursos económicos, está privada educacionalmente o acaba de integrarse en la comunidad.

TABLE 31–1 Common Chronic Illnesses | **TABLA 31–1 Enfermedades crónicas comunes**

English	Spanish	Pronunciation
arthritis	**artritis**	*(ahr-tree-tees)*
asthma	**asma**	*(ahs-mah)*
diabetes	**diabetes**	*(dee-ah-beh-tees)*
epilepsy	**epilepsia**	*(eh-pee-lehp-see-ah)*
gout	**gota**	*(goh-tah)*
hypertension	**hipertensión**	*(ee-pehr-tehn-see-ohn)*
mental retardation	**retraso mental**	*(reh-trah-soh mehn-tahl)*
obesity	**obesidad**	*(oh-beh-see-dahd)*

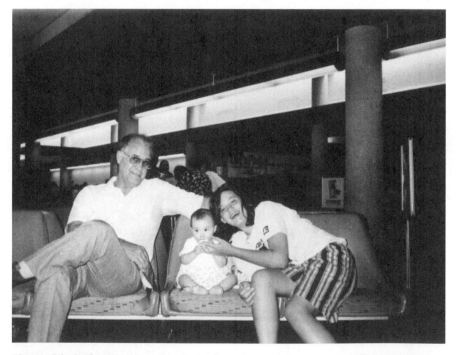

Figure 31–3 The American family is changing. It is important to determine family composition during your interview with the patient.

Unit 6

Unidad 6

Chapter Thirty-two — Capítulo treinta y dos

The Alphabet — El abecedario

The alphabet consists of a series of letters in a language in alphabetical order. It is also used as a manual for deaf and mute persons who use it with finger signals so they can be understood. In 1994, authors at the Royal Spanish Academy omitted the separate use of Ch, Ll, and Rr and incorporated them into the C, L, and R sections in dictionaries. These letters are included here only to facilitate their pronunciation.

El abecedario es una serie de letras de un idioma en orden alfabético. También se usa como un manual en personas sordomudas que lo emplean con signos en los dedos de sus manos para darse a entender con las personas. En 1994, los autores de la Real Academia Española omitieron el uso separado de las letras Ch, Ll, y Rr y las incorporaron a las secciones C, L, y R en los diccionarios. Estas letras se incuyen aquí sólo para facilitar la pronunciación.

A	B	C	Ch	D	E
ah (arm)	*beh* (bell)	*seh* (casette)	*Cheh* (change)	*deh* (day)	*eh* (bet)
F	**G**	**H**	**I**	**J**	**K**
eh-feh (efeminate)	*heh* (hen)	*ah-cheh*	*ee* (dear)	*hoh-tah* (holly)	*kah* (car)
L	**Ll**	**M**	**N**	**Ñ**	**O**
eh-leh (electric)	*eh-yeh*	*eh-meh* (emeritus)	*eh-neh* (energy)	*eh-nyeh*	*oh* (opera)
P	**Q**	**R**	**Rr**	**S**	**T**
peh (pay)	*koo* (cook)	*eh-reh* (air)	*doh-bleh* *eh-reh*	*eh-seh* (esence)	*teh* (tell)

U	V	W	X	Y	Z
oo	*beh* (verdict)	*doh-bleh oo*	*eh-kees*	*ee gree-eh-gah*	*seh-tah* (gazette)

Rules for Pronunciation *Reglas para la pronunciación*

Spanish is pronounced as it is written. Pay special attention to the five vowel sounds:

El español se escribe como se pronuncia. Ponga atención particularmente a los cinco sonidos de las vocales:

A *(ah)*	**asma** ***(ahs-mah)***	asthma
E *(eh)*	**vena** ***(beh-nah)***	vein
I *(ee)*	**herida** ***(eh-ree-dah)***	wound
O *(oh)*	**obeso** ***(oh-beh-soh)***	fat
U *(oo)*	**úlcera** ***(ool-seh-rah)***	ulcer

Now pay attention to the consonants:
Ahora ponga atención a las consonantes:

C	**célula** ***(seh-loo-lah)***	cell
C	**ciencia** ***(see-ehn-see-ah)***	science
C	**cama** ***(kah-mah)***	bed
C	**comer** ***(koh-mehr)***	to eat
C	**cuerpo** ***(koo-ehr-poh)***	body
C	**crisis** ***(kree-sees)***	crisis
CH	**chancro** ***(chahn-kroh)***	chancre
D	**dosis** ***(doh-sees)***	dose
F	**fiebre** ***(fee-eh-breh)***	fever
G	**genital** ***(heh-nee-tahl)***	genital
G	**gingivitis** ***(heen-hee-bee-tees)***	gingivitis
G	**gangrena** ***(gahn-greh-nah)***	gangrene
G	**gota** ***(goh-tah)***	gout
G	**gusto** ***(goos-toh)***	taste
G	**glaucoma** ***(glah-oo-koh-mah)***	glaucoma
H*	**hernia** ***(ehr-nee-ah)***	hernia
J	**jeringa** ***(heh-reen-gah)***	syringe
K	**kilogramo** ***(kee-loh-grah-moh)***	kilogram
L	**laringitis** ***(lah-reen-hee-tees)***	laryngitis

*Note that the *h* is always silent.

LL	**llorar** *(yoh-rahr)*	to cry
M	**meningitis** *(meh-neen-hee-tees)*	meningitis
N	**náusea** *(nah-oo-seh-ah)*	nausea
Ñ	**baño** *(bah-nyoh)*	bath
P	**palpitación** *(pahl-pee-tah-see-ohn)*	palpitation
Q	**quejar** *(keh-hahr)*	to complain
R	**curar** *(koo-rahr)*	to cure
RR	**carro** *(kah-roh)*	car
	hemorragia *(eh-moh-rah-hee-ah)*	hemorrhage
S	**síntomas** *(seen-toh-mahs)*	symptoms
T	**tensión** *(tehn-see-ohn)*	tension
V	**vértigo** *(behr-tee-goh)*	vertigo
W	**watusi** *(oo-ah-too-see)*	watusi
X	**extra** *(ehx-trah)*	extra
Y	**y** *(ee)*	and
Y	**yodo** *(yoh-doh)*	iodine
Z	**zumbido** *(soom-bee-doh)*	buzzing

Chapter Thirty-three **Capítulo treinta y tres**

Accents / Acentos

The acute accent is the only mark of its kind in Spanish. It is a small oblique line (**á**) that is drawn from right to left and specifies a syllable that has a stronger sound when pronouncing it. Accents are used generally to distinguish words written alike and identical in form with other parts of speech, but with a different meaning. For example: **papá** (*father*), **papa** (*vegetable*); **monté** (*mounted*), **monte** (*large hill*). Accents are sometimes omitted from capital letters.

El acento es la mayor intensidad con que se marca determinada sílaba al pronunciar una palabra. Es una rayita oblicua (á) que se escribe de derecha a izquierda y se coloca en ciertos casos sobre la vocal de la sílaba en que se carga la pronunciación. En español es muy necesario acentuar las palabras para darles el significado correcto que llevan. Por ejemplo: papá (padre), papa (vegetal); monté (verbo), monte (terreno elevado).

I love	**amo**	*(ah-moh)*
he loved	**él amó**	*(ehl ah-moh)*
the owner	**el dueño/amo**	*(ehl doo-eh-nyoh/ah-moh)*
road	**el camino**	*(ehl kah-mee-noh)*
he walked	**él caminó**	*(ehl kah-mee-noh)*
copper	**cobre**	*(koh-breh)*
I charged	**yo cobré**	*(yoh koh-breh)*
volumes	**volúmenes**	*(boh-loo-meh-nehs)*
never	**jamás**	*(hah-mahs)*
pencil	**lápiz**	*(lah-pees)*

Chapter Thirty-four — Capítulo treinta y cuatro

Gender of Nouns — Género de los sustantivos

In Spanish, the gender of a noun corresponds to sex. The name of any male being is masculine; that of a female being is feminine. The grammatical gender of an inanimate object must simply be memorized: a bone (**el hueso**) is masculine, the head (**la cabeza**) is feminine, and so on.

En español, el género de los sustantivos corresponde al sexo. El nombre de un hombre es masculino, el de una mujer es femenino. El género gramatical de un objeto inanimado se debe memorizar: un hueso es masculino, la cabeza es femenina y así sucesivamente.

All Spanish nouns must be masculine or feminine.

The definite article *the* has the following singular and plural forms in Spanish.

el (singular masculine)	**la** (singular feminine)
los (plural masculine)	**las** (plural feminine)

The indefinite article *a* or *an* has the following forms in Spanish.

un (singular masculine)	**una** (singular feminine)
unos (plural masculine)	**unas** (plural feminine)

Masculine nouns require a masculine article; feminine nouns require a feminine article.

the man	**el hombre**	***(ehl ohm-breh)***
the woman	**la mujer**	***(lah moo-hehr)***
the boy	**el muchacho**	***(ehl moo-chah-choh)***
the back	**la espalda**	***(lah ehs-pahl-dah)***
the friend	**el amigo**	***(ehl ah-mee-goh)***
a rib	**una costilla**	***(oo-nah kohs-tee-yah)***
the eye	**el ojo**	***(ehl oh-hoh)***
the bladder	**la vejiga**	***(lah beh-hee-gah)***

a skeleton	**un esqueleto**	*(oon ehs-keh-leh-toh)*
the clavicle	**la clavícula**	*(lah klah-bee-koo-lah)*

Nouns ending in **-al, -ante, -ador,** and **-ón** are usually masculine.

An important exception is **la mano.** In spite of the ending *o,* la mano is feminine.

the hospital	**el hospital**	*(ehl ohs-pee-tahl)*
the tranquilizer	**el tranquili-zante**	*(ehl trahn-kee-lee-sahn-teh)*
the worker	**el trabajador**	*(ehl trah-bah-hah-dohr)*
the heart	**el corazón**	*(ehl koh-rah-sohn)*

The days of the week, months of the year, and the names of languages are masculine.

Wednesday	**el miércoles**	*(ehl mee-ehr-koh-lehs)*
the month of April	**el mes de abril**	*(ehl mehs deh ah-breel)*
Spanish	**el español**	*(ehl ehs-pah-nyohl)*

Nouns ending in **-tad, -dad, -ción, -sión, -ez, -ie, -ud,** and **-umbre** are usually feminine.

the dehydration	**la deshidra-tación**	*(lah deh-see-drah-tah-see-ohn)*
the habit	**la costumbre**	*(lah kohs-toom-breh)*
the age	**la edad**	*(lah eh-dahd)*
the friendship	**la amistad**	*(lah ah-mees-tahd)*
the series	**la serie**	*(lah seh-ree-eh)*
the health	**la salud**	*(lah sah-lood)*

Nouns ending in **-e** should be memorized with the definite article.

the blood	**la sangre**	*(lah sahn-greh)*
the penis	**el pene**	*(ehl peh-neh)*

Plural of Nouns

A noun ending in a vowel forms the plural by adding **-s;** those ending in a consonant add **-es.**

the physician	**el médico**	*(ehl meh-dee-koh)*
the physicians	**los médicos**	*(lohs meh-dee-kohs)*
the doctor	**el doctor**	*(ehl dohk-tohr)*
the doctors	**los doctores**	*(lohs dohk-toh-rehs)*

A noun ending in **-z** changes to **-c** and then adds **-es.**

the nose	**la nariz**	*(lah nahr-ees)*
the noses	**las narices**	*(lahs nahr-ee-sehs)*

Nouns ending in a stressed vowel form the plural by adding **-es.**

the ruby	**el rubí**	*(ehl roo-bee)*
the rubies	**los rubíes**	*(lohs roo-bee-ehs)*

Nouns ending in unstressed **-es** or **-is** are considered to be both singular and plural. Number is expressed by the article.

Thursday	**el jueves**	*(ehl hoo-eh-behs)*
Thursdays	**los jueves**	*(lohs hoo-eh-behs)*

Special Uses of Articles

The definite article is used in Spanish, but omitted in English as follows.

1. Before the names of languages, except after **hablar, en,** or **de:**

   Spanish is important. — **El español es importante.** *(Ehl ehs-pah-nyohl ehs eem-pohr-tahn-teh)*

   My friend speaks French. — **Mi amigo habla francés.** *(Mee ah-mee-goh ah-blah frahn-sehs)*

   The whole book is in German. — **Todo el libro está en alemán.** *(Toh-doh ehl lee-broh ehs-tah ehn ah-leh-mahn)*

2. Before titles, except when addressing the person:

   Mr. Gomez left yesterday. — **El señor Gómez salió ayer.** *(Ehl seh-nyohr Goh-mehs sah-lee-oh ah-yehr)*

   How are you, Mrs. García? — **¿Cómo está, señora García?** *(Koh-moh ehs-tah, seh-nyoh-rah Gahr-see-ah)*

   The article is omitted before **don, doña, Santo, Santa, San.**

3. With parts of the body or personal possessions (clothing, etc.):

   He has black hair. — **El tiene pelo negro.** *(Ehl tee-eh-neh peh-loh neh-groh)*

Mary has a broken foot. — **María tiene el pie quebrado.** *(Mah-ree-ah tee-eh-neh ehl pee-eh keh-brah-doh)*

4. With the time of day (**la hora,** *the hour;* **las horas,** *the hours*):

It is one o'clock. — **Es la una.** *(Ehs lah oo-nah)*

I go to sleep at eleven. — **Me duermo a las once.** *(Meh doo-ehr-moh ah lahs ohn-seh)*

5. With the names of seasons:

I like summer. — **Me gusta el verano.** *(Meh goos-tah ehl beh-rah-noh)*

6. With the days of the week, except after the verb **ser** (*to be*):

I go downtown (on) Tuesdays. — **Los martes voy al centro.** *(Lohs mahr-tehs boy ahl sehn-troh)*

Today is Monday. — **Hoy es lunes.** *(Oh-ee ehs loo-nehs)*

7. Before certain geographic areas:

Canada — **el Canadá** *(ehl Kah-nah-dah)*

Argentina — **la Argentina** *(lah Ahr-hehn-tee-nah)*

Neuter Article Lo

1. The neuter article **lo** precedes an adjective used as a noun to express a quality or an abstract idea.

I like red (that which is red). — **Me gusta lo rojo.** *(Meh goos-tah loh roh-hoh)*

I think the same as you. — **Pienso lo mismo que usted.** *(Pee-ehn-soh loh mees-moh keh oos-tehd)*

2. **Lo** + adjective or adverb + **que** = *how.*

I see how good she is.	**Ya veo lo buena que es.** *(Yah beh-oh loh boo-eh-nah keh ehs)*

Since the article **lo** is neuter, it has no plural form. Therefore, **lo** is used whether the adjective is masculine or feminine, singular or plural.

Omission of Articles

1. The definite article is omitted in the following cases.
   A. Before nouns in a position:
   Austin, the capital of Texas, is at the center of the state.
   Austin, capital de Texas, está en el centro del estado.
   B. Before numerals expressing the numerical order of rulers:

Charles the Fifth	**Carlos Quinto** *(Kahr-lohs Keen-toh)*
Mary the Second	**María Segunda** *(Mah-ree-ah Seh-goon-dah)*

2. The indefinite article is omitted before predicate nouns denoting a class or group (social class, occupation, nationality, religion, etc.):

He is a barber.	**Es barbero.** *(Ehs bahr-beh-roh)*
I am Mexican.	**Soy mexicana.** *(Soh-ee meh-hee-kah-nah)*
I want to be a nurse.	**Quiero ser enfermera.** *(Kee-eh-roh sehr ehn-fehr-meh-rah)*

If the predicate noun is modified, the indefinite article is stated:

He is a hard-working barber.	**Es un barbero muy trabajador.** *(Ehs oon bahr-beh-roh moo-ee trah-bah-hah-dohr)*
I want to be a good nurse.	**Quiero ser una buena enfermera.** *(Kee-eh-roh sehr oo-nah boo-eh-nah ehn-fehr-meh-rah)*

Chapter Thirty-five — Capítulo treinta y cinco

Adjectives and Pronouns — Adjetivos y pronombres

Adjectives describe nouns and pronouns. In Spanish, adjectives are placed after the noun. They agree in number and gender with the noun they modify.

ADJECTIVES ENDING IN -O

Masculine singular:	The patient is happy. **El paciente está contento.** ***(Ehl pah-see-ehn-teh ehs-tah kohn-tehn-toh)***
Feminine singular:	She is happy. **Ella está contenta.** ***(Eh-yah ehs-tah kohn-tehn-tah)***
Masculine plural:	They are happy. **Ellos están contentos.** ***(Eh-yohs ehs-tahn kohn-tehn-tohs)***
Feminine plural:	They are happy. **Ellas están contentas.** ***(Eh-yahs ehs-tahn kohn-tehn-tahs)***

ADJECTIVES ENDING IN -E

Masculine singular:	He is sad. **El está triste.** ***(Ehl ehs-tah trees-teh)***
Feminine singular:	She is sad. **Ella está triste.** ***(Eh-yah ehs-tah trees-teh)***
Masculine plural:	They are sad. **Ellos están tristes.** ***(Eh-yohs ehs-tahn trees-tehs)***
Feminine plural:	They are sad. **Ellas están tristes.** ***(Eh-yahs ehs-tahn trees-tehs)***

ADJECTIVES ENDING IN A CONSONANT

Masculine singular:	The procedure is difficult. **El procedimiento es difícil.** ***(Ehl proh-seh-dee-mee-ehn-toh ehs dee-fee-seel)***
Feminine singular:	The measurement is difficult. **La medida es difícil.** ***(Lah meh-dee-dah ehs dee-fee-seel)***
Masculine plural:	The exams are difficult. **Los exámenes son difíciles.** ***(Lohs ehx-ah-meh-nehs sohn dee-fee-see-lehs)***
Feminine plural:	The measurements are difficult. **Las medidas son difíciles.** ***(Lahs meh-dee-dahs sohn dee-fee-see-lehs)***

Demonstrative adjectives precede the nouns they modify and agree with them in number and gender.

this book	**este libro**	***(ehs-teh lee-broh)***
these pens	**estas plumas**	***(ehs-tahs ploo-mahs)***

Este (*this*) refers to what is near or directly concerns me.
Esos (*those*) refers to what is near or directly concerns you.
Aquel (*that*) refers to what is remote to the speaker or the person addressed.

This pencil is red.	**Este lápiz es rojo.** ***(Ehs-teh lah-pees ehs roh-hoh)***
John, give me that bone.	**Juan, déme aquel hueso.** ***(Hoo-ahn, deh-meh ah-kehl oo-eh-soh)***

TABLE 35–1
Feminine and Masculine Adjectives

TABLA 35–1
Adjetivos femeninos y masculinos

Adjective	Feminine	Masculine
this	esta *(ehs-tah)*	este *(ehs-teh)*
these	estas *(ehs-tahs)*	estos *(ehs-tohs)*
that	esa *(eh-sah)*	ese *(eh-seh)*
those	esas *(eh-sahs)*	esos *(eh-sohs)*
that	aquella *(ah-keh-yah)*	aquel *(ah-kehl)*
those	aquellas *(ah-keh-yahs)*	aquellos *(ah-keh-yohs)*

TABLE 35–2 Personal Pronouns		**TABLA 35–2 Pronombres personales**	
Singular		**Plural**	
I	**yo** *(yoh)*	we (masculine)	**nosotros** *(noh-soh-trohs)*
		we (feminine)	**nosotras** *(noh-soh-trahs)*
you (familiar)	**tú** *(too)*	you	**vosotros/as** *(boh-soh-trohs/ahs)*
you (formal)	**usted** *(oos-tehd)*	you	**ustedes** *(oos-teh-dehs)*
he	**él** *(ehl)*	they (masculine)	**ellos** *(eh-yohs)*
she	**ella** *(eh-yah)*	they (feminine)	**ellas** *(eh-yahs)*

SOME COMMON LIMITING ADJECTIVES

all, everything	**todo**	*(toh-doh)*
bad	**malo**	*(mah-loh)*
better	**mejor**	*(meh-hohr)*
big (*age*)	**grande**	*(grahn-deh)*
first	**primero**	*(pree-meh-roh)*
fourth	**cuarto**	*(koo-ahr-toh)*
good	**bueno**	*(boo-eh-noh)*
less	**menos**	*(meh-nohs)*
little, few	**poco**	*(poh-koh)*
more	**mucho, más**	*(moo-choh, mahs)*
nothing	**nada**	*(nah-dah)*
one, a, an	**un**	*(oon)*
small (*age, fit*)	**pequeño/ chico**	*(peh-keh-nyoh/ chee-koh)*

Possessive Pronouns

	SINGULAR	**PLURAL**
mine	**el mío, la mía** *(ehl mee-oh, lah mee-ah)*	**los míos, las mías** *(lohs mee-ohs, lahs mee-ahs)*

yours	**el tuyo, la tuya** *(ehl too-yoh, lah too-yah)*	**los tuyos, las tuyas** *(lohs too-yohs, lahs too-yahs)*
his, hers, theirs	**el suyo, la suya** *(ehl soo-yoh, lah soo-yah)*	**los suyos, las suyas** *(lohs soo-yohs, lahs soo-yahs)*
ours	**el nuestro, la nuestra** *(ehl noo-ehs-troh, lah noo-ehs-trah)*	**los nuestros, las nuestras** *(lohs noo-ehs-trohs, lahs noo-ehs-trahs)*

Possessive pronouns are formed by the definite article + the long form of the possessive adjective.

My nose is prettier than yours.	**Mi nariz es más bonita que la tuya.** *(Mee nah-rees ehs mahs boh-nee-tah keh lah too-yah)*

After the verb **ser,** the article preceding the possessive pronoun is generally omitted.

The bones are mine.	**Los huesos son míos** *(Lohs oo-eh-sohs soh mee-ohs)*
That gown is yours.	**Aquella bata es suya.** *(Ah-keh-yah bah-tah ehs soo-yah)*
These books are mine.	**Estos libros son míos.** *(Ehs-tohs lee-brohs sohn mee-ohs)*

Possession is expressed by **de** + the possessor. This corresponds to *'s* or *s'* in English.

his pens and yours	**sus plumas y las de usted** *(soos ploo-mahs ee lahs deh oos-tehd)*
Martin's pencil	**el lápiz de Martín** *(ehl lah-pees deh Mahr-teen)*
my book and Louisa's	**mi libro y el de Luisa** *(mee lee-broh ee ehl deh Loo-ee-sah)*
our patient	**nuestro paciente** *(noo-ehs-troh pah-see-ehn-teh)*
her rings	**sus anillos** *(soos ah-nee-yohs)*
a friend of theirs	**un amigo de ellos** *(oon ah-mee-goh deh eh-yohs)*

Whose?

The interrogative pronoun *whose?* is expressed in Spanish by **¿de quién es?**

Whose pen is it?	**¿De quién es la pluma?** *(Deh kee-ehn ehs lah ploo-mah)*
It belongs to the doctor.	**Es del doctor.** *(Ehs dehl dohk-tohr)*
Whose card is it?	**¿De quién es la tarjeta?** *(Deh kee-ehn ehs lah tahr-heh-tah)*
Mr. García's.	**Del señor García.** *(Dehl seh-nyohr Gahr-see-ah)*
Whose X-rays are these?	**¿De quién son estas radiografías?** *(Deh kee-ehn sohn ehs-tahs rah-dee-oh-grah-fee-ahs)*
They are Mrs. Luna's.	**Son de la señora Luna.** *(Sohn deh lah seh-nyoh-rah Loo-nah)*

SOME COMMON PREPOSITIONS

about	**acerca de**	*(ah-sehr-kay deh)*
according	**según**	*(seh-goon)*
after	**después de**	*(dehs-poo-ehs deh)*
against	**contra**	*(kohn-trah)*
among, between	**entre**	*(ehn-treh)*
around	**alrededor de**	*(ahl-reh-deh-dohr deh)*
before	**antes de**	*(ahn-tehs deh)*
behind	**detrás de**	*(deh-trahs deh)*
beneath, under	**debajo de**	*(deh-bah-hoh deh)*
beside	**además de**	*(ah-deh-mahs deh)*
during	**durante**	*(doo-rahn-teh)*
far	**lejos de**	*(leh-hohs deh)*
for	**para**	*(pah-rah)*
for, by, therefore	**por**	*(pohr)*
from, of	**de**	*(deh)*
in, or	**en**	*(ehn)*
in front of	**enfrente de**	*(ehn-frehn-teh deh)*
in front of	**delante de**	*(deh-lahn-teh deh)*
near	**cerca de**	*(sehr-kah deh)*
outside of	**fuera de**	*(foo-eh-rah deh)*
over, above	**sobre**	*(soh-breh)*

since	**desde**	*(dehs-deh)*
to, at	**a**	*(ah)*
toward	**hacia**	*(ah-see-ah)*
until	**hasta**	*(ahs-tah)*
with	**con**	*(kohn)*
within	**dentro de**	*(dehn-troh deh)*

Chapter Thirty-six | Capítulo treinta y seis

Simple Questions, Interrogatives, Exclamations

Preguntas sencillas, interrogativas, exclamaciones

Simple questions are used most frequently. They are used in short form to ask a question or give a command. Note that in the Spanish language the questions must be accompanied by an inverted mark before (¿) and a regular one after it (?). We use questions to let the patient tell us what they know

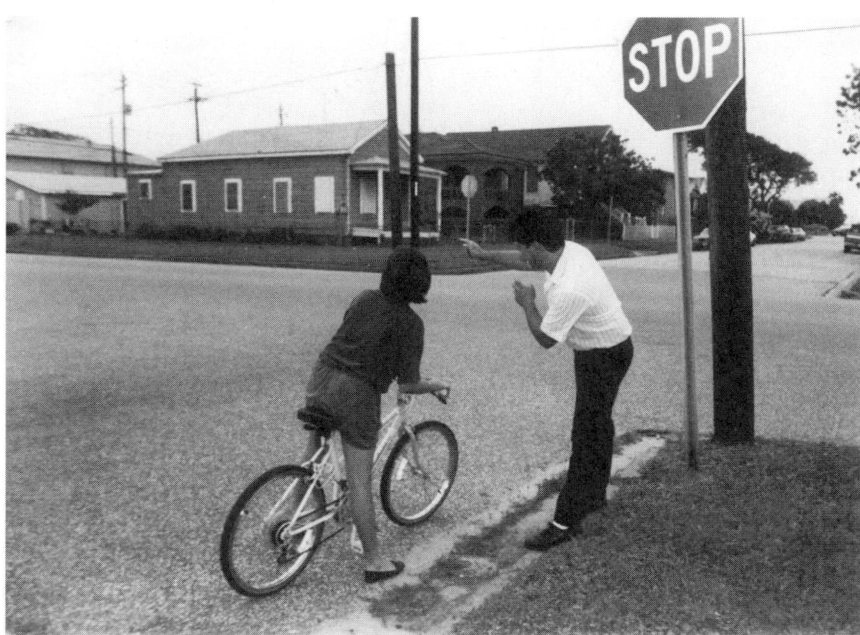

Figure 36–1 Simple questions are used frequently. Remember to give simple answers.

or how they feel. The exclamation points indicate emotion or the mood that the patient is in and are used before and after the statement (¡!).

Las preguntas sencillas son las que usamos con mayor frecuencia. Se usan en forma corta ya sea interrogando o exclamando. Note que las preguntas en la lengua española se deben de acompañar por signo de interrogación invertido (¿) al inicio y al final como lo conocemos (?). Las interrogativas son preguntas que se hacen para que nos respondan lo que saben o sienten en ese momento. Las exclamaciones reflejan una emoción o estado de ánimo de la persona y se usan antes y después de la expresión (¡!).

what?	**¿qué?/¿qué tal?**	*(keh/keh tahl)*
when?	**¿cuándo?**	*(koo-ahn-doh)*
where?	**¿dónde?**	*(dohn-deh)*
why?	**¿por qué?**	*(pohr keh)*
for whom?	**¿para quién?**	*(pah-rah kee-ehn)*
for what?	**¿para qué?**	*(pah-rah keh)*
which?	**¿cuál?**	*(koo-ahl)*
who?	**¿quién?**	*(kee-ehn)*
how many?	**¿cuántos?**	*(koo-ahn-tohs)*
how much?	**¿cuánto?**	*(koo-ahn-toh)*

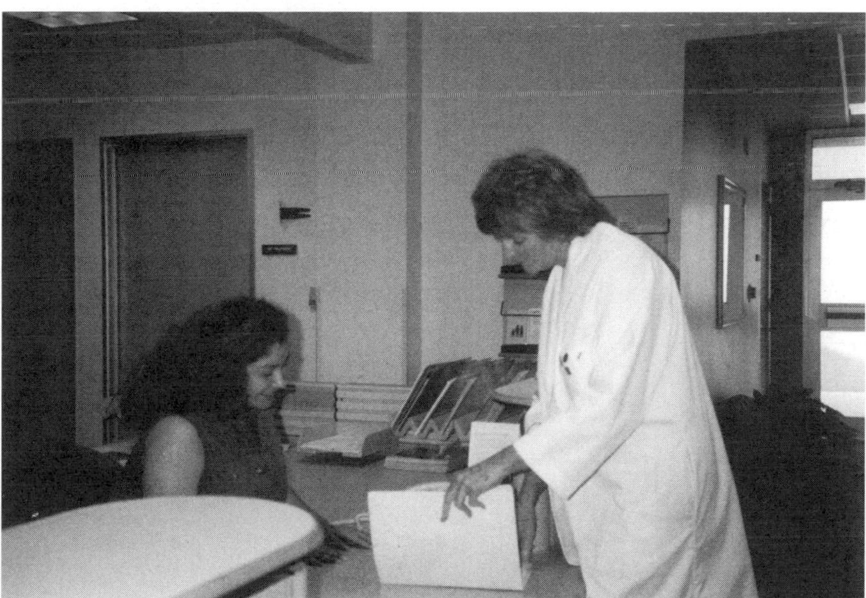

Figure 36–2 Questions are often asked to clarify messages.

What is it?	**¿Qué es?**	*(Keh ehs)*
What happens?	**¿Qué pasa?**	*(Keh pah-sah)*
What's going on?	**¿Qué pasa?**	*(Keh pah-sah)*
Why not?	**¿Por qué no?**	*(Pohr keh noh)*
Since when?	**¿Desde cuándo?**	*(Dehs-deh koo-ahn-doh)*
Do you understand?	**¿Comprende?/ ¿Entiende?**	*(Kohm-prehn-deh/Ehn-tee-ehn-deh)*
Always!	**¡Siempre!**	*(See-ehm-preh)*
Never!	**¡Nunca!**	*(Noon-kah)*
None!	**¡Ninguno!**	*(Neen-goo-noh)*
Do you want the bedpan?	**¿Quiere el pato/el bacín?**	*(Kee-eh-reh ehl pah-toh/ ehl bah-seen)*
Do you wish to pass urine?	**¿Quiere orinar?**	*(Kee-eh-reh oh-ree-nahr)*
Do you wish to have a bowel movement?	**¿Quiere evacuar/ hacer del baño?**	*(Kee-eh-reh eh-bah-koo-ahr/ah-sehr dehl bah-nyoh)*
Do you want:	**¿Quiere:**	*(Kee-eh-reh)*
a glass of water?	**un vaso de agua?**	*(oon bah-soh deh ah-goo-ah)*
a glass of juice?	**un vaso de jugo?**	*(oon bah-soh deh hoo-goh)*
Do you want:	**¿Quiere:**	*(Kee-eh-reh)*
something to eat?	**algo de comer?**	*(ahl-goh deh koh-mehr)*
something to drink?	**algo de tomar/ beber?**	*(ahl-goh deh toh-mahr/ beh-behr)*
something to read?	**algo de leer?**	*(ahl-goh deh leh-ehr)*
Are you cold?	**¿Tiene frío?**	*(Tee-eh-neh free-oh)*
Are you hot?	**¿Tiene calor?**	*(Tee-eh-neh kah-lohr)*
Are you hungry?	**¿Tiene hambre?**	*(Tee-eh-neh ahm-breh)*
Are you sleepy?	**¿Tiene sueño?**	*(Tee-eh-neh soo-eh-nyoh)*
Are you thirsty?	**¿Tiene sed?**	*(Tee-eh-neh sehd)*
Is that enough?	**¿Es suficiente?**	*(Ehs soo-fee-see-ehn-teh)*
Is that a lot?	**¿Es mucho?**	*(Ehs moo-choh)*
Is that too much?	**¿Es demasiado?**	*(Ehs deh-mah-see-ah-doh)*
Are you comfortable?	**¿Está cómoda?**	*(Ehs tah koh-moh-dah)*
Can you feel this?	**¿Siente esto?**	*(See-ehn-teh ehs-toh)*
Don't worry!	**¡No se preocupe!**	*(Noh seh preh-oh-koo-peh)*
Be patient!	**¡Tenga paciencia!**	*(Tehn-gah pah-see-ehn-see-ah)*

Chapter Thirty-seven | Capítulo treinta y siete

Negatives, Affirmatives | Negativos, afirmativos

The principal negative words and their affirmative opposites are:
Las principales palabras negativas y sus opuestas afirmativas son:

NEGATIVE		AFFIRMATIVE	
no, not	**no** *(noh)*	yes	**sí** *(see)*
no one, nobody	**nadie** *(nah-dee-eh)*	someone, somebody	**alguien** *(ahl-gee-ehn)*
nothing	**nada** *(nah-dah)*	something	**algo** *(ahl-goh)*
never, not ever	**nunca, jamás** *(noon-kah, hah-mahs)*	always	**siempre** *(see-ehm-preh)*
neither	**tampoco** *(tahm-poh-koh)*	also	**también** *(tahm-bee-ehn)*
neither . . . nor	**ni...ni** *(nee...nee)*	either . . . or	**o...o** *(oh...oh)*
not one, not any	**ninguno** *(neen-goo-noh)*	some, any	**alguno** *(ahl-goo-noh)*
without	**sin** *(seen)*	with	**con** *(kohn)*

EXAMPLES	EJEMPLOS
You do not know the plan.	**Usted no sabe el plan.** *(Oos-tehd noh sah-beh ehl plahn)*
I see no one here.	**No veo a nadie aquí.** *(Noh beh-oh ah nah-dee-eh ah-kee)*
I have neither paper nor pencil.	**No tengo ni papel ni lápiz.** *(Noh tehn-goh nee pah-pehl nee lah-pees)*
He left without saying anything.	**Salió sin decir nada.** *(Sah-lee-oh seen deh-seer nah-dah)*

But — *Pero/Sino*

Though both **pero** (*but, nevertheless*) and **sino** (*on the contrary*) are translated as *but,* their use differs as follows: **Sino** is used only if the first clause of the sentence is negative and the second clause is in direct contrast to the first. **Pero** is used in all other cases where *but* is required.

Aunque *pero* **y** *sino* **se traducen** *but,* **su uso se distingue como lo siguiente:** *sino* **se usa sólo si la primera cláusula de la oración es negativa y la segunda cláusula está en contraste directo con la primera.** *Pero* **se usa en todos los otros casos cuando se requiere.**

He doesn't speak English, but Spanish.	**No habla inglés, sino español.** ***(Noh ah-blah een-glehs, see-noh ehs-pah-nyohl)***
He is not wearing a green shirt, but a blue one.	**No usa camisa verde, sino azul.** ***(Noh oo-sah kah-mee-sah behr-deh, see-noh ah-sool)***
I don't like to study, but (rather) to go to the theater.	**No me gusta estudiar, sino ir al teatro.** ***(Noh meh goos-tah ehs-too-dee-ahr, see-noh eer ahl teh-ah-troh)***

Chapter Thirty-eight / Capítulo treinta y ocho

Verbs / Verbos

Verbs are to a sentence what the spinal cord is to the body. Verbs give structure to a sentence because they tell us what is being done and when it is being done; for example: I *talk* to the nurse (present), I *talked* to the nurse (past), I *will talk* to the nurse (future).

Los verbos son para una oración lo que la espina dorsal es para el cuerpo. Los verbos dan estructura a una oración al indicar qué es lo que se está haciendo y cuándo se está haciendo; por ejemplo: Yo *hablo* con la enfermera (presente), Yo *hablé* con la enfermera ayer (pasado), Yo *hablaré* con la enfermera mañana (futuro).

Regular verbs end in **-ar, -er,** or **-ir** in Spanish. They are easy to conjugate because you usually take the stem of the verb and add the endings: **o, as, a, amos, an.** See Table 38–1.

Los verbos regulares tienen la terminación *-ar, -er, o -ir* en español. Son fáciles de conjugarse ya que usualmente se toma la raíz del verbo y se le agrega la terminación: *o, as, a, amos, -an.* Vea la Tabla 38–1.

TABLE 38–1 Regular Verb / TABLA 38–1 Verbo regular

Verb	Stem	Endings	Persons
to live **vivir** *(bee-beer)*	viv	o	yo vivo *(yoh bee-boh)*
		es	tú vives *(too bee-behs)*
		e	el/ella vive *(ehl/eh-yah bee-beh)*
		imos	nosotros vivimos *(noh-soh-trohs bee-bee-mohs)*
		en	ellos/ellas viven *(eh-yohs/eh-yahs bee-behn)*

to auscultate	**auscultar**	*(ah-oos-kool-tahr)*
to be born	**nacer**	*(nah-sehr)*
to become ill	**enfermar**	*(ehn-fehr-mahr)*
to bring near	**acercar**	*(ah-sehr-kahr)*
to call	**llamar**	*(yah-mahr)*
to die	**morir**	*(moh-reer)*
to eat	**comer**	*(koh-mehr)*
to examine	**examinar**	*(ehx-ah-mee-nahr)*
to get better	**mejorar**	*(meh-hoh-rahr)*
to heal	**sanar**	*(sah-nahr)*
to hear	**oír**	*(oh-eer)*
to hurt	**doler**	*(doh-lehr)*
to leave (behind)	**dejar**	*(deh-hahr)*
to listen	**escuchar**	*(ehs-koo-chahr)*
to live	**vivir**	*(bee-beer)*
to name	**nombrar**	*(nohm-brahr)*
to operate	**operar**	*(oh-peh-rahr)*
to palpate	**palpar**	*(pahl-pahr)*
to revise	**revisar**	*(reh-bee-sahr)*
to see	**ver**	*(behr)*
to vomit	**vomitar**	*(boh-mee-tahr)*

TABLE 38–2
Present and Past Tense

TABLA 38–2
Tiempo presente y pasado

VERB: to eat **comer** *(koh-mehr)*

	Present Tense	**Tiempo presente**
I eat	**yo como**	*(yoh koh-moh)*
you eat	**tú comes**	*(too koh-mehs)*
he/she eats	**él/ella come**	*(ehl/eh-yah koh-meh)*
we eat	**nosotros comemos**	*(noh-soh-trohs koh-meh-mohs)*
they eat	**ellos/ellas comen**	*(eh-yohs/eh-yahs koh-mehn)*
	Past Tense	**Tiempo pasado**
I ate	**yo comí**	*(yoh koh-mee)*
you ate	**tú comiste**	*(too koh-mees-teh)*
he/she ate	**él/ella comió**	*(ehl/eh-yah koh-mee-oh)*
we ate	**nosotros comimos**	*(noh-soh-trohs koh-mee-mohs)*
they ate	**ellos/ellas comieron**	*(eh-yohs/eh-yahs koh-mee-eh-rohn)*

to agree	**acordar**	*(ah-kohr-dahr)*
to bore	**aburrir**	*(ah-boo-reer)*
to come	**venir**	*(beh-neer)*
to deserve	**merecer**	*(meh-reh-sehr)*
to finish	**acabar**	*(ah-kah-bahr)*
to go out	**salir**	*(sah-leer)*
to let go	**soltar**	*(sohl-tahr)*
to need	**necesitar**	*(neh-seh-see-tahr)*
to reach	**alcanzar**	*(ahl-kahn-sahr)*
to remain	**quedar**	*(keh-dahr)*
to stop	**parar**	*(pah-rahr)*
to take out	**sacar**	*(sah-kahr)*
to walk	**caminar**	*(kah-mee-nahr)*

Personal pronouns designate who is performing the action. Many times it is not necessary to include the personal pronouns when conjugating a verb or using it in a sentence.

Los pronombres personales designan a las personas. Muchas veces no es necesario usar la persona al conjugar verbos o al usarlos en una oración.

Personal Pronouns

I	**yo**	*(yoh)*
you (*informal*)	**tú**	*(too)*
he/she/you	**él/ella/usted**	*(ehl/eh-yah/oos-tehd)*
we	**nosotros**	*(noh-soh-trohs)*
they/you (*plural*)	**ellos/ellas/ ustedes**	*(eh-yohs/eh-yahs/oos-teh-dehs)*

TO FEEL	**SENTIR**	**(SEHN-TEER)**
I feel	**siento**	*(see-ehn-toh)*
you feel	**sientes**	*(see-ehn-tehs)*
he/she feels; you feel	**siente**	*(see-ehn-teh)*
we feel	**sentimos**	*(sehn-tee-mohs)*
they feel	**sienten**	*(see-ehn-tehn)*

TO SIT DOWN	**SENTARSE**	**(SEHN-TAHR-SEH)**
I sit	**me siento**	*(meh see-ehn-toh)*
you sit	**te sientas**	*(teh see-ehn-tahs)*

he/she sits; you sit	**se sienta**	*(seh see-ehn-tah)*
we sit	**nos sentamos**	*(nohs sehn-tah-mohs)*
they sit	**se sientan**	*(seh see-ehn-tahn)*

The reflexive pronouns change the verb's action.
Los pronombres reflexivos cambian la acción del verbo.

MOVER (TO MOVE)

ACTION ON SELF	ACTION ON OBJECT
yo me muevo *(yoh meh moo-eh-boh)*	**yo muevo** *(yoh moo-eh-boh)*
tú te mueves *(too teh moo-eh-behs)*	**tú mueves** *(too moo-eh-behs)*
él/ella se mueve *(ehl/eh-yah seh moo-eh-beh)*	**él/ella mueve** *(ehl/eh-yah moo-eh-beh)*
nosotros nos movemos *(noh-soh-trohs nohs moh-beh-mohs)*	**nosotros movemos** *(noh-soh-trohs moh-beh-mohs)*
ellos/ellas se mueven *(eh-yohs/eh-yahs seh moo-eh-behn)*	**ellos/ellas mueven** *(eh-yohs/eh-yahs moo-eh-behn)*

to advise	**aconsejar**	*(ah-kohn-seh-hahr)*
to ask	**preguntar**	*(preh-goon-tahr)*
to bathe	**bañar**	*(bah-nyahr)*
to be afraid	**temer**	*(teh-mehr)*
to believe	**creer**	*(kreh-ehr)*
to boil	**hervir**	*(ehr-beer)*
to break	**romper**	*(rohm-pehr)*
to build	**construir**	*(kohns-troo-eer)*
to carry	**llevar**	*(yeh-bahr)*
to change	**cambiar**	*(kahm-bee-ahr)*
to clean	**limpiar**	*(leem-pee-ahr)*
to communicate	**comunicar**	*(koh-moo-nee-kahr)*
to complain	**quejar**	*(keh-hahr)*
to conduct	**conducir**	*(kohn-doo-seer)*
to confuse	**confundir**	*(kohn-foon-deer)*
to cook	**cocinar**	*(koh-see-nahr)*
to cover	**cubrir**	*(koo-breer)*
to cry	**llorar**	*(yoh-rahr)*

to cut	**cortar**	*(kohr-tahr)*
to deny	**negar**	*(neh-gahr)*
to destroy	**destruir**	*(dehs-troo-eer)*
to disappear	**desaparecer**	*(deh-sah-pah-reh-sehr)*
to discover, find	**descubrir**	*(dehs-koo-breer)*
to do/make	**hacer**	*(ah-sehr)*
to drink	**beber**	*(beh-behr)*
to eat breakfast	**desayunar**	*(deh-sah-yoo-nahr)*
to embrace	**abrazar**	*(ah-brah-sahr)*
to employ	**emplear**	*(ehm-pleh-ahr)*
to feel	**sentir**	*(sehn-teer)*
to fill	**llenar**	*(yeh-nahr)*
to find	**hallar**	*(ah-yahr)*
to fix	**componer**	*(kohm-poh-nehr)*
to fly	**volar**	*(boh-lahr)*
to get up, raise	**levantar**	*(leh-bahn-tahr)*
to give	**dar**	*(dahr)*
to go	**ir**	*(eer)*
to go to bed, lie down	**acostar**	*(ah-kohs-tahr)*
to have	**haber**	*(ah-behr)*
to hunt	**cazar**	*(kah-sahr)*
to joke, kid	**bromear**	*(broh-meh-ahr)*
to jump	**saltar**	*(sahl-tahr)*
to kiss	**besar**	*(beh-sahr)*
to know	**conocer**	*(koh-noh-sehr)*
to lose	**perder**	*(pehr-dehr)*
to marry	**casar**	*(kah-sahr)*
to paint	**pintar**	*(peen-tahr)*
to point	**señalar**	*(seh-nyah-lahr)*
to promise	**prometer**	*(proh-meh-tehr)*
to receive	**recibir**	*(reh-see-beer)*
to recognize	**reconocer**	*(reh-koh-noh-sehr)*
to remember	**acordar/ recordar**	*(ah-kohr-dahr/ reh-kohr-dahr)*
to respond	**responder**	*(rehs-pohn-dehr)*
to return	**regresar/ volver**	*(reh-greh-sahr/ bohl-behr)*
to scream	**gritar**	*(gree-tahr)*
to see	**ver**	*(behr)*
to sell	**vender**	*(behn-dehr)*
to serve	**servir**	*(sehr-beer)*
to shake	**temblar**	*(tehm-blahr)*

to sit	**sentar**	*(sehn-tahr)*
to sleep	**dormir**	*(dohr-meer)*
to speak	**hablar**	*(ah-blahr)*
to start	**comenzar**	*(koh-mehn-sahr)*
to step	**pisar**	*(pee-sahr)*
to suffer	**sufrir**	*(soo-freer)*
to take	**tomar**	*(toh-mahr)*
to thank for	**agradecer**	*(ah-grah-deh-sehr)*
to try	**tratar**	*(trah-tahr)*
to turn	**voltear**	*(bohl-teh-ahr)*
to turn off	**apagar**	*(ah-pah-gahr)*
to want	**querer**	*(keh-rehr)*
to wash	**lavar**	*(lah-bahr)*
to wish	**desear**	*(deh-seh-ahr)*
to work	**trabajar**	*(trah-bah-hahr)*

TABLE 38–3
Verb Tenses

TABLA 38–3
Tiempo de los verbos

Verb	**Present Tense**	**Tiempo presente**
speak	hablar	*(ah-blahr)*
I speak	**yo hablo**	*(yoh ah-bloh)*
you speak	**tú hablas**	*(too ah-blahs)*
he/she speaks	**él/ella habla**	*(ehl/eh-yah ah-blah)*
we speak	**nosotros hablamos**	*(noh-soh-trohs ah-blah-mohs)*
they speak	**ellos/ellas hablan**	*(eh-yohs/eh-yahs ah-blahn)*
	Past Tense	**Tiempo pasado**
I spoke	**yo hablé**	*(yoh ah-bleh)*
you spoke	**tú hablaste**	*(too ah-blahs-teh)*
he/she spoke	**él/ella habló**	*(ehl/eh-yah ah-bloh)*
we spoke	**nosotros hablamos**	*(noh-soh-trohs ah-blah-mohs)*
they spoke	**ellos/ellas hablaron**	*(eh-yohs/eh-yahs ah-blah-rohn)*
	Future Tense	**Tiempo futuro**
I will speak	**yo hablaré**	*(yoh ah-blah-reh)*
you will speak	**tú hablarás**	*(too ah-blah-rahs)*
he/she will speak	**él/ella hablará**	*(ehl/eh-yah ah-blah-rah)*
we will speak	**nosotros hablaremos**	*(noh-soh-trohs ah-blah-reh-mohs)*
they will speak	**ellos/ellas hablarán**	*(eh-yohs/eh-yahs ah-blah-rahn)*

to accept	**aceptar**	*(ah-sehp-tahr)*
to activate	**activar**	*(ahk-tee-bahr)*
to administer	**administrar**	*(ahd-mee-nees-trahr)*
to authorize	**autorizar**	*(ah-oo-toh-ree-sahr)*
to beat, knock	**golpear**	*(gohl-peh-ahr)*
to bleed	**sangrar**	*(sahn-grahr)*
to conserve	**conservar**	*(kohn-sehr-bahr)*
to control	**controlar**	*(kohn-troh-lahr)*
to evaluate	**evaluar**	*(eh-bah-loo-ahr)*
to hit	**pegar**	*(peh-gahr)*
to inform	**informar**	*(een-fohr-mahr)*
to interpret	**interpretar**	*(een-tehr-preh-tahr)*
to present	**presentar**	*(preh-sehn-tahr)*
to protect	**protejer**	*(proh-teh-hehr)*
to provoke	**provocar**	*(proh-boh-kahr)*
to reduce	**reducir**	*(reh-doo-seer)*
to revise	**revisar**	*(reh-bee-sahr)*
to select	**seleccionar**	*(seh-lehk-see-oh-nahr)*
to separate	**separar**	*(seh-pah-rahr)*
to suspend	**suspender**	*(soos-pehn-dehr)*
to write	**escribir**	*(ehs-kree-beer)*

The verbs **ser** and **estar** both translate in English as *to be*, but they are not interchangeable. Both are irregular in the present and the past tense.

Los verbos *ser* y *estar* se traducen al inglés *to be*, **pero no se intercambian. Los dos verbos son irregulares en el tiempo presente y en el pasado.**

	SER	**ESTAR**
I am	**yo soy** *(yo soh-ee)*	**yo estoy** *(yoh ehs-tohy)*
you are	**usted es/tú eres** *(oos-tehd ehs/ too eh-rehs)*	**usted está/tú estás** *(oos-tehd ehs-tah/too ehs-tahs)*
he/she/it is	**él/ella/eso es** *(ehl/eh-yah/ eh-soh ehs)*	**él/ella/eso está** *(ehl/eh-yah/eh-soh ehs-tah)*
we are	**nosotros somos** *(noh-soh-trohs soh-mohs)*	**nosotros estamos** *(noh-soh-trohs ehs-tah-mohs)*

they are	**ellos/ellas son** *(eh-yohs/eh-yahs sohn)*	**ellos/ellas están** *(eh-yohs/eh-yahs ehs-tahn)*

Uses of ser — *Usos de ser*

Ser expresses a relatively permanent quality.

age:	You are old.	**Usted *es* viejo.**
characteristic:	The snow is cold.	**La nieve *es* fría.**
color:	The urine is yellow.	**La orina *es* amarilla.**
shape:	The glass is round.	**El vaso *es* redondo.**
size:	You are tall.	**Usted *es* alto.**
possession:	The pencil is mine.	**El lápiz *es* mío.**
wealth:	The man is rich.	**El hombre *es* rico.**

Ser is used with predicate nouns, pronouns, or adjectives.

He is a dentist.	**El *es* dentista**
Who am I?	**¿Quién *soy* yo?**
We are protestant.	**Nosotros *somos* protestantes.**

Ser indicates material, origin, or ownership.

material:	The needle is metal.	**La aguja *es* de metal.**
origin:	The doctor is from Texas.	**El doctor *es* de Tejas.**
ownership:	The dentures are mine.	**Las dentaduras *son* mías.**

Ser tells time.

It is one o'clock.	***Es* la una.**
It is 10 o'clock.	***Son* las diez.**

Uses of Estar — *Usos de estar*

Estar expresses location (permanent and temporary).

Dallas is in Texas. — **Dallas *está* en Tejas.**
I am in the room. — **Yo *estoy* en el cuarto.**

Estar expresses status of health.

How are you? — **¿Cómo *está* usted?**
I am fine. — ***Estoy* bien.**
We are sick. — ***Estamos* enfermos.**

Estar expresses a temporary characteristic or quality.

He is nervous. — **El *está* nervioso.**
I am ready. — ***Estoy* lista.**
You are far away. — **Usted *está* lejos.**

Unit 7

Unidad 7

Chapter Thirty-nine　　Capítulo treinta y nueve

A Cultural Perspective

Hispanic is a term often used to identify people who speak Spanish and who have Cuban, Central and South American, Mexican, or Puerto Rican backgrounds. Currently, Mexican Americans and Puerto Ricans are the two largest Hispanic groups in the United States. The movement of Hispanics into the United States seems to have occurred in phases. In 1910 many Mexicans entered the United States with permanent visas. In the early 1940s, the "Bracero" program (source of cheap agricultural labor) increased the Mexican population in the United States. During the 1950s Puerto Ricans were recruited to work as laborers in the United States. In the 1960s many Cubans and Latin Americans migrated to the United States in an attempt to better their social and economic status. A second influx of Cubans occurred in the early 1970s when entire families were ousted from or chose to leave communist Cuba. Living conditions in Mexico and South and Central America have fluctuated considerably over the years, forcing many people to immigrate or to settle illegally in the United States year after year. Although one can find Hispanics throughout the United States, the largest groups are in Arizona, California, Colorado, Florida, New Mexico, New York, and Texas.

As a group, Hispanics have certain similarities. They are young (median age ranges from 17 to 28 years), their median level of education ranges from 9 to 12 years, they are mostly employed in blue-collar jobs (well over 50%), and their median annual income is about $15,000. If one relates the socioeconomic conditions of a group to their level of health, then one can agree that Hispanics (with the preceding statistics), in general, are at risk for health problems. This risk doubles when Hispanics are not able to communicate with health care providers due to language barriers. The use of interpreters is not uncommon. In major university hospitals, where Hispanic patient populations are large, bilingual staff members often act as interpreters. Very often, hospitals refuse to hire interpreters who would facilitate communication; instead, housekeepers,

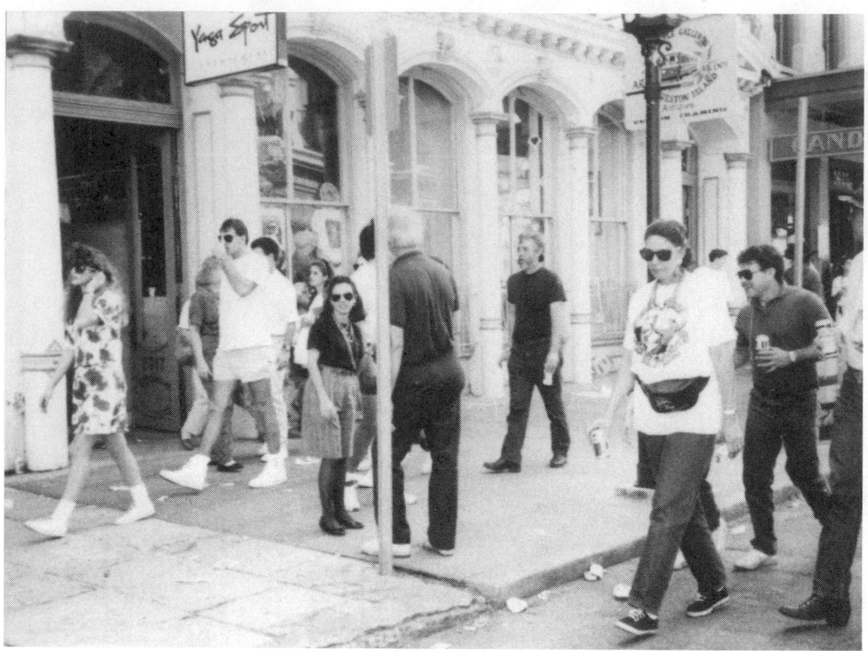

Figure 39–1 Hispanics have many similar characteristics.

orderlies, physical plant, or transportation employees are burdened with this additional task. The medical staff who are not able to communicate in Spanish are at a disadvantage because they cannot verify whether the information that the patient is receiving is being translated adequately.

Hispanics have lived in the United States for decades. Many members of the third and fourth generations may not have retained Spanish as their primary language. However, in large cities where Hispanics concentrate, one commonality is evident: the use of Spanish, especially among teenagers and the elderly, is still practiced. Perhaps the current use of Spanish among the young relates to a new influx of Hispanic immigrants.

Hispanics tend to cluster, as do other cultural groups who share similar ethnicity, socioeconomic level, or belief systems. Because Hispanics value camaraderie and rely on familiar support systems, they frequently gather in large numbers when one of the members is sick in the hospital. This is often annoying to staff who have to complete myriads of documents, deal with multiple services, and do not understand why so many people insist on visiting the patient even when the crisis is over. Determining the severity of the condition of the patient, reviewing the hospital's policies and procedures, and identifying the benefits/liabilities of having family members present, may help to alleviate the medical staff's confusion caused by the many visitors.

The concept of health varies in many cultures. For most Hispanics being healthy means being free from pain. It also means being able to perform all daily activities. Many think that health is a gift from God and that there is very little that one can do to avoid illness. In all cultures, behavior is learned; and as it is shared through the years, it tends to change and new behaviors are added. For some Hispanics, being sick is viewed as a punishment. Penance may include going to confession, making a long pilgrimage to a church, wearing a habit for a prescribed number of days, or keeping a **promesa** or **mandas** (*promise*) made to a patron saint. Some people kneel and "walk" on their knees several blocks to church, thus helping the illness disappear.

Music plays an important role in Hispanic lives. One often hears popular ballads while traveling through Hispanic communities. It is not unusual for hospitalized patients to ask to see a favorite Spanish program.

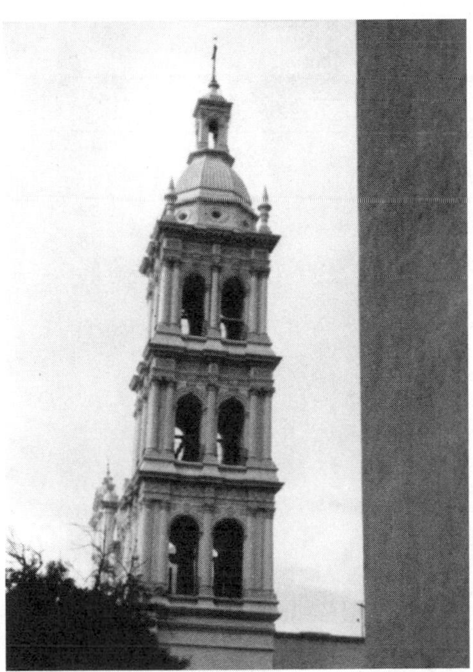

Figure 39–2 Consideration must be given to the cultural and religious habits of people.

Again, this is not only observed in the elder population, but also in the younger population (teenagers).

Catholicism is predominant in many Hispanic groups. However, other religions such as Baptist, Jehovah's Witness, and Methodist claim to have large numbers of Hispanic members. It is not unusual to see that some patients may take candles (**veladoras**) or their favorite religious medals to the hospital. Understanding the importance of religion (for any ethnic group) will facilitate the care and treatment of the patient.

Vibrant colors in clothes, jewelry, and make-up are trademarks of Hispanics. These, along with what appear to be loud intonations, rapid speech, and hand movements, often confuse medical staff who may not be aware of Hispanic cultural characteristics. It is extremely important to assess the patient's cultural background before diagnosing the unusual behavior or mannerisms.

Hospital food, traditionally, would not win any awards. Besides not being hot (temperature) it is often too bland (not enough condiments/ spices) for Hispanic (and many other) tastes. It is important to communicate the availability of foods to the patient. It is also helpful to assist in

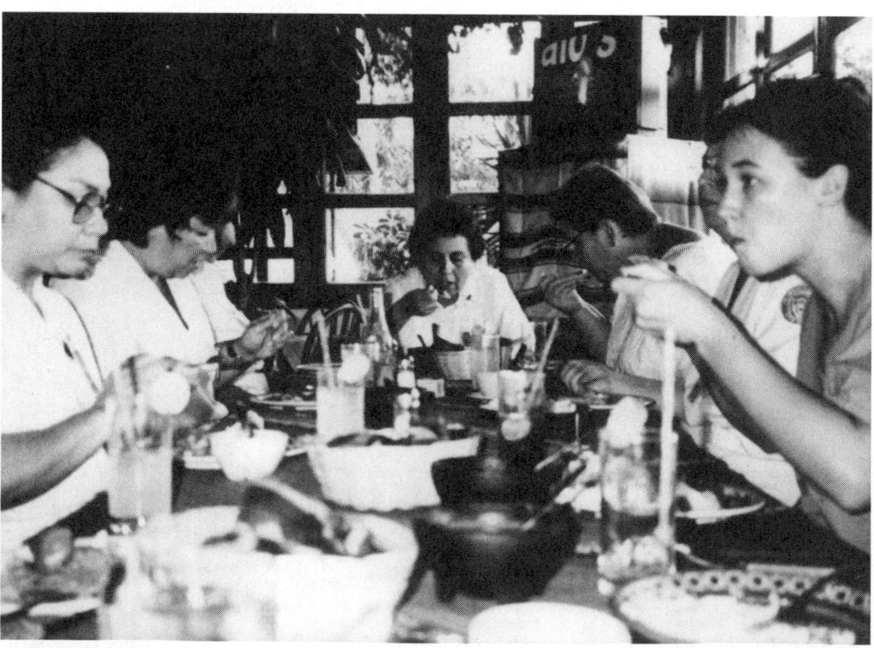

Figure 39–3 Patients have food likes and dislikes. It is necessary to assess cultural tendencies.

the decision-making process when selecting a menu. Often the patient's religion, ethnicity, age, and illness make it difficult to choose a menu.

Acculturation to a different group is often difficult. While parents may resent having to change, young members of an ethnic group may embrace the new groups' ideologies and way of living. This often causes stress within the family and outside the family. Careful assessment must be made by medical staff who may not be aware of the degree of acculturation of Hispanic patients. This is a great opportunity to provide anticipatory guidance and teaching related to assimilation to a new group.

REFERENCES

Andrews, M. A. & Boyle, J. S. (1995). *Transcultural Concepts in Nursing Care.* (2nd. ed.). Philadelphia: Lippincott.

Bonuck, K. & Arno, P. (1992). What is access and what does it mean for nursing? *Scholarly Inquiry for Nursing Practice.* 6(3), 211–216.

Clark, M. J. (1999). *Nursing in the Community.* (3rd. ed.). Stamford, Connecticut: Appleton & Lange.

Clemon-Stone, S. A., Eigsti, D. G., & McGuire, S. L. (1991). *Comprehensive Family and Community Health Nursing* (3rd. ed.). New York: Mosby Year Book, Inc.

Dancy, B. & Logan, B. (1994). In Bolander, V. (ed.). *Sorensen and Luckmann's Basic Nursing* (3rd. ed.). Culture and Ethnicity. Philadelphia: W. B. Saunders Co., 331–342.

Friedman, M. M. (1998). *Family Nursing: Theory and Practice* (4th. ed.). East Norwalk, Connecticut: Appleton & Lange.

Giger, J. N. & Davidhizar, R. E. (1995). *Transcultural Nursing: Assessment and Intervention.* St. Louis: Mosby.

Lester, M. A. (1998). Cultural competence: a nursing dialogue. *American Journal of Nursing.* 98:9, pp. 26–33.

Purnell, L. D. & Paulanka, B. J. (1998). *Transcultural Health Care.* Philadelphia: F. A. Davis Company.

Rooda, L. A. (1993). Knowledge and attitudes of nurses towards culturally different patients: Implications for nursing education. *Journal of Nursing Education.* 32(5). 209–213.

Santiago, J. M. (1993). Taking issue. *Hospital and Community Psychiatry.* 44(7). 613.

Smith, C. M. & Maurer, F. A. (1995). *Community Health Nursing, Theory and Practice.* Philadelphia: W. B. Saunders Company.

Spector, R. E. (1996). *Cultural Diversity in Health and Illness.* (4th. ed.). Stamford, Connecticut: Appleton & Lange.

Stewart, M. (1998). Nurses need to strengthen cultural competence for the next century to ensure quality patient care. *American Nurse.* 30, 1, pp. 26–27, January.

United States Department of Health and Human Services (1991). Health status of minorities and low-income groups (3rd. ed.). Washington, D.C.: U.S. Government Printing Office.

U.S. Census Bureau: Census Data, Washington, D.C. U.S. Government Printing Office, 1990.

Williams, S. R. (1999). *Essentials of Nutrition and Diet Therapy.* (7th. ed.). St. Louis: Mosby.

Zuckerman, M. (1990). Some dubious premises in research and theory on racial differences: Scientific, social and ethical issues. American Psychologist, 45(19), 1297–1303.

Chapter Forty | Capítulo cuarenta

Home Cures and Popular Beliefs

Data about many cultures have been collected by anthropologists, nursing scientists, sociologists, psychologists, and others with interest in studying behaviors exhibited by different ethnic groups. Since behaviors are learned from generation to generation, it is beneficial to understand a patient's cultural background in order to understand his or her behavior.

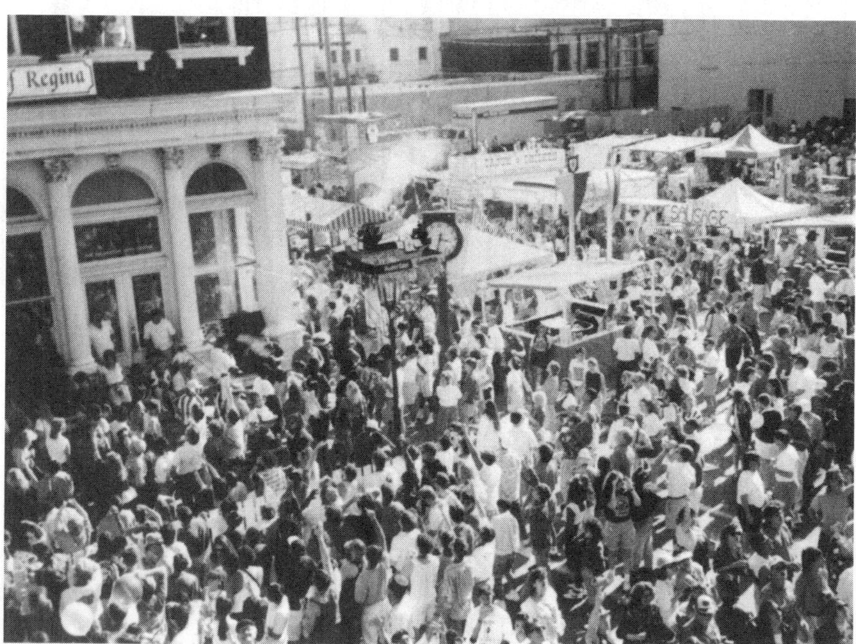

Figure 40–1 People in a society have diverse customs and beliefs.

In times of crisis or physical distress a patient may revert to treatment modalities used during childhood. It is not uncommon during the initial interview to find that Hispanic patients favor a variety of home treatment modalities even when complying with Western medical regimes. It is imperative that the health care provider be nonjudgmental regarding these differences in beliefs and practices because it is the patient's perception of the illness that governs his or her behavior. Failure to assess the use of treatment modalities may result in frustration both for the patient and for the health care provider. It is also important not to stereotype patients, even within a specific culture. Ideally, each patient must be viewed as a unique individual with care plans that incorporate his or her beliefs and practices.

For years, medicinal plants have been used throughout the world. According to Dr. Hero Gali (1985) there are over 20,000 plants being used for medicinal purposes in Mexico. It is not difficult to find **hierberías** in open market places where vendors are allowed to recommend dried herbs that have been successful in alleviating certain ailments. Along the Texas–Mexico border, in rural areas, and in larger cities where a high concentra-

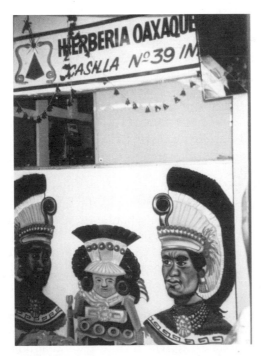

Figure 40–2 Home remedies have been used for centuries.

tion of Mexican Americans is found, many (especially the older generations) still tend to shop at **hierberías** and have specific prescriptions made for their ailments. Popular among Hispanics is the use of herbal teas. Chamomile (**manzanilla**), mint (**hierba buena**), eucalyptus (**eucalipto**), ginger (**jengibre**), vanilla (**vainilla**), and olive (**olivo**) are often used for common ailments such as colic, colds, cough, and indigestion.

Some folk medicine beliefs and practices can be traced to ancient Greece. These beliefs were elaborated on by the Arabs and brought to Spain by the Moslems. Eventually, those beliefs were transmitted to America at the time of the Spanish conquest of Mexico. The combination of Spanish–Catholic tradition in Mexico with the Indian heritage (Aztecs, Mayans, etc.) yields the practice of **curanderismo** as it is observed today.

Expensive and time-consuming treatment is avoided by the lower socioeconomic groups when they visit a **curandero.** The **curandero** successfully integrates concepts and practices from diverse sources. He combines psycho-therapeutic skills and ritualistic herbal remedies. Many of the **curandero's** tools are religious in nature. In his "office" he usually has a large number of crosses and pictures of saints. He centers his thinking about illness on Christ and encourages patients to feel that they are doing what Christ did: suffer on earth. The **curandero** is usually sought for minor illnesses and chronic untreatable conditions that are feared to be supernatural. He is also seen for febrile conditions in children, convulsions, apathy, and disruptive behavior. Most **curanderos** do not charge for their services but they accept donations. The practitioners of **curanderismo** offer no barriers to care and have no waiting lists. This makes it attractive to many patients who do not have insurance or who find the health care system inaccessible. Other Hispanic groups rely on health care providers similar to the **curandero. Sobadoras** (female healers) are very popular in Puerto Rico. They use oils (**aceite de culebra, aceite de olivo**) in their treatment of patients. The **sobadoras** combine their listening skills with massage skills to assist the patient.

Acculturation and assimilation of persons of Hispanic origin has been slowed by various social mechanisms of the larger society that tend to keep massive numbers of people separate (in vast housing projects) and by a tendency on their part to separate themselves from the larger community by living in **barrios.** This isolation is not unusual. People tend to group because they find commonalities, acceptance, and comfort within the group. This sociocultural isolation results in the preservation of many folk beliefs of Spanish origin.

Prominent among health disease concepts are **mal de ojo** (*evil eye*), **empacho** (*surfeit/indulgence*), and **susto** (*fright*).

Mal de ojo is an illness to which children and adults are susceptible. When a person with stronger vision looks at another admiringly, but does

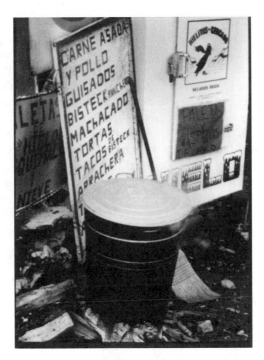

Figure 40–3 Many customs prevail through the years. It is important to assess a patient's degree of acculturation and assimilation.

not touch him, he or she gives the person **mal de ojo.** Symptoms of fever, headaches, restlessness, crying, and vomiting are most commonly reported. When the stronger vision person actually touches the other one the symptoms disappear. When the person is not available to touch the other, the treatment of choice is "sweeping." To sweep (**barrer**) means both to pass an unbroken raw egg over the body without touching, or actually rub the body with the egg. Prayers are recited during the sweeping. After the sweeping, to extract the fever from the patient's body and transmit it to the egg, the egg is broken and placed in a bowl of water. The bowl is placed under the head of the patient's bed. The egg is said to absorb the fever and, by morning, it should be "cooked." The cooked egg is a sign that the patient had **ojo.**

Empacho is caused by a bolus of poorly digested or uncooked food sticking to the wall of the stomach. This is a disease primarily seen in children and attributed to overeating foods such as bread and bananas. Most common symptoms are lack of appetite, stomachache, diarrhea, and vomiting. Other reported symptoms include fever, crying, and restlessness in children. The treatment includes rubbing the stomach and rubbing and pinching the back. In order to dislodge the bolus, grasp a fold of skin on the back, pull it up, and release it. This procedure is done with both hands at least three times before breakfast. The patient is then administered a tea made with **estafiate** (larkspur) or **manzanilla** (chamomile). It is important to determine how long the child has been ill and what procedures have been performed. There could be intestinal blockage that may lead to toxic megacolon if medical attention is not sought.

Susto is the result of a traumatic experience that may be anything from a simple scare at night (lightning, loud noises) to witnessing an accident. Children are more susceptible than adults, but groups of individuals may develop symptoms at the same time. The most common symptom of **susto** is sleeping. Also, anorexia, insomnia, hallucinations, or weakness often accompany this condition. Treatment of **susto** involves sweeping. The sweeping of the body is generally done by the healer (usually a grandmother) with orange or lemon tree branches or with palm leaves while reciting or chanting prayers. An herbal tea is usually administered after the sweeping.

Hispanics tend to use the "hot and cold" theory of disease. This theory is often used to explain the cause of an ailment and to choose a form of treatment. When a person has a "hot" disease he or she may refuse to eat hot foods, medicines, or hot teas because he or she may think that the condition will worsen. Cold treatments and cold beverages are assumed to be beneficial in this case. On the other hand, when a person has a "cold" disease, he or she may ingest hot teas to alleviate his or her symptoms. Hot and cold diseases are often labeled differently by different cultural groups (Hispanic, Chinese, etc.). It is pertinent to ask a patient, during the history-taking phase of the visit, if he or she has determined to what category a certain disease belongs.

There is a widespread fatalistic attitude among many Hispanics, specifically those in the low-income, low-education segments. Because of a lack of education related to health promotion and health prevention, many Hispanics leave their health status "up to God." Many also believe that the hospital is the place where one goes to die. Mr. T., one of our diabetic patients, believed that his son was "murdered" by doctors who gave him too much medicine and thus refused to go to the hospital when he needed help.

Many Hispanics may secure health information and treatment from many sources including relatives, magazines, radio, religion, and tradition. Given a choice, they often consult medical doctors but they may be ingesting their own home remedies. It is appropriate to ask what treatment modalities they have been using prior to the visit. It is important to respect cultural and value differences, and when possible, attempt to incorporate these treatments in the plan of care. Perhaps, if this is done, patient compliance with medical treatment will increase.

REFERENCES

Clark, M. J. (1999). *Nursing in the Community.* (3rd. ed). Connecticut: Appleton & Lange.

Ellis J. R. & Hartley, C. L. (1992). *Nursing in Today's World.* (4th. ed.). New York: J. B. Lippincott Company.

Friedman, M. M. (1998). *Family Nursing: Theory and Practice.* (4th. ed.). East Norwalk, Connecticut: Appleton & Lange.

Gali, H. (1985). *Las Hierbas del Indio.* Mexico: Gomez Gomez Hnos.

Giger, J. N. & Davidhizar, R. E. (1995). *Transcultural Nursing: Assessment and Intervention.* St. Louis: Mosby.

Purnell, L. D. & Paulanka, B. J. (1998). *Transcultural Health Care.* Philadelphia: F. A. Davis Company.

Spector, R. E. (1996). *Cultural Diversity in Health and Illness.* (4th. ed.). Connecticut: Appleton & Lange.

Torres, E. (1989a). *Green Medicine.* Kingsville: Nieves Press.

Torres, E. (1989b). *The Folk Healer.* Kingsville: Nieves Press.

Phrase and Sentence Index

A bowel movement.
Hacer del baño.
(Ah-sehr dehl bah-nyoh)

A friend of theirs.
Un amigo de ellos.
(Oon ah-mee-goh deh eh-yohs)

A nurse will see you.
Una enfermera la atenderá.
(Ooh-nah ehn-fehr-meh-rah lah ah-tehn-deh-rah)
Un enfermero lo atenderá.
(Oon ehn-fehr-meh-roh loh ah-tehn-deh-rah)

A standard schedule is used.
Se usa un horario estándar.
(Seh oo-sah oon oh-rah-ree-oh ehs-tahn-dahr)

A standard procedure is used.
Se usa un procedimiento estándar.
(Seh oo-sah oon proh-seh-dee-mee-ehn-toh ehs-tahn-dahr)

A virus known as HIV . . .
El virus causal del SIDA se conoce cómo VIH . . .
(Ehl bee-roos kah-oo-sahl dehl see-dah seh koh-noh-seh koh-moh VIH)

About 31% of infected individuals will develop AIDS within six to seven years.
Cerca del 31 por ciento de individuos infectados desarrollan SIDA dentro de seis a siete años.
(Sehr-kah dehl treh-een-tah ee oon pohr-see-ehn-toh deh een-dee-bee-doo-ohs een-fehk-tah-dohs deh-sah-roh-yahn see-dah dehn-troh deh seh-ees ah see-eh-teh ah-nyohs)

About 85% of AIDS patients have had one or both . . .
Cerca del 85 por ciento de pacientes con SIDA han tenido una o ambas. . .
(Sehr-kah dehl oh-chehn-tah ee seen-koh pohr see-ehn-toh deh pah-see-ehn-tehs kohn see-dah ahn teh-nee-doh oo-nah oh ahm-bahs)

About 99 degrees today.
Cerca de noventa y nueve grados hoy.
(Sehr-kah deh noh-behn-tah ee noo-eh-beh grah-dohs oh-ee)

About your baby.
En cuanto a su bebé.
(Ehn koo-ahn-toh ah soo beh-beh)

According to . . .
De acuerdo con . . .
(Deh ah-koo-ehr-doh kohn)

Activities are part of the plan.
Las actividades son parte del plan.
(Lahs ahk-tee-bee-dah-dehs sohn pahr-teh dehl plahn)

After meals.
Después de las comidas.
(Dehs-poo-ehs deh lahs koh-mee-dahs)

After you finish brushing, we will practice flossing.
Después de terminar de cepillar practicaremos usando el hilo dental.
(Dehs-poo-ehs deh tehr-mee-nahr deh seh-pee-yahr prahk-tee-kah-reh-mohs oo-sahn-doh ehl ee-loh dehn-tahl)

Again.
Otra vez.
(Oh-trah behs)

AIDS has a high fatality rate approaching 100%.
El SIDA tiene una tasa cercana al 100 por ciento de mortalidad.
(Ehl see-dah tee-eh-neh oo-nah tah-sah sehr-kah-nah ahl see-ehn pohr-see-ehn-toh deh mohr-tah-lee-dahd)

All of a sudden . . .
De golpe . . .
(Deh gohl-peh)

Almost always the technician comes at six in the morning.
Casi siempre el técnico viene a las seis de la mañana.
(Kah-see see-ehm-preh ehl tehk-nee-koh bee-eh-neh ah lahs seh-ees deh lah mah-nyah-nah)

Also, I have a headache.
También, tengo dolor de cabeza.
(Tahm-bee-ehn, tehn-goh doh-lohr deh kah-beh-sah)

Always!
¡Siempre!
(See-ehm-preh)

Among the vegetables that we serve are . . .
Entre los vegetales/verduras que servimos hay . . .
(Ehn-treh lohs beh-heh-tah-lehs/behr-doo-rahs keh sehr-bee-mohs ah-ee)

And how old are you?
¿Y cuántos años tiene?
(Ee koo-ahn-tohs ah-nyohs tee-eh-neh)

Another for a serology test.
Otro para una prueba serológica.
(Oh-troh pah-rah oo-nah proo-eh-bah seh-roh-loh-hee-kah)

Answer "yes" or "no."
Conteste "sí" o "no."
(Kohn-tehs-teh "see" oh "noh")

Anything else?
¿Alguna otra cosa?
(Ahl-goo-nah oh-trah koh-sah)

Are there elevators?
¿Hay elevadores?
(Ah-ee eh-leh-bah-doh-rehs)

Are there ramps?
¿Hay rampas?
(Ah-ee rahm-pahs)

Are you a housewife?
¿Es ama de casa?
(Ehs ah-mah deh kah-sah)

Are you a widow/widower?
¿Es usted viuda(o)?
(Ehs oos-tehd bee-oo-dah[doh])

Are you allergic to anything?
¿Es alérgico a alguna cosa?
(Ehs ah-lehr-hee-koh ah ahl-goo-nah koh-sah)

Are you allergic to drugs?
¿Es alérgico a drogas?
(Ehs ah-lehr-hee-koh ah droh-gahs)

Are you allergic to foods?
¿Es alérgico a comidas?
(Ehs ah-lehr-hee-koh ah koh-mee-dahs)

Are you allergic to plants?
¿Es alérgico a plantas?
(Ehs ah-lehr-hee-koh ah plahn-tahs)

Are you bleeding?
¿Está sangrando?
(Ehs-tah sahn-grahn-doh)

Are you cold?
¿Tiene frío?
(Tee-eh-neh free-oh)

Are you comfortable?
¿Está cómoda?
(Ehs-tah koh-moh-dah)

Are you constipated?
¿Está estreñido?
(Ehs-tah ehs-treh-nyee-doh)

Are you diabetic?
¿Es diabética?
(Ehs dee-ah-beh-tee-kah)

Are you divorced?
¿Es usted divorciado(a)?
(Ehs oos-tehd dee-bohr-see-ah doh[dah])

Are you dizzy?
¿Tiene mareos?
(Tee-eh-neh mah-reh-ohs)

Are you employed?
¿Trabaja usted?
(Trah-bah-hah oos-tehd)

Are you feeling a contraction?
¿Está sintiendo una contracción?
(Ehs-tah seen-tee-ehn-doh oo-nah kohn-trahk-see-ohn)

Are you from this area?
¿Es usted de esta área?
(Ehs oos-tehd deh ehs-tah ah-reah)

Are you having problems breathing?
¿Tiene problemas al respirar?
(Tee-eh-neh proh-bleh-mahs ahl rehs-pee-rahr)

Are you hot?
¿Tiene calor?
(Tee-eh-neh kah-lohr)

Are you hungry?
¿Tiene hambre?
(Tee-eh-neh ahm-breh)

Are you hurting?
¿Tiene dolor?
(Tee-eh-neh doh-lohr)

Are you in a hurry?
¿Tiene prisa?
(Tee-eh-neh pree-sah)

Are you mad because you are going to O.T.?
¿Está enojado porque va a O.T.?
(Ehs-tah eh-noh-hah-doh pohr-keh bah ah O.T.)

Are you married?
¿Está casada?
(Ehs-tah kah-sah-dah)

Are you nauseated?
¿Está nauseado?/¿Tiene náuseas?
(Ehs-tah nah-oo-seh-ah-doh/Tee-eh-neh nah-oo-seh-ahs)

Are you okay?
¿Está bien?/¿Se siente bien?
(Ehs-tah bee-ehn/Seh see-ehn-teh bee-ehn)

Are you on vacation?
¿Está de vacaciones?
(Ehs-tah deh bah-kah-see-oh-nehs)

Are you pregnant?
¿Está embarazada?
(Ehs-tah ehm-bah-rah-sah-dah)

Are you related?
¿Es pariente?
(Ehs pah-ree-ehn-teh)

Are you single?
¿Es usted soltero(a)?
(Ehs oos-tehd sohl-teh-roh[rah])

Are you sleepy?
¿Tiene sueño?
(Tee-eh-neh soo-eh-nyoh)

Are you taking antidepressants?
¿Está tomando antidepresivos?
(Ehs-tah toh-mahn-doh ahn-tee-deh-preh-see-bohs)

Are you taking any medications?
¿Está tomando algunas medicinas?
(Ehs-tah toh-mahn-doh ahl-goo-nahs meh-dee-see-nahs)

Are you taking nitroglycerin?
¿Está tomando nitroglicerina?
(Ehs-tah toh-mahn-doh nee-troh-glee-seh-ree-nah)

Are you taking steroids?
¿Está tomando esteroides?
(Ehs-tah toh-mahn-doh ehs-teh-roh-ee-dehs)

Are you taking your medicines?
¿Está tomando sus medicinas?
(Ehs-tah toh-mahn-doh soos meh-dee-see-nahs)

Are you the patient?
¿Es usted el/la paciente?
(Ehs oos-tehd ehl/lah pah-see-ehn-teh)

Are you thirsty?
¿Tiene sed?
(Tee-eh-neh sehd)

Are you under a doctor's care?
¿Está bajo el cuidado de un doctor?
(Ehs-tah bah-hoh ehl koo-ee-dah-doh deh oon dohk-tohr)

Are you working also?
¿Trabaja también?
(Trah-bah-hah tahm-bee-ehn)

Are your teeth sensitive to pain?
¿Son los dientes sensitivos al dolor?
(Sohn lohs dee-ehn-tehs sehn-see-tee-bohs ahl doh-lohr)

Are your teeth sensitive to cold?
¿Tiene sensibilidad al frio?
(Tee-eh-neh sehn-see-bee-lee-dahd ahl free-oh)

Are your teeth sensitive to shock?
¿Tiene sensibilidad a toques?
(Tee-eh-neh sehn-see-bee-lee-dahd ah toh-kehs)

Arm and hand.
Brazo y mano.
(Brah-soh ee mah-noh)

As a whole . . .
En conjunto . . ./En todo . . .
(Ehn kohn-hoon-toh/Ehn toh-doh)

As soon as you can, go to your doctor.
En cuanto pueda acuda a su médico.
(Ehn koo-ahn-toh poo-eh-dah ah-koo-dah ah soo meh-dee-koh)

Ask for unit Six A.
Pregunte por la unidad Seis A.
(Preh-goon-teh pohr lah oo-nee-dahd Seh-ees Ah)

Ask the receptionist for a number.
Pida un número a la recepcionista.
(Pee-dah oon noo-meh-roh ah lah reh-sehp-see-ohn-ees-tah)

At bedtime.
Al acostarse./A la hora de dormir.
(Ahl ah-kohs-tahr-seh/Ah lah oh-rah deh dohr-meer)

At eleven thirty.
A las once y media.
(Ah lahs ohn-seh ee meh-dee-ah)

At five P.M.
A las cinco de la tarde.
(Ah lahs seen-koh deh lah tahr-deh)

At least 30 minutes!
¡Al menos treinta minutos!
(Ahl meh-nohs treh-een-tah mee-noo-tohs)

At the same time, we take the X-rays.
Al mismo tiempo, tomamos los rayos X.
(Ahl mees-moh tee-ehm-poh, toh-mah-mohs lohs rah-yohs eh-kees)

At what hospital have you been treated?
¿En qué hospital lo han tratado?
(Ehn keh ohs-pee-tahl loh ahn trah-tah-doh?

At what time?
¿A qué hora?
(Ah keh oh-rah)

At what time do they close?
¿A qué hora cierran?
(Ah keh oh-rah see-eh-rahn)

At what time do you get up?
¿A qué hora se levanta?
(Ah keh oh-rah seh leh-bahn-tah)

At what time do you go to bed?
¿A qué hora se acuesta?
(Ah keh oh-rah seh ah-koo-ehs-tah)

At what time do you go to sleep?
¿A qué hora te acuestas a dormir?
(Ah keh oh-rah teh ah-koo-ehs-tahs ah dohr-meer)

Austin is at the center of the state.
Austin está en el centro del estado.
(Aoos-teen ehs-tah ehn ehl sehn-troh dehl ehs-tah-doh)

Avoid sunlight.
Evite asolearse/los rayos del sol.
(Eh-bee-teh ah-soh-leh-ahr-seh/lohs rah-yohs dehl sohl)

Back pain?
¿Dolor de espalda?
(Doh-lohr deh ehs-pahl-dah)

Backward.
Atrás.
(Ah-trahs)

Bad breath?
¿Mal aliento?
(Mahl ah-lee-ehn-toh)

Bathe him every day.
Báñelo diariamente.
(Bah-nyeh-loh dee-ah-ree-ah-mehn-teh)

Be patient!
¡Tenga paciencia!
(Tehn-gah pah-see-ehn-see-ah)

Be still!
¡Quieto!
(Kee-eh-toh)

Before meals.
Antes de las comidas.
(Ahn-tehs deh lahs koh-mee-dahs)

Bend!
¡Doble!
(Doh-bleh)

Bend it.
Dóblala.
(Doh-blah-lah)

Bend over!
¡Agáchese!
(Ah-gah-cheh-seh)

Bend the elbow.
Doble el codo.
(Doh-bleh ehl koh-doh)

Bend the wrist.
Doble la muñeca.
(Doh-bleh lah moo-nyeh-kah)

Bend your hip.
Dobla tu cadera.
(Doh-blah too kah-deh-rah)

Bend your knees!
¡Doble las piernas!
(Doh-bleh lahs pee-ehr-nahs)

Bend your shoulder.
Dobla tu hombro.
(Doh-blah too ohm-broh)

Bend your toes.
Dobla tus dedos.
(Doh-blah toos deh-dohs)

Besides your cholesterol, are there any other medical problems?
Además de su colesterol, ¿tiene otros problemas médicos?
(Ah-deh-mahs deh soo koh-lehs-teh-rohl, tee-eh-neh oh-throhs proh-bleh-mahs meh-dee-kohs)

Bite!
¡Muerda!
(Moo-ehr-dah)

Blood banks and other centers use sterile equipment and disposable needles.
Los bancos de sangre y otros centros usan equipos estériles y agujas desechables.
(Lohs bahn-kohs deh sahn-greh ee oh-trohs sehn-trohs oo-sahn eh-kee-pohs ehs-teh-ree-lehs ee ah-goo-hahs deh-seh-chah-blehs)

Boil the water he drinks.
Hierva el agua que toma.
(Ee-ehr-bah ehl ah-goo-ah keh toh-mah)

Breast feed or give bottle every three hours.
Déle pecho o biberón cada tres horas.
(Deh-leh peh-choh oh bee-beh-rohn kah-dah trehs oh-rahs)

Breathe, deep!
¡Respire, hondo/profundo!
(Rehs-pee-reh oon-doh/proh-foon-doh)

Breathe deep; let it out slowly.
Respira hondo; déjalo ir despacio.
(Rehs-pee-rah oon-doh; deh-hah-loh eer dehs-pah-see-oh)

Breathe in!
¡Respire!
(Rehs-pee-reh)

Breathe out!
¡Exhale!/¡Respire!
(Ehx-ah-leh/Rehs-pee-reh)

Breathe regularly.
Respire regular/normal.
(Rehs-pee-reh reh-goo-lahr/nohr-mahl)

Breathe through the mouth.
Respire por la boca.
(Rehs-pee-reh pohr lah boh-kah)

Brush your teeth!
¡Cepille los dientes!
(Seh-pee-yeh lohs dee-ehn-tehs)

But I don't have a pencil.
Pero no tengo un lápiz.
(Peh-roh noh tehn-goh oon lah-pees)

But we will give you something to drink.
Pero le daremos algo que tomar.
(Peh-roh leh dah-reh-mohs ahl-goh keh toh-mahr)

Buzzing in the ears . . .
Zumbido en los oídos . . .
(Soom-bee-doh ehn lohs oh-ee-dohs)

Call!
¡Llame!
(Yah-meh)

Call if you need help.
Llame si necesita ayuda.
(Yah-meh see neh-seh-see-tah ah-yoo-dah)

Call your friends.
Llame a sus amigos.
(Yah-meh ah soos ah-mee-gohs)

Call your physician.
Llame a su médico.
(Yah-meh ah soo meh-dee-koh)

Can casual contact cause AIDS?
¿Los contactos eventuales pueden causar SIDA?
(Lohs kohn-tahk-tohs eh-behn-too-ah-lehs poo-eh-dehn kah-oo-sahr see-dah)

Can I join you?
¿Te puedo acompañar?
(Teh poo-eh-doh ah-kohm-pah-nyahr)

Can you . . . ?
¿Puede usted . . . ?
(Poo-eh-deh oos-tehd . . .)

Can you breathe?
¿Puede respirar?
(Poo-eh-deh rehs-pee-rahr)

Can you do house chores?
¿Puede hacer los quehaceres?
(Poo-eh-deh ah-sehr lohs keh-ah-seh-rehs)

Can you feel this?
¿Siente esto?
(See-ehn-teh ehs-toh)

Can you get out of bed?
¿Puede salir de la cama?
(Poo-eh-deh sah-leer deh lah kah-mah)

Can you give me directions?
¿Me puede dar direcciones?
(Meh poo-eh-deh dahr dee-rehk-see-ohn-ehs)

Can you go with me?
¿Puede ir conmigo?
(Poo-eh-deh eer kohn-mee-goh)

Can you hear me?
¿Puede oírme?
(Poo-eh-deh oh-eer-meh)

Can you read?
¿Puede leer?
(Poo-eh-deh leh-ehr)

Can you see the blackboard well?
¿Puede ver bien la pizarra/el pizarrón?
(Poo-eh-deh behr bee-ehn lah pee-sah-rah/ ehl pee-sah-rohn)

Can you see the fire extinguisher?
¿Ve el extinguidor de fuego?
(Beh ehl ehx-teen-ghee-dohr deh foo-eh-goh)

Can you see the places that are stained?
¿Puede ver los lugares que están dañados?
(Poo-eh-deh behr lohs loo-gah-rehs keh ehs-tahn dah-nah-dohs)

Can you take off work?
¿Puede faltar al trabajo?
(Poo-eh-deh fahl-tahr ahl trah-bah-hoh)

Can you take vacation?
¿Puede tomar vacaciones?
(Poo-eh-deh toh-mahr bah-kah-see-ohn-ehs)

Can you talk?
¿Puede hablar?
(Poo-eh-deh ah-blahr)

Can you tell me what kind of diet you have?
¿Puede decirme qué dieta tiene?
(Poo-eh-deh deh-seer-meh keh dee-eh-tah tee-eh-neh)

Can you write?
¿Puede escribir usted?
(Poo-eh-deh ehs-kree-beer oos-tehd)

Can you write the name?
¿Puede escribir el nombre?
(Poo-eh-deh ehs-kree-beer ehl nohm-breh)

Car accidents?
¿Accidentes de auto?
(Ahk-see-dehn-tehs deh ah-oo-toh)

Change into this gown.
Póngase esta bata.
(Pohn-gah-seh ehs-tah bah-tah)

Choose!
¡Escoja!
(Ehs-koh-hah)

Clean your breast thoroughly.
Lave muy bien sus senos/pechos.
(Lah-beh moo-ee bee-ehn soohs seh-nohs/ peh-chohs)

Clean your nipples before you breast feed.
Lave sus pezones antes de dar pecho.
(Lah-beh soos peh-sohn-ehs ahn-tehs deh dahr peh-choh)

Close it.
Ciérrala(lo).
(See-eh-rah-lah[-loh])

Close your books, please.
Cierren sus libros, por favor.
(See-eh-rehn soos lee-brohs, pohr fah-bohr)

Close your eyes!
¡Cierre los ojos!
(See-eh-reh lohs oh-hohs)

Close your mouth!
¡Cierre la boca!
(See-eh-reh lah boh-kah)

Come in.
Pase/Entre usted.
(Pah-seh/Ehn-treh oos-tehd)

Common-law wife/husband?
¿Unión libre?
(Oo-nee-ohn lee-breh)

Cough!
¡Tose!
(Toh-seh)

Cough deeply.
Tosa más fuerte.
(Toh-sah mahs foo-ehr-teh)

Cross your arms.
Cruza tus brazos.
(Kroo-sah toos brah-sohs)

Cross your legs.
Cruza tus piernas.
(Kroo-sah toos pee-ehr-nahs)

Curve the floss into a "C."
Ponga el hilo en forma de una "C".
(Pohn-gah ehl ee-loh ehn fohr-mah deh oo-nah "C")

Dial 9, wait for the tone, then dial the number you want to call.
Marque el nueve, espere el tono, luego marque el número que quiera llamar.
(Mahr-keh ehl noo-eh-beh, ehs-peh-reh ehl toh-noh, loo-eh-goh mahr-keh ehl noo-meh-roh keh kee-eh-rah yah-mahr)

Did anyone treat you prior to our arrival?
¿Lo trató alguien antes de nuestra llegada?
(Loh trah-toh ahl-gee-ehn ahn-tehs deh noo-ehs-trah yeh-gah-dah)

Did you arrive in a wheel chair?
¿Llegó en silla de ruedas?
(Yeh-goh ehn see-yah deh roo-eh-dahs)

Did you bring a hearing aid?
¿Trajo un aparato para oír?
(Trah-hoh oon ah-pah-rah-toh pah-rah oh-eer)

Did you bring an artificial eye?
¿Trajo un ojo artificial?
(Trah-hoh oon oh-hoh ahr-tee-fee-see-ahl)

Did you bring an artificial limb?
¿Trajo un prostético?
(Trah-hoh oon prohs-teh-tee-koh)

Did you bring contact lenses?
¿Trajo lentes de contacto?
(Trah-hoh lehn-tehs deh kohn-tahk-toh)

Did you bring dentures?
¿Trajo una dentadura postiza?
(Trah-hoh oon-ah dehn-tah-doo-rah pohs-tee-sah)

Did you bring glasses?
¿Trajo anteojos/lentes?
(Trah-hoh ahn-teh-oh-hohs/lehn-tehs)

Did you bring jewelry? / cash?
¿Trajo joyas?/dinero?
(Trah-hoh hoh-yahs/dee-neh-roh)

Did you bring valuables?
¿Trajo algo de valor?
(Trah-hoh ahl-goh deh bah-lohr)

Did you call anyone?
¿Llamó a alguien?
(Yah-moh ah ahl-ghee-ehn)

Did you come by car?
¿Vino en carro?
(Bee-noh ehn kah-roh)

Did you faint?
¿Se desmayó?
(Seh dehs-mah-yoh)

Did you fall?
¿Se cayó?
(Seh kah-yoh)

Did you feel warm water run out of your vagina?
¿Sintió qué salió agua tibia de su vagina?
(Seen-tee-oh keh sah-lee-oh ah-goo-ah tee-bee-ah deh soo bah-hee-nah)

Did you have a bowel movement?
¿Hizo del baño/caca?/¿Evacuó? ¿Obró?
(Ee-soh dehl bah-nyoh/kah-kah/eh-bah-koo-oh/oh-broh)

Did you have a miscarriage?
¿Tuvo un niño nacido muerto?
(Too-boh oon nee-nyoh nah-see-doh moo-ehr-toh)

Did you have an ectopic [tubal] pregnancy?
¿Tuvo un embarazo fuera de la matriz o en las trompas?
(Too-boh oon ehm-bah-rah-soh foo-eh-rah deh lah mah-trees oh ehn lahs trohm-pahs)

Did you hit the windshield / steering wheel?
¿Se pegó contra el parabrisas/volante?
(Seh peh-goh kohn-trah ehl pah-rah-bree-sahs/boh-lahn-teh)

Did you lose consciousness?
¿Perdió el conocimiento?/¿Se desmayó?
(Pehr-dee-oh ehl koh-noh-see-mee-ehn-toh/seh dehs-mah-yoh)

Did you see blood in the urine?
¿Vió sangre en la orina?
(Bee-oh sahn-greh ehn lah oh-ree-nah)

Did you see how the accident happened?
¿Vió cómo pasó el accidente?
(Bee-oh koh-moh pah-soh ehl ahk-see-dehn-teh)

Did you take drugs or alcohol in the last 3 hours?
¿Tomó drogas o alcohol en las últimas tres horas?
(Toh-moh droh-gahs oh ahl-kohl ehn lahs ool-tee-mahs trehs oh-rahs)

Did you take medications today? When?
¿Tomó sus medicinas hoy? ¿Cuándo?
(Toh-moh soos meh-dee-see-nahs oh-ee) (Koo-ahn-do)

Did you understand?
¿Entendió?
(Ehn-tehn-dee-oh)

Did you walk?
¿Caminó?
(Kah-mee-noh)

Difficulty in swallowing . . .
Dificultad al tragar . . .
(Dee-fee-kool-tahd ahl trah-gahr)

Do all go to school?
¿Todos van a la escuela?
(Toh-dohs bahn ah lah ehs-koo-eh-lah)

Do any of your children have asthma?
¿Algunos de sus niños tienen asma?
(Ahl-goo-nohs deh soos nee-nyohs tee-eh-nehn ahs-mah)

Do any of your children have bad coordination?
¿Algunos de sus niños tienen mala coordinación?
(Ahl-goo-nohs deh soos nee-nyohs tee-eh-nehn mah-lah kohr-dee-nah-see-ohn)

Do any of your children have chickenpox?
¿Algunos de sus niños tienen viruelas?
(Ahl-goo-nohs deh soos nee-nyohs tee-eh-nehn bee-roo-eh-lahs)

Do any of your children have a cold?
¿Algunos de sus niños tienen resfriado?
(Ahl-goo-nohs deh soos nee-nyohs tee-eh-nehn rehs-free-ah-doh)

Do any of your children have convulsions?
¿Algunos de sus niños tienen convulsiones?
(Ahl-goo-nohs deh soos nee-nyohs tee-eh-nehn kohn-bool-see-ohn-ehs)

Do any of your children have delayed speech?
¿Algunos de sus niños tienen tardío el lenguaje?
(Ahl-goo-nohs deh soos nee-nyohs tee-eh-nehn tahr-dee-oh ehl lehn-goo-ah-heh)

Do any of your children have diphtheria?
¿Algunos de sus niños tienen difteria?
(Ahl-goo-nohs deh soos nee-nyohs tee-eh-nehn deef-teh-ree-ah)

Do any of your children have hearing defects?
¿Algunos de sus niños tienen defectos del oído?
(Ahl-goo-nohs deh soos nee-nyohs tee-eh-nehn deh-fehk-tohs dehl oh-ee-doh)

Do any of your children have measles?
¿Algunos de sus niños tienen sarampión?
(Ahl-goo-nohs deh soos nee-nyohs tee-eh-nehn sah-rahm-pee-ohn)

Do any of your children have mumps?
¿Algunos de sus niños tienen paperas?
(Ahl-goo-nohs deh soos nee-nyohs tee-eh-nehn pah-peh-rahs)

Do any of your children have nausea and vomiting?
¿Algunos de sus niños tienen náusea y vómitos?
(Ahl-goo-nohs deh soos nee-nyohs tee-eh-nehn nah-oo-seh-ah ee boh-mee-tohs)

Do any of your children have pneumonia?
¿Algunos de sus niños tienen pulmonía?
(Ahl-goo-nohs deh soos nee-nyohs tee-eh-nehn pool-moh-nee-ah)

Do any of your children have visual defects?
¿Algunos de sus niños tienen defectos de la vista?
(Ahl-goo-nohs deh soos nee-nyohs tee-eh-nehn deh-fehk-tohs deh lah bees-tah)

Do exercise number . . .
Hagan el ejercicio número . . .
(Ah-gahn ehl eh-hehr-see-see-oh noo-meh-roh)

Do I have time?
¿Tengo tiempo?
(Tehn-goh tee-ehm-poh)

Do not bend your leg!
¡No doble la pierna!
(Noh doh-bleh lah pee-ehr-nah)

Do not drink alcohol with this medicine.
No tome alcohol con esta medicina.
(No toh-meh ahl-kohl kohn ehs-tah meh-dee-see-nah)

Do not drive!
¡No maneje/conduzca!
(Noh mah-neh-heh/kohn-doos-kah)

Do not eat or drink anything for thirty minutes.
No coma o beba nada por treinta minutos.
(Noh koh-mah oh beh-bah nah-dah pohr treh-een-tah mee-noo-tohs)

Do not get up!
¡No se levante!
(Noh seh leh-bahn-teh)

Do not hold on to the wall.
No se agarre de la pared.
(Noh seh ah-gah-reh deh lah pah-rehd)

Do not lift more than ten pounds of weight.
No levante más de diez libras de peso.
(Noh leh-bahn-teh mahs deh dee-ehs lee-brahs deh peh-soh)

Do not move!
¡No se mueva!
(Noh seh moo-eh-bah)

Do not move the patient!
¡No muevas al paciente!
(Noh moo-eh-vahs ahl pah-see-ehn-teh)

Do not operate machinery!
¡No maneje/opere una máquina/maquinaria!
(Noh mah-neh-heh/oh-peh-reh oo-nah mah-kee-nah/mah-kee-nah-ree-ah)

Do not put on plastic panties.
No le ponga calzones de plástico.
(Noh leh pohn-gah kahl-sohn-ehs deh plahs-tee-koh)

Do they live close to you?
¿Viven cerca de usted?
(Bee-behn sehr-kah deh oos-tehd)

Do you dribble?
¿Se orina sin sentir?
(Seh oh-ree-nah seen sehn-teer)

Do you drink alcohol?
¿Toma bebidas alcohólicas?
(Toh-mah beh-bee-dahs ahl-koh-lee-kahs)

Do you drink coffee?
¿Toma café?
(Toh-mah kah-feh)

Do you eat breakfast/brunch?
¿Tomas desayuno/almuerzo?
(Toh-mahs deh-sah-yoo-noh/ahl-moo-ehr-soh)

Do you engage in protected sex?
¿Practica el sexo seguro?
(Prahk-tee-kah ehl sehx-oh seh-goo-roh)

Do you feed every three hours?
¿Le da de comer cada tres horas?
(Leh dah deh koh-mehr kah-dah trehs oh-rahs)

Do you feel all right?
¿Se siente bien?
(Seh see-ehn-teh bee-ehn)

Do you feel dizzy?
¿Se siente mareado?
(Seh see-ehn-teh mah-reh-ah-doh)

Do you feel nauseated?
¿Se siente nauseado?
(Seh see-ehn-teh nah-oo-seh-ah-doh)

Do you feel weak?
¿Se siente débil?
(Seh see-ehn-teh deh-beel)

Do you get distracted easily?
¿Te distraes fácilmente?
(Teh dees-trah-ehs fah-seel-mehn-teh)

Do you get headaches?
¿Tiene dolor de cabeza?
(Tee-eh-neh doh-lohr deh kah-beh-sah)

Do you get tired easily?
¿Se cansa con facilidad?
(Seh kahn-sah kohn fah-see-lee-dahd)

Do you have a driver's license?
¿Tiene licencia para manejar?
(Tee-eh-neh lee-sehn-see-ah pah-rah mah-neh-hahr)

Do you have a family doctor?
¿Tiene un doctor familiar?
(Tee-eh-neh oon dohk-tohr fah-mee-lee-ahr)

Do you have a hospital card?
¿Tiene usted tarjeta de hospital?
(Tee-eh-neh oos-tehd tahr-heh-tah deh ohs-pee-tahl)

Do you have a husband?
¿Tiene esposo?
(Tee-eh-neh ehs-poh-soh)

Do you have a pacemaker?
¿Tiene marcapasos?
(Tee-eh-neh mahr-kah-pah-sohs)

Do you have a phone?
¿Tiene teléfono?
(Tee-eh-neh teh-leh-foh-noh)

Do you have allergies?
¿Tiene alergias?
(Tee-eh-neh ah-lehr-hee-ahs)

Do you have asthma, high blood pressure, cardiac problems, diabetes?
¿Tiene asma, alta presión, problemas cardíacos, diabetes?
(Tee-eh-neh ahs-mah, ahl-tah preh-see-ohn, proh-bleh-mahs kahr-dee-ah-kohs, dee-ah-beh-tehs)

Do you have another car?
¿Tiene otro carro?
(Tee-eh-neh oh-troh kah-roh)

Do you have any blood disorders such as anemia or leukemia?
¿Tiene problemas de sangre como anemia o leucemia?
(Tee-eh-neh proh-bleh-mahs deh sahn-greh koh-moh ah-neh-mee-ah oh loo-seh-mee-ah)

Do you have any children?
¿Tiene niño[s]?
(Tee-eh-neh nee-nyoh[s])

Do you have any condition or disease not listed in this questionnaire?
¿Tiene problemas o condiciones de salud que no estén en este cuestionario?
(Tee-eh-neh proh-bleh-mahs oh kohn-dee-see-ohn-ehs deh sahl-ood keh noh ehs-tehn ehn ehs-teh koo-ehs-tee-oh-nah-ree-oh)

Do you have any further questions?
¿Tiene más preguntas que hacer?
(Tee-eh-neh mahs preh-goon-tahs keh ah-sehr)

Do you have any infectious disease now?
¿Tiene alguna enfermedad infecciosa ahora?
(Tee-eh-neh ahl-goo-nah ehn-fehr-meh-dahd een-fehk-see-oh-sah ah-oh-rah)

Do you have any questions?
¿Tiene preguntas?
(Tee-eh-neh preh-goon-tahs)

Do you have any symptoms: nausea, dizziness, or others?
¿Tiene algún síntoma como: náuseas, vértigo u otras?
(Tee-eh-neh ahl-goon seen-toh-mah koh-moh: nah-oo-seh-ahs, behr-tee-goh oo oh-trahs)

Do you have bad breath?
¿Tiene mal aliento?
(Tee-eh-neh mahl ah-lee-ehn-toh)

Do you have brothers / sisters?
¿Tiene hermanos/hermanas?
(Tee-eh-neh ehr-mah-nohs/ehr-mah-nahs)

Do you have cancer?
¿Tiene cáncer?
(Tee-eh-neh kahn-sehr)

Do you have car insurance?
¿Tiene seguro de carro?
(Tee-eh-neh seh-goo-roh deh kah-roh)

Do you have cardiac problems?
¿Tiene problemas cardíacos?
(Tee-eh-neh proh-bleh-mahs kahr-dee-ah-kohs)

Do you have chest pain?
¿Tiene dolor en el pecho?
(Tee-eh-neh doh-lohr ehn ehl peh-choh)

Do you have convulsions?
¿Tiene convulsiones?
(Tee-eh-neh kohn-bool-see-oh-nehs)

Do you have diabetes?
¿Tiene diabetes?
(Tee-eh-neh dee-ah-beh-tehs)

Do you have diarrhea?
¿Tiene diarrea?
(Tee-eh-neh dee-ah-reh-ah)

Do you have dizzy spells?
¿Tiene mareos?
(Tee-eh-neh mah-reh-ohs)

Do you have frequent blisters?
¿Tiene ampollas frecuentes?
(Tee-eh-neh ahm-poh-yahs freh-koo-ehn-tehs)

Do you have frequent ulcerations?
¿Tiene ulceraciones frecuentes?
(Tee-eh-neh ool-seh-rah-see-oh-nehs freh-koo-ehn-tehs)

Do you have health insurance?
¿Tiene seguro de salud?
(Tee-eh-neh seh-goo-roh deh sah-lood)

Do you have help at home?
¿Tiene ayuda en casa?
(Tee-eh-neh ah-yoo-dah ehn kah-sah)

Do you have her support in everything?
¿Tiene apoyo de ella en todo?
(Tee-eh-neh ah-poh-yoh deh eh-yah ehn toh-doh)

Do you have hesitancy?
¿Se corta el chorro de la orina?
(Seh kohr-tah ehl choh-roh deh lah oh-ree-nah)

Do you have high blood pressure?
¿Tiene la presión alta?
(Tee-eh-neh lah preh-see-ohn ahl-tah)

Do you have hospital insurance?
¿Tiene seguro de hospital?
(Tee-eh-neh seh-goo-roh deh ohs-pee-tahl)

Do you have insomnia?
¿Tiene insomnio?
(Tee-eh-neh een-sohm-nee-oh)

Do you have medical problems?
¿Tiene problemas médicos?
(Tee-eh-neh proh-bleh-mahs meh-dee-kohs)

Do you have Medicare?
¿Tiene Medicare?
(Tee-eh-neh Meh-dee-kehr)

Do you have pain?
¿Tiene dolor?
(Tee-eh-neh doh-lohr)

Do you have problems with starting to urinate?
¿Tiene dificultad para empezar a orinar?
(Tee-eh-neh dee-fee-kool-tahd pah-rah ehm-peh-sahr ah oh-ree-nahr)

Do you have problems with your teeth?
¿Tiene[s] problemas con los dientes?
(Tee-eh-neh[s] proh-bleh-mahs kohn lohs dee-ehn-tehs)

Do you have problems you want the nurse to know?
¿Tiene problemas que quiere decirle a la enfermera?
(Tee-eh-neh proh-bleh-mahs keh kee-eh-reh deh-seer-leh ah lah ehn-fehr-meh-rah)

Do you have questions?
¿Tiene[s] preguntas?
(Tee-eh-neh[s] preh-goon-tahs)

Do you have relatives/friends?
¿Tiene parientes/amigos?
(Tee-eh-neh pah-ree-ehn-tehs/ah-mee-gohs)

Do you have relatives with cardiac problems?
¿Tiene familiares con problemas cardíacos?
(Tee-eh-neh fah-mee-lee-ah-rehs kohn proh-bleh-mahs kahr-dee-ah-kohs)

Do you have special problems?
¿Tiene problemas especiales?
(Tee-eh-neh proh-bleh-mahs ehs-peh-see-ah-lehs)

Do you have time?
¿Tiene[s] tiempo?
(Tee-eh-neh[s] tee-ehm-poh)

Do you have trouble making friends at work?
¿En su trabajo tiene dificultad para hacer amistades?
(Ehn soo trah-bah-hoh tee-eh-neh dee-fee-kool-tahd pah-rah ah-sehr ah-mees-tah-dehs)

Do you have tuberculosis?
¿Tiene tuberculosis?
(Tee-eh-neh too-behr-koo-loh-sees)

Do you have vision problems?
¿Tiene[s] problemas con la visión?
(Tee-eh-neh[s] proh-bleh-mahs kohn lah bee-see-ohn?)

Do you have your Medicare card?
¿Tiene usted su tarjeta de Medicare?
(Tee-eh-neh oos-tehd soo tahr-heh-tah deh Meh-dee-kehr)

Do you know?
¿Sabe?
(Sah-beh)

Do you know him/her?
¿Lo/la conoce?
(Loh/lah koh-noh-seh)

Do you know his/her phone number?
¿Sabe su teléfono?
(Sah-beh soo teh-leh-foh-noh)

Do you know how to return?
¿Sabe cómo regresar?
(Sah-beh koh-moh re-greh-sahr)

[Do you know] the day today?
¿Qué día es hoy?
(Keh dee-ah ehs oh-ee)

Do you know the day of the week?
¿Sabe el día de la semana?
(Sah-beh ehl dee-ah deh lah seh-mah-nah)

Do you know the hospital name?
¿Sabe el nombre del hospital?
(Sah-beh ehl nohm-breh dehl ohs-pee-tahl)

Do you know the street name?
¿Sabe el nombre de la calle?
(Sah-beh ehl nohm-breh deh lah kah-yeh)

Do you know where you are?
¿Sabe dónde está?
(Sah-beh dohn-deh ehs-tah)

Do you know why?
¿Sabe por qué?
(Sah-beh pohr keh)

Do you like going to school?
¿Te/le gusta ir a la escuela?
(Teh/leh goos-tah eer ah lah ehs-koo-eh-lah)

Do you like them hot/cold?
¿Le gustan calientes/fríos?
(Leh goos-tahn kah-lee-ehn-tehs/free-ohs)

Do you live by yourself?
¿Vive solo?
(Bee-beh soh-loh)

Do you live here?
¿Vive aquí?
(Bee-beh ah-kee)

Do you live with your husband?
¿Vive con su esposo?
(Bee-beh kohn soo ehs-poh-soh)

Do you miss school a lot?
¿Falta[s] mucho a la escuela?
(Fahl-tah[s] moo-choh ah lah ehs-koo-eh lah)

Do you need help?
¿Necesita ayuda?
(Neh-seh-see-tah ah-yoo-dah)

Do you need help with school work?
¿Necesita[s] ayuda con la tarea?
(Neh-seh-see-tah[s] ah-yoo-dah kohn lah tah-reh-ah)

Do you need ice?
¿Necesita hielo?
(Neh-seh-see-tah ee-eh-loh)

Do you need more pillows?
¿Necesita más almohadas?
(Neh-seh-see-tah mahs ahl-moh-ah-dahs)

Do you need the headboard up?
¿Necesita levantar más la cabecera?
(Neh-seh-see-tah leh-bahn-tahr mahs lah kah-beh-seh-rah)

Do you need to call a taxi?
¿Necesita llamar un taxi/carro de sitio?
(Neh-seh-see-tah yah-mahr oon tahx-ee/kah-roh deh see-tee-oh)

Do you need to see a social worker?
¿Necesita ver a la trabajadora social?
(Neh-seh-see-tah behr ah lah trah-bah-hah-doh-rah soh-see-ahl)

Do you need to see a dietitian?
¿Necesita ver a la dietista?
(Neh-seh-see-tah behr ah lah dee-eh-tees-tah)

Do you participate in homosexual relations?
¿Participa en relaciones homosexuales?
(Pahr-tee-see-pah ehn reh-lah-see-ohn-ehs oh-moh-sex-oo-ahl-ehs)

Do you play sports?
¿Juega[s] deportes?
(Hoo-eh-gah[s] deh-pohr-tehs)

Do you prefer to call your doctor?
¿Prefiere llamar a su doctor?
(Preh-fee-eh-reh yah-mahr ah soo dohk-tohr)

Do you remember me?
¿Se acuerda de mí?
(Seh ah-koo-ehr-dah deh mee)

Do you remember the street?
¿Recuerda la calle?
(Reh-koo-ehr-dah lah kah-yeh)

Do you sleep during the day?
¿Duerme durante el día?
(Doo-ehr-meh doo-rahn-teh ehl dee-ah)

Do you smoke?
¿Fuma usted?
(Foo-mah oos-tehd)

Do you smoke or drink alcohol?
¿Fuma o toma alcohol?
(Foo-mah oh toh-mah ahl-kohl)

Do you speak English?
¿Habla usted inglés?
(Ah-blah oos-tehd een-glehs)

Do you speak Spanish?
¿Habla usted español?
(Ah-blah oos-tehd ehs-pah-nyohl)

Do you take a special diet?
¿Toma dieta especial?
(Toh-mah dee-eh-tah ehs-peh-see-ahl)

Do you take any drugs?
¿Toma drogas?
(Toh-mah droh-gahs)

Do you take any medications?
¿Toma algunas medicinas?
(Toh-mah ahl-goo-nahs meh-dee-see-nahs)

Do you take any narcotics?
¿Toma narcóticos?
(Toh-mah nahr-koh-tee-kohs)

Do you take drugs from habit?
¿Tiene vicio de tomar drogas?
(Tee-eh-neh bee-see-oh deh toh-mahr droh-gahs)

Do you try to relax to forget your anxiety?
¿Procura distraerse para olvidar su ansiedad?
(Proh-koo-rah dees-trah-ehr seh pah-rah ohl-bee-dahr soo ahn-see-eh-dahd)

Do you understand?
¿Comprende?/¿Entiende?
(Kohm-prehn-deh?/Ehn-tee-ehn-deh)

Do you use drugs / medicine?
¿Usa drogas/medicamento?
(Oo-sah droh-gahs/meh-dee-kah-mehn-toh)

Do you wake up at night?
¿Se despierta en la noche?
(Seh dehs-pee-ehr-tah ehn lah noh-cheh)

Do you walk to school?
¿Camina[s] a la escuela?
(Kah-mee-nah[s] ah lah ehs-koo-eh-lah)

Do you want a cup of coffee?
¿Quiere una taza de café?
(Kee-eh-reh oo-nah tah-sah deh kah-feh)

Do you want a glass of juice?
¿Quiere un vaso con jugo?
(Kee-eh-reh oon bah-soh kohn hoo-goh)

Do you want a glass of water?
¿Quiere un vaso con agua?
(Kee-eh-reh oon bah-soh kohn ah-goo-ah)

Do you want something to drink?
¿Quiere algo de tomar/beber?
(Kee-eh-reh ahl-goh deh toh-mahr/beh-behr)

Do you want something to eat?
¿Quiere algo de comer?
(Kee-eh-reh ahl-goh deh koh-mehr)

Do you want to go home?
¿Quiere ir a su casa?
(Kee-eh-reh eer ah soo kah-sah)

Do you want to have a bowel movement?
¿Quiere evacuar? ¿Quiere obrar?
(Kee-eh-reh eh-bah-koo-ahr/Kee-eh-reh oh-brahr)

Do you want to pass urine?
¿Quiere orinar?
(Kee-eh-reh oh-ree-nahr)

Do you want to read?
¿Quiere leer?
(Kee-eh-reh leh-ehr)

Do you want to see a priest?
¿Necesita ver al sacerdote?
(Neh-seh-see-tah behr ahl sah-sehr-doh-teh)

Do you want to see our doctor?
¿Quiere ver a nuestro doctor?
(Kee-eh-reh behr ah noo-ehs-troh dohk-tohr)

Do you want to take the stairs?
¿Quiere tomar la escalera?
(Kee-eh-reh toh-mahr lah ehs-kah-leh-rah)

Do you want the bedpan?
¿Quiere el pato/el bacín?
(Kee-eh-reh ehl pah-toh/ehl bah-seen)

Do you want water?
¿Quiere agua?
(Kee-eh-reh ah-goo-ah)

Do you wear glasses?
¿Usas anteojos/lentes?
(Oo-sahs ahn-teh-oh-hohs?/lehn-tehs)

Do you work?
¿Trabaja usted?
(Trah-bah-hah oos-tehd)

Do you work everyday?
¿Trabaja todos los días?
(Trah-bah-hah toh-dohs lohs dee-ahs)

Do your gums bleed?
¿Le sangran las encías?
(Leh sahn-grahn lahs ehn-see-ahs)

Doctor, I think I am infected with AIDS.
Doctor, pienso que estoy infectado de SIDA.
(Dohk-tohr, pee-ehn-so keh ehs-toh-ee een-fek-tah-doh deh see-dah)

Doctor, I have had pain for the last five hours.
Doctor, desde hace cinco horas tengo dolor.
(Dohk-tohr, dehs-deh ah-seh seen-koh oh-rahs tehn-goh doh-lohr)

Doctor's name.
Nombre del doctor.
(Nohm-breh dehl dohk-tohr)

Does he/she cough only at night?
¿Tose sólo de noche?
(Toh-seh soh-loh deh noh-cheh)

Does he/she cry a lot?
¿Llora mucho?
(Yoh-rah moo-choh)

Does he/she go to school?
¿Va a la escuela?
(Bah ah lah ehs-koo-eh-lah)

Does he/she have: fever/diarrhea/colic?
¿Tiene: fiebre/diarrea/cólico?
(Tee-eh-neh: fee-eh-breh/dee-ah-re-ah/koh-lee-koh)

Does he/she have any friends?
¿Tiene amigos?
(Tee-eh-neh ah-mee-gohs)

Does he/she play outdoors?
¿Juega afuera de la casa?
(Joo-eh-gah ah-foo-eh-rah deh lah kah-sah)

Does he/she sleep well?
¿Duerme bien?
(Doo-ehr-meh bee-ehn)

Does he/she speak English?
¿Él/Ella habla inglés?
(Ehl/Eh-yah ah-blah een-glehs)

Does he/she wet the bed?
¿Moja la cama?
(Moh-hah lah kah-mah)

Does it come and go?
¿Va y viene?
(Bah eeh bee-eh-neh)

Does it have undigested food?
¿Tiene restos de comida?
(Tee-eh-neh rehs-tohs deh koh-mee-dah)

Does it hurt to breathe?
¿Te duele al respirar?
(Teh doo-eh-leh ahl rehs-pee-rahr)

Does it hurt to cough?
¿Te duele al toser?
(Teh doo-eh-leh ahl toh-sehr)

Does it hurt when you chew very hard?
¿Le duele al masticar con fuerza?
(Leh doo-eh-leh ahl mahs-tee-kahr kohn foo-ehr-sah)

Does it smell bad?
¿Huele mal?
(Oo-eh-leh mahl)

Does it still hurt?
¿Todavía le duele?
(Toh-dah-bee-ah leh doo-eh-leh)

Does the baby sleep all night?
¿Duerme el bebé toda la noche?
(Doo-ehr-meh ehl beh-beh toh-dah lah noh-cheh)

Does the cough produce vomit?
¿La tos le produce vómito?
(Lah tohs leh proh-doo-seh boh-mee-toh)

Does the pain get better if you stop and rest?
¿Se mejora el dolor si se detiene y descansa?
(Seh meh-hoh-rah ehl doh-lohr see seh deh-tee-eh-neh ee dehs-kahn-sah)

Does the pain move from one place to another?
¿El dolor se mueve de un lugar a otro?
(Ehl doh-lohr seh moo-eh-beh deh oon loo-gahr ah oh-troh)

Does the school have complaints about him?
¿Tiene quejas de la escuela?
(Tee-eh-neh keh-hahs deh lah ehs-koo-eh-lah)

Does the vomit have blood?
¿Tiene sangre el vómito?
(Tee-eh-neh sahn-greh ehl boh-mee-toh)

Does the wind hurt your teeth?
¿Le molesta el aire?
(Leh moh-lehs-tah ehl ah-ee-reh)

Don't be afraid!
¡No tenga miedo!
(Noh tehn-gah mee-eh-doh)

Don't breathe!
¡No respire!
(Noh rehs-pee-reh)

Don't change clothes.
No se cambie de ropa.
(Noh seh kahm-bee-eh deh roh-pah)

Don't get constipated.
No se deje estreñir.
(Noh seh deh-heh ehs-treh-nyeer)

Don't get up!
¡No se levante!
(Noh seh leh-bahn-teh)

Don't hold on!
¡No se agarre!
(Noh seh ah-gahr-reh)

Don't hold the rail.
No agarre el barandal.
(Noh ah-gah-reh ehl bah-rahn-dahl)

Don't laugh!
¡No se ría!
(Noh seh ree-ah)

Don't let him put dirt in his mouth.
No deje que se meta tierra en la boca.
(Noh deh-heh keh seh meh-tah tee-eh-rah ehn lah boh-kah)

Don't let me bend it.
No dejes que la doble.
(Noh deh-hehs keh lah doh-bleh)

Don't let me close them.
No me dejes cerrarlos.
(Noh meh deh-hehs seh-rahr-lohs)

Don't let me extend it.
No me dejes extenderlo.
(Noh meh deh-hehs ehx-tehn-dehr-loh)

Don't let the baby sleep more than three hours during the day.
No deje que el bebé duerma más de tres horas durante el día.
(Noh deh-heh keh ehl beh-beh doo-ehr-mah mahs deh trehs oh-rahs doo-rahn-teh ehl dee-ah)

Don't lie down!
¡No se acueste!
(Noh seh ah-koo-ehs-teh)

Don't lift more than 5 pounds.
No levante más de cinco libras.
(Noh leh-bahn-teh mahs deh seen-koh lee-brahs)

Don't move!
¡No se mueva!
(Noh seh moo-eh-bah)

Don't sit!
¡No se siente!
(Noh seh see-ehn-teh)

Don't talk!
¡No hable!
(Noh ah-bleh)

Don't touch anything!
¡No toques nada!
(Noh toh-kehs nah-dah)

Don't turn.
No voltee.
(Noh bohl-teh-eh)

Don't walk barefoot.
No camine descalzo.
(Noh kah-mee-neh dehs-kahl-soh)

Don't worry!
¡No se preocupe!
(Noh seh preh-oh-koo-peh)

Dosage?
¿Dosis?
(Doh-sees)

Dress the baby with few clothes.
Vista al bebé con poca ropa.
(Bees-tah ahl beh-beh kohn poh-kah roh-pah)

Dress him/her with loose clothes.
Póngale ropa cómoda.
(Pohn-gah-leh roh-pah koh-moh-dah)

Drink!
¡Beba!/¡Tome!
(Beh-bah/Toh-meh)

Drink a lot of water and juices.
Tome mucha agua y jugos.
(Toh-meh moo-chah ah-goo-ah ee hoo-gohs)

Drug carts are checked for quantity, number, and expiration dates on all items.
Los carros de drogas se revisan para notar cantidad, número y fecha de caducidad en todos los artículos.
(Lohs kah-rohs deh droh-gahs seh reh-bee-sahn pah-rah noh-tahr kahn-tee-dahd, noo-meh-roh ee feh-chah deh kah-doo-see-dahd ehn toh-dohs lohs ahr-tee-koo-lohs)

Drugs are dispensed only upon the order of a physician.
Los medicamentos son distribuidos solamente por órdenes de un doctor.
(Lohs meh-dee-kah-mehn-tohs sohn dees-tree-boo-ee-dohs sohl-ah-mehn-teh pohr ohr-dehn-ehs deh oon dohk-tohr)

Each hour.
Cada hora.
(Kah-dah oh-rah)

Eat!
¡Coma!
(Koh-mah)

Eat soft foods.
Coma alimentos blandos.
(Koh-mah ah-lee-mehn-tohs blahn-dohs)

Every time you go to the bathroom to void, you must place the urine in the container.
Cada vez que vaya al baño a orinar, debe poner la orina en el recipiente.
(Kah-dah behs keh bah-yah ahl bah-nyoh ah oh-ree-nahr, deh-beh poh-nehr lah oh-ree-nah ehn ehl reh-see-pee-ehn-teh)

Every two hours.
Cada dos horas.
(Kah-dah dohs oh-rahs)

Everybody experiences some anxiety.
Todo el mundo pasa por cierta ansiedad.
(Toh-doh ehl moon-doh pah-sah pohr see-ehr-tah ahn-see-eh-dahd)

Everything will be all right.
Todo saldrá con éxito.
(Toh-doh sahl-drah kohn ehx-ee-toh)

Excuse me!
¡Excúseme!
(Ehx-koo-seh-meh)

Exit to the right/left.
Salga a la derecha/izquierda.
(Sahl-gah ah lah deh-reh-chah/ees-kee-ehr-dah)

Expiration date.
Caducidad.
(Kah-doo-see-dahd)

Expired items on the unit are returned to the pharmacy.
Los artículos con fecha vencida se devuelven a la farmacia.
(Lohs ahr-tee-koo-lohs kohn feh-chah behn-see-dah seh deh-boo-ehl-behn ah lah fahr-mah-see-ah.

Extend it.
Extiéndelo.
(Ehx-tee-ehn-deh-loh)

Extend your arm.
Extiende tu brazo.
(Ehx-tee-ehn-deh too brah-soh)

Extend your leg and foot.
Extiende tu pierna y pie.
(Ehx-tee-ehn-deh too pee-ehr-nah ee pee-eh)

Extend your wrist.
Extiende tu muñeca.
(Ehx-tee-ehn-deh too moo-nyeh-kah)

Family history of cancer?
¿Hay historia de cáncer en la familia?
(Ah-ee ees-toh-ree-ah deh kahn-sehr ehn lah fah-mee-lee-ah)

Fetus of infected mothers.
Fetos de madres contaminadas.
(Feh-tohs deh mah-drehs kohn-tah-mee-nah-dahs)

Fever?
¿Fiebre?
(Fee-eh-breh)

Fifteen per day.
Quince al día.
(Keen-seh ahl dee-ah)

Flex it!
¡Dóblalo!
(Doh-blah-loh)

Flex the foot upward.
Dobla el pie para arriba.
(Doh-blah ehl pee-eh pah-rah ah-ree-bah)

Flex your arm.
Dobla tu brazo.
(Doh-blah too brah-soh)

Flex your arm; don't let me extend it.
Dobla tu brazo; no me dejes extenderlo.
(Doh-blah too brah-soh; noh meh deh-hehs ehx-tehn-dehr-loh)

Flex your knee and turn to the middle.
Dobla tu rodilla y voltea al medio.
(Doh-blah too roh-dee-yah ee bohl-teh-ah ahl meh-dee-oh)

Follow my finger.
Siga mi dedo.
(See-gah mee deh-doh)

Follow the green line.
Siga la línea verde.
(See-gah lah lee-nee-ah behr-deh)

Follow the instructions carefully.
Siga las instrucciones con cuidado.
(See-gah lahs eens-trook-see-ohn-ehs kohn koo-ee-dah-doh)

Follow the red arrows.
Siga las flechas rojas.
(See-gah lahs fleh-chahs roh-hahs)

Foods you may not eat:
Comidas que no debe comer:
(Koh-mee-dahs keh noh deh-beh koh-mehr)

For now, change into this gown.
Por ahora, póngase esta bata.
(Pohr ah-oh-rah, pohn-gah-seh ehs-tah bah-tah)

For the birth control plan that you wish to have.
Para el control de fertilidad que desee.
(Pah-rah ehl kohn-trohl deh fehr-tee-lee-dahd keh deh-seh-eh)

For the most part . . .
Por la mayor parte . . .
(Pohr lah mah-yohr pahr-teh)

For what purpose?
¿Para qué?
(Pah-rah keh)

For what reason?
¿Cuál es la razón?
(Koo-ahl ehs lah rah-sohn)

For whom?
¿Para quién?
(Pah-rah kee-ehn)

Forty-five years old.
Cuarenta y cinco años.
(Koo-ah-rehn-tah ee seen-koh ah-nyohs)

Forward.
Adelante.
(Ah-deh-lahn-teh)

Four times.
Cuatro veces.
(Koo-ah-troh beh-sehs)

Four times a day.
Cuatro veces al día.
(Koo-ah-troh beh-sehs ahl dee-ah)

Frequent blisters?
¿Ulceraciones frecuentes?
(Ool-seh-rah-see-oh-nehs freh-koo-ehn-tehs)

From here, turn to the left, then turn right.
De aquí, dé vuelta a la izquierda, luego voltee a la derecha.
(Deh ah-kee, deh boo-ehl-tah ah lah ees-kee-ehr-dah, loo-eh-goh bohl-teh-eh ah lah deh-reh-chah)

From time to time . . .
De vez en cuando . . .
(Deh behs ehn koo-ahn-doh)

From what height did he/she fall?
¿De qué altura cayó?
(Deh keh ahl-too-rah kah-yoh)

Gas producing foods.
Comidas que producen gas.
(Koh-mee-dahs keh proh-doo-sehn gahs)

Get!
¡Consiga!
(Kohn-see-gah)

Get out!
¡Fuera!
(Foo-eh-rah)

Get up!
¡Levántese!
(Leh-bahn-teh-seh)

Give him/her the medicine every four hours.
Déle la medicina cada cuatro horas.
(Deh-leh lah meh-dee-see-nah kah-dah koo-ah-troh oh-rahs)

Give it to the clerk.
Déselo a la secretaria.
(Deh-seh-loh ah lah seh-kreh-tah-ree-ah)

Give the medicine with a dropper.
Dé la medicina con gotero.
(Deh lah meh-dee-see-nah kohn goh-teh-roh)

Give the patient a hand mirror and toothbrush.
Déle al paciente un espejo de mano y un cepillo de dientes.
(Deh-leh ahl pah-see-ehn-teh oon ehs-peh-hoh deh mah-noh ee oon seh-pee-yoh deh dee-ehn-tehs)

Go immediately to the hospital!
¡Vaya inmediatamente/en seguida al hospital!
(Bah-yah een-meh-dee-ah-tah-mehn-teh/ ehn seh-ghee-dah ahl ohs-pee-tahl)

Go on, please.
Continúe/Siga, por favor.
(Kohn-tee-noo-eh/See-gah, pohr fah-bohr)

Go to the glass doors.
Vaya a las puertas de vidrio.
(Bah-yah ah lahs poo-ehr-tahs deh bee-dree-oh)

Go to the hospital right away.
Acuda inmediatamente al hospital.
(Ah-koo-dah een-meh-dee-ah-tah-mehn-teh ahl ohs-pee-tahl)

Good!
¡Bueno!
(Boo-eh-noh)

Good afternoon!
¡Buenas tardes!
(Boo-eh-nahs tahr-dehs)

Good afternoon, Miss González.
Buenas tardes, señorita González.
(Boo-eh-nahs tahr-dehs, seh-nyoh-ree-tah Gohn-sah-lehs)

Good evening! / Good night!
¡Buenas noches!
(Boo-eh-nahs noh-chehs)

Good luck!
¡Buena suerte!
(Boo-eh-nah soo-ehr-teh)

Good morning!
¡Buenos días!
(Boo-eh-nohs dee-ahs)

Good morning, doctor!
¡Buenos días, doctor!
(Boo-eh-nohs dee-ahs, dohk-tohr)

Has anything changed in your life?
¿Ha cambiado algo en su vida?
(Ah kahm-bee-ah-doh ahl-goh ehn soo bee-dah)

Has the child been ill?
¿Ha estado enfermo el niño?
(Ah ehs-tah-doh ehn-fehr-moh ehl nee-nyoh)

Has the pain gotten worse or gotten better?
¿Se ha puesto el dolor peor o mejor?
(Seh ah poo-ehs-toh ehl doh-lohr peh-ohr oh meh-hohr)

Has this happened to you before?
¿Le ha pasado esto antes?
(Leh ah pah-sah-doh ehs-toh ahn-tehs)

Has this problem happened before?
¿Le ha pasado antes este problema?
(Leh ah pah-sah-doh ahn-tehs ehs-teh proh-bleh-mah)

Have a good day!
¡Pase un buen día!
(Pah-seh oon boo-ehn dee-ah)

Have you been a patient before?
¿Ha sido un paciente antes?
(Ah see-doh oon pah-see-ehn-teh ahn-tehs)

Have you been exposed to any infectious diseases?
¿Ha estado expuesto a enfermedades infecciosas?
(Ah ehs-tah-doh ex-poo-ehs-toh ah ehn-fehr-meh-dah-dehs een-fek-see-oh-sahs)

Have you been here before?
¿Ha estado aquí antes?
(Ah ehs-tah-doh ah-kee ahn-tehs)

Have you been in this hospital?
¿Ha estado en este hospital?
(Ah ehs-tah-doh ehn ehs-teh ohs-pee-tahl)

Have you been sick?
¿Ha estado enfermo(a)?
(Ah ehs-tah-doh ehn-fehr-moh[mah])

Have you eaten?
¿Ha comido?
(Ah koh-mee-doh)

Have you ever been to the emergency room?
¿Ha estado en el cuarto de emergencia/ urgencias?
(Ah ehs-tah-doh ehn ehl koo-ahr-toh deh eh-mehr-hehn-see-ah/ oor-hehn-see-ahs)

Have you ever had a heart attack or pains in your heart?
¿Ha tenido ataque al corazón o dolor en el pecho?
(Ah teh-nee-doh ah-tah-keh ahl koh-rah-sohn oh doh-lohr ehn ehl peh-choh)

Have you ever had a sexually transmitted disease?
¿Ha tenido enfermedades transmitidas sexualmente?
(Ah teh-nee-doh ehn-fehr-meh-dah-dehs trahns-mee-tee-dahs sehx-oo-ahl-mehn-teh)

Have you ever had allergic reaction to a local anesthetic?
¿Ha tenido alergia a la anestesia local?
(Ah teh-nee-doh ah-lehr-hee-ah ah lah ah-nehs-teh-see-ah loh-kahl)

Have you ever had cancer?
¿Ha tenido cáncer?
(Ah teh-nee-doh kahn-sehr)

Have you ever had chemotherapy treatment?
¿Ha tenido tratamiento de quimioterapia?
(Ah the-nee-doh trah-tah-mee-ehn-toh deh kee-mee-oh-tehr-ah-pee-ah)

Have you ever had hepatitis or cirrhosis?
¿Ha tenido hepatitis o cirrosis?
(Ah teh-nee-doh eh-pah-tee-tees oh see roh-sees)

Have you ever had tuberculosis / lung problems?
¿Ha tenido tuberculosis/problemas con los pulmones?
(Ah teh-nee-doh too-behr-koo-lohs-ees/ proh-bleh-mahs kohn lohs pool-moh-nehs)

Have you had a blood transfusion?
¿Ha tenido transfusiones de sangre?
(Ah teh-nee-doh trahns-foo-see-ohn-ehs deh sahn-greh)

Have you had an abortion?
¿Ha tenido aborto?
(Ah teh-nee-doh ah-bohr-toh)

Have you had any accidents?
¿Ha tenido algún accidente?
(Ah teh-nee-doh ahl-goon ahk-see-dehn-teh)

Have you had any bleeding, swelling, or bruising?
¿Ha tenido sangrados, hinchazón o moretones?
(Ah teh-nee-doh sahn-grah-dohs, een-chah-sohn oh moh-reh-toh-nehs)

Have you had any hard blows to your head or chest?
¿Se ha golpeado fuerte la cabeza o el tórax?
(Seh ah gohl-peh-ah-doh foo-ehr-teh lah kah-beh-zah oh ehl toh-rahx)

Have you had anything broken?
¿Ha tenido algo quebrado?
(Ah teh-nee-doh ahl-goh keh-brah-doh)

Have you had blood drawn before?
¿Le han tomado muestras antes?
(Leh ahn toh-mah-doh moo-ehs-trahs ahn-tehs)

Have you had blood transfusions?
¿Ha tenido transfusiones de sangre?
(Ah teh-nee-doh trahns-foo-see-ohn-ehs deh sahn-greh)

Have you had broken bones?
¿Ha tenido huesos rotos/fracturados?
(Ah teh-nee-doh oo-eh-sohs roh-tohs/ frahk-too-rah-dohs)

Have you had cancer?
¿Ha tenido cáncer?
(Ah teh-nee-doh kahn-sehr)

Have you had headaches?
¿Ha tenido dolor de cabeza?
(Ah teh-nee-doh doh-lohr deh kah-beh-sah)

Have you had neck pain?
¿Ha tenido dolor en el cuello?
(Ah teh-nee-doh doh-lohr ehn ehl koo-eh-yoh)

Have you had pain in the left arm?
¿Ha sentido dolor en el brazo izquierdo?
(Ah sehn-tee-doh doh-lohr ehn ehl brah-soh ees-kee-ehr-doh)

Have you had reaction to transfusions?
¿Ha tenido reacción a transfusiones?
(Ah teh-nee-doh reh-ahk-see-ohn ah trahns-foo-see-ohn-ehs)

Have you had rheumatic fever?
¿Ha tenido fiebre reumática?
(Ah teh-nee-doh fee-eh-breh reh-oo-mah-tee-kah)

Have you had sexual relations?
¿Ha tenido relaciones sexuales?
(Ah teh-nee-doh reh-lah-see-oh-nehs sehx-oo-ah-lehs)

Have you had surgeries?
¿Ha tenido operaciones?
(Ah teh-nee-doh oh-peh-rah-see-ohn-ehs)

Have you had swelling?
¿Ha tenido hinchazón?
(Ah teh-nee-doh een-chah-sohn)

Have you had swelling in the ankles?
¿Ha tenido hinchazón en los tobillos?
(Ah teh-nee-doh een-chah-sohn ehn lohs toh-bee-yohs)

Have you had swelling in the eyelids?
¿Ha tenido hinchazón en los párpados?
(Ah teh-nee-doh een-chah-sohn ehn lohs pahr-pah-dohs)

Have you had swelling on your feet?
¿Ha tenido hinchazón en los pies?
(Hah teh-nee-doh een-chah-sohn ehn lohs pee-ehs)

Have you had this happen before?
¿Le ha pasado esto antes?
(Leh ah pah-sah-doh ehs-toh ahn-tehs)

Have you had X-rays?
¿Le han tomado rayos X?
(Leh ahn toh-mah-doh rah-yohs eh-kees)

Have you passed out?
¿Se ha desmayado?
(Seh ah dehs-mah-yah-doh)

Have you seen blood in the urine?
¿Ha visto sangre en la orina?
(Ah bees-toh sahn-greh ehn lah oh-ree-nah)

Having continuous anxiety may cause serious problems.
El tener ansiedad continua puede llevar a problemas serios.
(Ehl teh-nehr ahn-see-eh-dahd kohn-tee-noo-ah poo-eh-deh yeh-bahr ah proh-bleh-mahs seh-ree-ohs)

He assigns a dosage schedule to the order in the computer.
El asigna un horario de dosis a la orden en la computadora.
(Ehl ah-seeg-nah oon oh-rah-ree-oh deh doh-sees ah lah ohr-dehn ehn lah kohm-poo-tah-doh-rah)

He bought me the book.
Me compró el libro.
(Meh kohm-proh ehl lee-broh)

He collected the money from me.
Me cobró el dinero.
(Meh koh-broh ehl dee-neh-roh)

He doesn't speak English, but Spanish.
No habla inglés, sino español.
(Noh ah-blah een-glehs, see-noh ehs-pah-nyohl)

He gave me the money.
Me dió el dinero.
(Meh dee-oh ehl dee-neh-roh)

He had high cholesterol and surgery.
Tenía colesterol alto y le hicieron cirugía.
(Teh-nee-ah koh-lehs-teh-rohl ahl-toh ee leh ee-see-eh-rohn see-roo-hee-ah)

He has black hair.
El tiene el pelo negro.
(Ehl tee-ehn-eh ehl peh-loh neh-groh)

He is a barber.
Es barbero.
(Ehs bahr-beh-roh)

He is a hard-working barber.
Es un barbero muy trabajador.
(Ehs oon bahr-beh-roh moo-ee trah-bah-hah-dohr)

He is content.
El está contento.
(Ehl ehs-tah kohn-tehn-toh)

He is happy.
El es [está] alegre.
(Ehl ehs [ehs-tah] ah-leh-greh)

He is not wearing a white shirt, but a blue one.
No usa camisa blanca, sino azul.
(Noh oo-sah kah-mee-sah blahn-kah, see-noh ah-sool)

He is sad.
El es [está] triste.
(Ehl ehs [ehs-tah] trees-teh)

He keeps track of my cholesterol.
El me controla el colesterol.
(Ehl meh kohn-troh-lah ehl koh-lehs-teh-rohl)

He left without saying anything.
Salió sin decir nada.
(Sah-lee-oh seen deh-seer nah-dah)

He loved . . .
El amó . . .
(Ehl ah-moh)

He takes the temperature. It is 100 degrees.
Le toma la temperatura. Es de cien grados.
(Leh toh-mah lah tehm-peh-rah-too-rah. Ehs deh see-ehn grah-dohs)

He tells her that she will be discharged tomorrow.
Le comunica que mañana será dada de alta.
(Leh koh-moo-nee-kah keh mah-nyah-nah seh-rah dah-dah deh ahl-tah)

He will take you.
El lo llevará.
(Ehl loh yeh-bah-rah)

He will talk to you.
El hablará con usted.
(Ehl ah-blah-rah kohn oos-tehd)

Hello.
Hola.
(Oh-lah)

Hello, I am the nurse in charge.
Hola, yo soy la enfermera encargada.
(Oh-lah, yoh soh-ee lah ehn-fehr-meh-rah ehn-kahr-gah-dah)

Hello, I'm John Goodguy.
Hola, soy John Goodguy.
(Oh-lah, soh-ee John Goodguy)

Hello, Mr. Garza! Tell me, what is wrong?
¡Hola, señor Garza! Dígame, ¿qué le pasa?
(Oh-lah, seh-nyohr Gahr-sah! Dee-gah-meh, keh leh pah-sah)

Hello, Mrs. Garza. I am here to draw your blood.
Hola, señora Garza. Estoy aquí para sacarle una muestra de sangre.
(Oh-lah, seh-nyoh-rah Gahr-sah. Ehs-tohy ah-kee pah-rah sah-kahr-leh oo-nah moo-ehs-trah deh sahn-greh)

Hello, Mrs. Mora.
Hola, señora Mora.
(Oh-lah, seh-nyoh-rah Moh-rah)

Hello, Mrs. Vargas. I need to take your temperature and blood pressure.
Hola, señora Vargas. Necesito tomarle la temperatura y presión de la sangre.
(Oh-lah, seh-nyoh-rah Bahr-gahs. Neh-seh-see-toh toh-mahr-leh lah tehm-peh-rah-too-rah ee preh-see-ohn deh lah sahn-greh)

Help him to burp.
Póngalo a repetir/eructar.
(Pohn-gah-loh ah reh-peh-teer/eh-rook-tahr)

Her rings.
Sus anillos.
(Soos ah-nee-yohs).

Here, below the sternum.
Aquí, debajo del esternón.
(Ah-kee deh-bah-hoh dehl ehs-tehr-nohn)

Here is a glasss of water to rinse with.
Aquí está un vaso de agua para que se enjuague.
(Ah-kee ehs-tah oon bah-soh deh ah-goo-ah pah-rah keh seh ehn-hoo-ah-geh)

Here is the bell.
Aquí está la campana.
(Ah-kee ehs-tah lah kahm-pah-nah)

Here is the toilet paper.
Aquí está el papel del baño/higiénico.
(Ah-kee ehs-tah ehl pah-pehl dehl bah-nyoh/ee-hee-eh-nee-koh)

Hi!
¡Hola!
(Oh-lah)

HIV is not transmissible by casual contact.
El VIH no es transmitido en forma casual.
(Ehl VIH noh ehs trahns-mee-tee-doh ehn fohr-mah kah-soo-ahl)

HIV is not transmissible by living in the same house as infected persons.
El VIH no es transmitido al vivir en la misma casa con personas infectadas.
(Ehl VIH noh ehs trahns-mee-tee-doh ahl bee-beer ehn lah mees-mah kah-sah kohn pehr-soh-nahs een-fehk-tah-dahs)

Hold it!
¡Deténlo!
(Deh-tehn-loh)

Hold my finger.
Detén mi dedo.
(Deh-tehn mee deh-doh)

Hold your breath!
¡No respire!
(Noh rehs-pee-reh)

Hospital policy.
Regla del hospital.
(Reh-glah dehl ohs-pee-tahl)

How?
¿Cómo?
(Koh-moh)

How are you?
¿Cómo está?
(Koh-moh ehs-tah)

How bad is it?
¿Qué tan mal está?
(Keh tahn mahl ehs-tah)

How close are your contractions?
¿Cada cuánto tiempo tiene las contracciones?
(Kah-dah koo-ahn-toh tee-ehm-poh tee-eh-neh lahs kohn-trahk-see-ohn-ehs)

How did he/she fall?
¿Cómo se cayó?
(Koh-moh seh kah-yoh)

How did this injury happen?
¿Cómo ocurrió esta lesión?
(Koh-moh oh-koo-ree-oh ehs-tah leh-see-ohn)

How did you?
¿Cómo hizo?
(Koh-moh ee-soh)

How did you get here?
¿Cómo llegó aquí?
(Koh-moh yeh-goh ah-kee)

How did you move the victim?
¿Cómo movió a la víctima?
(Koh-moh moh-bee-oh ah lah beek-tee-mah)

How do you feel?
¿Cómo te sientes?
(Koh-moh teh see-ehn-tehs)

How do you feel now?
¿Cómo se siente ahora?
(Koh-moh seh see-ehn-teh ah-oh-rah?

How do you get along with your peers?
¿Cómo se lleva usted con sus compañeros?
(Koh-moh seh yeh-bah oos-tehd kohn soos kohm-pah-nyeh-rohs)

How do you like hot dogs?
¿Cómo le gustan los emparedados de salchicha?
(Koh-moh leh goos-tahn lohs ehm-pah-reh-dah-dohs deh sahl-chee-chah)

How do you like the eggs fixed?
¿Cómo le gustan los huevos?
(Koh-moh leh goos-tahn lohs oo-eh-bohs)

How do you like your coffee?
¿Cómo le gusta el café?
(Koh-moh leh goos-tah ehl kah-feh)

How do you spend the day?
¿Cómo pasa el día?
(Koh-moh pah-sah ehl dee-ah)

How far?
¿Qué tan lejos?
(Keh tahn leh-hohs)

How is AIDS diagnosed?
¿Cómo se diagnostica el SIDA?
(Koh-moh seh dee-ahg-nohs-tee-kah ehl see-dah)

How is it done?
¿Cómo se hace?
(Koh-moh seh ah-seh)

How long ago?
¿Cuánto tiempo hace?
(Koo-ahn-toh tee-ehm-poh ah-seh)

How long did it last?
¿Cuánto duró?
(Koo-ahn-toh doo-roh)

How long have you been sick?
¿Desde cuándo está enfermo[a]?
(Dehs-deh koo-ahn-doh ehs-tah ehn-fehr-moh[ah])

How long have you felt depressed?
¿Désde cuándo se siente deprimido?
(Dehs-deh koo-ahn-doh seh see-ehn-teh deh-pree-mee-doh)

How many?
¿Cuántos?/Cuántas?
(Koo-ahn-tohs/Koo-ahn-tahs)

How many boys/girls?
¿Cuántos niños?/¿Cuántas niñas?
(Koo-ahn-tohs nee-nyohs/Koo-ahn-tahs nee-nyahs)

How many cars crashed?
¿Cuántos carros chocaron?
(Koo-ahn-tohs kah-rohs choh-kah-rohn)

How many children do you have?
¿Cuántos niños tiene?
(Koo-ahn-tohs nee-nyohs tee-eh-neh)

How many cigarettes per day?
¿Cuántos cigarrillos por día?
(Koo-ahn-tohs see-gah-ree-yohs pohr dee-ah)

How many cups per day?
¿Cuántas tazas diarias?
(Koo-ahn-tahs tah-sahs dee-ah-ree-ahs)

How many diapers have you changed since yesterday?
¿Cuántos pañales le ha cambiado desde ayer?
(Koo-ahn-tohs pah-nyah-lehs leh ah kahm-bee-ah-doh dehs-deh ah-yehr)

How many friends do you have?
¿Cuántos amigos tienes?
(Koo-ahn-tohs ah-mee-gohs tee-eh-nehs)

How many glasses of water do you drink?
¿Cuántos vasos de agua toma?
(Koo-ahn-tohs bah-sohs deh ah-goo-ah toh-mah)

How many hours do you sleep?
¿Cuántas horas duermes?
(Koo-ahn-tahs oh-rahs doo-ehr-mehs)

How many hours do you work?
¿Cuántas horas trabaja?
(Koo-ahn-tahs oh-rahs trah-bah-hah)

How many months pregnant?
¿Cuántos meses tiene de embarazo?
(Koo-ahn-tohs meh-sehs tee-eh-neh deh ehm-bah-rah-soh)

How many ounces does he take?
¿Cuántas onzas toma?
(Koo-ahn-tahs ohn-sahs toh-mah)

How many people were in the car/bus/truck?
¿Cuántas personas estaban en el carro/autobús/camioneta?
(Koo-ahn-tahs pehr-soh-nahs ehs-tab-bahn ehn ehl kah-roh/ah-oo-toh-boohs/kah-mee-oh-neh-tah)

How many persons in your family?
¿Cuántas personas forman su familia?
(Koo-ahn-tahs pehr-soh-nahs fohr-mahn soo fah-mee-lee-ah)

How many pounds have you gained?
¿Cuántas libras ha aumentado?
(Koo-ahn-tahs lee-brahs ah ah-oo-mehn-tah-doh)

How many pregnancies have you had?
¿Cuántos embarazos ha tenido?
(Koo-ahn-tohs ehm-bah-rah-sohs ah teh-nee-doh)

How many times a day?
¿Cuántas veces al día?
(Koo-ahn-tahs beh-sehs ahl dee-ah)

How many times do you eat per day?
¿Cuántas veces come por día?
(Koo-ahn-tahs beh-sehs koh-meh pohr dee-ah)

How many times does he wake up?
¿Cuántas veces se despierta?
(Koo-ahn-tahs beh-sehs seh dehs-pee-ehr-tah)

How many times has he vomited?
¿Cuántas veces ha vomitado?
(Koo-ahn-tahs beh-sehs ah boh-mee-tah-doh)

How many years did you go to school?
¿Cuántos años fue a la escuela?
(Koo-ahn-tohs ah-nyohs foo-eh ah lah ehs-koo-eh-lah)

How much?
¿Cuánto?
(Koo-ahn-toh)

How much do you drink per day?
¿Cuánto alcohol toma por día?
(Koo-ahn-toh ahl-kohl toh-mah pohr dee-ah)

How much medicine did you take?
¿Cuánta medicina tomó?
(Koo-ahn-tah meh-dee-see-nah toh-moh)

How much water do you drink?
¿Cuánta agua toma?
(Koo-ahn-tah ah-goo-ah toh-mah)

How often do you feed the baby?
¿Qué tan a menudo alimenta al bebé?
(Keh tahn ah meh-noo-doh ah-lee-mehn-tah ahl beh-beh)

How often do you have the pain?
¿Qué tan seguido tiene el dolor?
(Keh tahn seh-gee-doh tee-eh-neh ehl doh-lohr)

How often do you urinate?
¿Cuántas veces orina?
(Koo-ahn-tahs beh-sehs oh-ree-nah)

How old are you / they?
¿Cuántos años tiene/tienen?
(Koo-ahn-tohs ah-nyohs tee-eh-neh/tee-ehn-ehn)

How serious is AIDS?
¿Qué tan serio es el SIDA?
(Keh tahn seh-ree-oh ehs ehl see-dah)

How severe is the pain?
¿Qué tan severo es el dolor
(Keh tahn seh-beh-roh ehs ehl doh-lohr)

I also need a urine sample.
También necesito una muestra de orina.
(Tahm-bee-ehn neh-seh-see-toh oo-nah moo-ehs-trah deh oh-ree-nah)

I am . . .
Yo soy . . .
(Yoh soh-ee)

I am 53 years old.
Tengo cincuenta y tres años.
(Tehn-goh seen-koo-ehn-tah ee trehs ah-nyos)

I am a paramedic.
Soy paramédico.
(Soh-ee pahr-ah-meh-dee-koh)

I am afraid to get lost.
Tengo miedo de perderme.
(Tehn-goh mee-eh-doh deh pehr-dehr-meh)

I am back.
Ya regresé.
(Yah reh-greh-seh)

I am continuously . . .
Continuamente estoy . . .
(Kohn-tee-noo-ah-mehn-teh ehs-tohy)

I am Dr. Blanco.
Yo soy el doctor Blanco.
(Yoh soh-ee ehl dohk-tohr Blahn-koh)

I am fine, doctor, thank you! I feel like new.
¡Muy bien, doctor, ¡gracias! Me siento como nuevo.
(Moo-ee bee-ehn, dohk-tohr, grah-see-ahs/ Meh see-ehn-toh koh-moh noo-eh-boh)

I am going to ask many questions!
¡Voy a hacerle muchas preguntas!
(Boy ah ah-sehr-leh moo-chahs preh-goon-tahs)

I am going to ask some questions.
Voy a hacerle unas preguntas.
(Boy ah ah-sehr-leh oo-nahs preh-goon-tahs)

I am going to call the radiologist.
Voy a llamar al radiólogo.
(Boy ah yah-mahr ahl rah-dee-oh-loh-goh)

I am going to clean your teeth.
Voy a limpiarle los dientes.
(Boy ah leem-pee-ahr-leh lohs dee-ehn-tehs)

I am going to cover you.
Lo voy a cubrir.
(Loh boy ah koo-breer)

I am going to cover you with a sheet.
Voy a cubrirlo con una sábana.
(Boy ah koo-breer-loh kohn oo-nah sah-bah-nah)

I am going to examine you.
Voy a examinarla.
(Boy ah ehx-ah-mee-nahr-lah)

I am going to explain how to collect the urine.
Le voy a explicar cómo juntar la orina.
(Leh boy ah ehx-plee-kahr koh-moh hoon-tahr lah oh-ree-nah)

I am going to explain the collection of urine.
Le voy a explicar la colección de orina.
(Leh boy ah ehx-plee-kahr lah koh-lehk-see-ohn deh oh-ree-nah)

I am going to get a wheel chair.
Voy a traer una silla de ruedas.
(Boy ah trah-ehr oo-nah see-yah deh roo-eh-dahs)

I am going to give you a list.
Voy a darle una lista.
(Boy ah dahr-leh oo-nah lees-tah)

I am going to give you a tour of the floor.
Voy a darle un recorrido por el piso.
(Boy ah dahr-leh oon reh-koh-ree-doh pohr ehl pee-soh)

I am going to help you lie down.
Voy a ayudarlo a acostarse.
(Boy ah ah-yoo-dahr-loh ah ah-kohs-tahr-seh)

I am going to help you lie on the stretcher.
Voy a ayudarlo a acostarse en la camilla.
(Boy ah ah-yoo-dahr-loh ah ah-kohs-tahr-seh ehn lah kah-mee-yah)

I am going to hit gently.
Voy a darle golpecitos.
(Boy-ee ah dahr-leh gohl-peh-see-tohs)

I am going to let you rest.
Voy a dejarlo descansar.
(Boy ah deh-hahr-loh dehs-kahn-sahr)

I am going to lift your sleeve.
Voy a levantar la manga.
(Boy ah leh-bahn-tahr lah mahn-gah)

I am going to listen to the baby's heartbeat.
Voy a escuchar el latido del corazón del bebé.
(Boy ah ehs-koo-chahr ehl lah-tee-doh dehl koh-rah-sohn dehl beh-beh)

I am going to order a general chemistry.
Voy a ordenar una química general.
(Boy ah ohr-deh-nahr oo-nah kee-mee-kah geh-neh-rahl)

I am going to polish your teeth now.
Ahora voy a pulir sus dientes.
(Ah-oh-rah boy ah poo-leer soos dee-ehn-tehs)

I am going to put a Band-Aid on you.
Voy a ponerle una cinta adhesiva/una curita/un bandaid.
(Boy ah poh-nehr-leh oo-nah seen-tah ah-deh-see-bah/oo-nah koo-ree-tah/oon bahn-dah-eed)

I am going to put a splint on the leg.
Voy a ponerle una tablilla en la pierna.
(Boy ah poh-nehr-leh oo-nah tah-blee-yah ehn lah pee-ehr-nah)

I am going to put some solution around all your teeth.
Voy a poner una solución alrededor de todos sus dientes.
(Boy ah poh-nehr oo-nah soh-loo-see-ohn ahl-reh-deh-dohr deh toh-dohs soos dee-ehn-tehs)

I am going to take X-rays.
Le tomaré radiografías.
(Leh toh-mah-reh rah-dee-oh-grah-fee-ahs)

I am going to take X-rays of the abdomen first.
Voy a tomar rayos X del abdomen primero.
(Boy ah toh-mahr rah-yohs eh-kees dehl ahb-doh-mehn pree-meh-roh)

I am going to use local anesthetic.
Voy a usar anestesia local.
(Boy-ee ah oo-sahr ah-nehs-teh-see-ah loh-kahl)

I am here to draw your blood.
Estoy aquí para tomarle una muestra de sangre.
(Ehs-tohy ah-kee pah-rah toh-mahr-leh oo-nah moo-ehs-trah deh sahn-greh)

I am here to examine the baby.
Estoy aquí para examinar al bebé.
(Ehs-tohy ah-kee pah-rah ehx-ah-mee-nahr ahl beh-beh)

I am hurting a lot.
Tengo mucho dolor.
(Tehn-goh moo-choh doh-lohr)

I am Mexican.
Soy mexicana.
(Soh-ee meh-hee-kah-nah)

I am not going today.
Hoy no voy a ir.
(Oh-ee noh boy ah eer)

I am pre-diabetic; I control it with diet.
Soy prediabética; me controlo con dieta.
(Soh-ee preh-dee-ah-beh-tee-kah; meh kohn-troh-loh kohn dee-eh-tah)

I am putting a cassette under your waist.
Estoy poniendo una casetera abajo de la cintura.
(Ehs-tohy poh-nee-ehn-doh oo-nah kah-seh-teh-rah ah-bah-hoh deh lah seen-too-rah)

I am putting in a temporary filling.
Le aplicaré empaste temporal.
(Leh ah-plee-kah-reh ehm-pahs-teh tehm-poh-rahl)

I am sorry, no toothpicks.
Lo siento, no hay palillos.
(Loh see-ehn-toh noh ah-ee pah-lee-yohs)

I am the dentist.
Yo soy el/la dentista.
(Yo soh-ee ehl/lah dehn-tees-tah)

I am the doctor.
Yo soy el/la doctor(a).
(Yoh soh-ee ehl/lah dohk-tohr[-rah])

I am the medical student.
Yo soy el/la estudiante de medicina.
(Yo soh-ee ehl/lah ehs-too-dee-ahn-teh deh meh-dee-see-nah)

I am the nurse.
Yo soy el/la enfermero(a).
(Yoh soh-ee ehl/lah ehn-fehr-meh-roh[-rah])

I am the social worker.
Yo soy el/la trabajador(a) social.
(Yo soh-ee ehl/lah trah-bah-hah-dohr[-dohra] soh-see-ahl)

I am the technician.
Yo soy el/la técnico(a).
(Yoh soh-ee ehl/lah tehk-nee-koh[ah])

I am the therapist.
Yo soy el/la terapista.
(Yoh soh-ee ehl/lah teh-rah-pees-tah)

I am through.
Ya terminé.
(Yah tehr-mee-neh)

I am very healthy!
¡Estoy muy sano!
(Ehs-toh-ee moo-ee sah-noh)

I can stop.
Puedo pararme.
(Poo-eh-doh pah-rahr-meh)

I cannot read English. Can you help me?
No puedo leer inglés. ¿Puede ayudarme?
(Noh poo-eh-doh leh-ehr een-glehs. Poo-eh-deh ah-yoo-dahr-meh)

I charged.
Yo cobré.
(Yoh koh-breh)

I checked your X-rays.
Revisé sus radiografías.
(Reh-bee-seh soos rah-dee-oh-grah-fee-ahs)

I do not like it.
No me gusta.
(Noh meh goos-tah)

I don't have a pen either.
Tampoco tengo una pluma.
(Tahm-poh-koh tehn-goh oo-nah ploo-mah)

I don't think so.
No lo creo.
(Noh loh kreh-oh)

I feel dizzy.
Me siento mareado.
(Meh see-ehn-toh mah-reh-ah-doh)

I feel overwhelmed, anxious.
Me siento abatido, ansioso.
(Meh see-ehn-toh ah-bah-tee-doh, ahn-see-oh-soh)

I go downtown [on] Tuesdays.
Los martes voy al centro.
(Lohs mahr-tehs boy ahl sehn-troh)

I go to sleep at eleven.
Me duermo a las once.
(Meh doo-ehr-moh ah lahs ohn-seh)

I guess this wasn't a planned activity for today!
¡Supongo que esta actividad no estaba planeada para hoy!
(Soo-pohn-goh keh ehs-tah ahk-tee-bee-dahd noh ehs-tah-bah plah-neh-ah-dah pah-rah oh-ee)

I have a gown.
Tengo una bata.
(Tehn-goh oo-nah bah-tah)

I have a piece of paper.
Tengo un pedazo de papel.
(Tehn-goh oon peh-dah-soh deh pah-pehl)

I have been sick all morning.
Me he sentido mal toda la mañana.
(Meh eh sehn-tee-doh mahl toh-dah lah mah-nyah-nah)

I have diarrhea and stomach pains.
Tengo diarrea y dolores de estómago.
(Tehn-goh dee-ah-reh-ah ee doh-loh-rehs deh ehs-toh-mah-goh)

I have finished the exam.
Terminé de revisarte.
(Tehr-mee-neh deh reh-bee-sahr-teh)

I have first-hand information.
Tengo información de primera.
(Tehn-goh een-fohr-mah-see-ohn deh pree-meh-rah)

I have looked at the information we discussed yesterday.
He revisado la información que discutimos ayer.
(Eh reh-bee-sah-doh lah een-fohr-mah-see-ohn keh dees-koo-tee-mohs ah-yehr)

I have nausea, vomiting, fever, and general malaise.
Tengo náuseas, vómito, fiebre y malestar general.

(Tehn-goh nah-oo-seh-ahs, boh-mee-toh, fee-eh-breh ee mahl-ehs-tahr heh-neh-rahl)

I have nausea and fever.
Tengo náusea y fiebre.
(Tehn-goh nah-oo-seh-ah ee fee-eh-breh)

I have neither paper nor pencil.
No tengo ni papel ni lápiz.
(Noh tehn-goh nee pah-pehl nee lah-pees)

I have noticed some difficulty breathing for the last two days.
Me he dado cuenta de alguna dificultad para respirar en los últimos dos días.
(Meh eh dah-doh koo-ehn-tah deh ahl-goo-nah dee-fee-kuhl-tahd pah-rah rehs-pee-rahr ehn lohs ool-tee-mohs dohs dee-ahs)

I have pain.
Tengo dolor.
(Tehn-goh doh-lohr)

I have the bedpan.
Tengo el bacín/pato.
(Tehn-goh ehl bah-seen/pah-toh)

I have to assess first.
Necesito evaluar primero.
(Neh-seh-see-toh eh-bah-loo-ahr pree-meh-roh)

I have to enter the information in the computer.
Tengo que poner la información en la computadora.
(Tehn-goh keh poh-nehr lah een-fohr-mah-see-ohn ehn lah kohm-poo-tah-doh-rah)

I hope you do well.
Que siga bien.
(Keh see-gah bee-ehn)

I like green [that which is green].
Me gusta lo verde.
(Meh goos-tah loh behr-deh)

I like summer.
Me gusta el verano.
(Meh goos-tah ehl beh-rah-noh)

I need better directions.
Necesito mejores direcciones.
(Neh-seh-see-toh meh-hoh-rehs dee-rehk-see-ohn-ehs)

I need for you to sign this permission slip so that the procedure might be done.
Necesito que firme usted el permiso, para realizar este estudio.
(Neh-seh-see-toh keh feer-meh oos-tehd ehl pehr-mee-soh, pah-rah reh-ah-lee-sahr ehs-teh ehs-too-dee-oh)

I need to ask you some questions.
Necesito hacerle unas preguntas.
(Neh-seh-see-toh ah-sehr-leh oo-nahs preh-goon-tahs)

I need to cut the pants.
Necesito cortar el pantalón.
(Neh-seh-see-toh kohr-tahr ehl pahn-tah-lohn)

I need to go to the surgery clinic.
Necesito ir a la clínica de cirugía.
(Neh-seh-see-toh eer ah lah klee-nee-kah deh see-roo-hee-ah)

I need to see Doctor White.
Necesito ver al doctor White.
(Neh-seh-see-toh behr ahl dohk-tohr White)

I need to see if you are hurt.
Necesito ver si está lastimado.
(Neh-seh-see-toh behr see ehs-tah lahs-tee-mah-doh)

I need to see the injured.
Necesito ver al accidentado.
(Neh-seh-see-toh behr ahl ahk-see-dehn-tah-doh)

I need to use a tourniquet.
Necesito usar un torniquete/una ligadura.
(Neh-seh-see-toh oo-sahr oon tohr-nee-keh-teh/oon-ah lee-gah-doo-rah)

I need two tubes of blood.
Necesito dos tubos de sangre.
(Neh-seh-see-toh dohs too-bohs deh sahn-greh)

I never have headaches!
¡Nunca tengo dolor de cabeza!
(Noon-kah tehn-goh doh-lohr deh kah-beh-sah)

I pulled your tooth.
Le saqué el diente.
(Leh sah-keh ehl dee-ehn-teh)

I see.
Ya veo.
(Yah beh-oh)

I see how good she is.
Ya veo lo buena que es.
(Yah beh-oh loh boo-eh-nah keh ehs)

I see no one.
No veo a nadie.
(Noh beh-oh ah nah-dee-eh)

I see no one here.
No veo a nadie aquí.
(Noh beh-oh ah nah-dee-eh ah-kee)

I think it is broken.
Creo que está rota.
(Kreh-oh keh ehs-tah roh-tah)

I think the same as you.
Pienso lo mismo que usted.
(Pee-ehn-soh loh mees-moh keh oos-tehd)

I want . . .
Yo quiero . . .
(Yoh kee-eh-roh . . .)

I want something to eat!
¡Yo quiero algo de comer!
(Yoh kee-eh-roh ahl-goh deh koh-mehr)

I want something to drink!
¡Yo quiero algo de tomar/beber!
(Yoh kee-eh-roh ahl-goh deh toh-mahr/ beh-behr)

I want something to read!
¡Yo quiero algo de leer!
(Yoh kee-eh-roh ahl-goh deh leh-ehr)

I want to be a nurse.
Quiero ser enfermera.
(Kee-eh-roh sehr ehn-fehr-meh-rah)

I want to examine the older child.
Quiero examinar al niño mayor.
(Kee-eh-roh ehx-ah-mee-nahr ahl nee-nyoh mah-yohr)

I want to see if the X-rays are good.
Quiero ver si los rayos X salieron bien.
(Kee-eh-roh behr see lohs rah-yohs eh-kees sah-lee-eh-rohn bee-ehn)

I want to take a sample of blood from your finger.
Quiero tomar una muestra de sangre del dedo.
(Kee-eh-roh toh-mahr oo-nah moo-ehs-trah deh sahn-greh del deh-doh)

I want to take a sample from your finger.
Quiero tomar una muestra del dedo.
(Kee-eh-roh toh-mahr oo-nah moo-ehs-trah dehl deh-doh)

I want to talk about bacterial plaque.
Quiero platicar acerca de la placa bacteriana.
(Kee-eh-roh plah-tee-kahr ah-sehr-kah deh lah plah-kah bahk-teh-ree-ah-nah)

I want to talk to you.
Quiero hablar con usted.
(Kee-eh-roh ah-blahr kohn oos-tehd)

I want to test the sugar level.
Quiero revisar el nivel de azúcar.
(Kee-eh-roh reh-bee-sahr ehl nee-behl deh ah-soo-kahr)

I want you to chew on them for four minutes.
Quiero que las mastique por cuatro minutos.
(Kee-eh-roh keh lahs mahs-tee-keh pohr koo-ah-troh mee-noo-tohs)

I want you to write your name and today's date.
Quiero que escriba su nombre y la fecha de hoy.
(Kee-eh-roh keh ehs-kree-bah soo nohm-breh ee lah feh-chah deh oh-ee)

I was doing nothing.
No estaba haciendo nada.
(Noh ehs-tah-bah ah-see-ehn-doh nah-dah)

I was just sitting, watching television when the pain started.
Solo estaba sentado, viendo televisión cuando comenzó el dolor.
(Soh-loh ehs-tah-bah sehn-tah-doh, bee-ehn-doh teh-leh-bee-see-ohn koo-ahn-doh koh-mehn-soh ehl doh-lohr)

I was told to come here.
Me dijeron que viniera aquí.
(Meh dee-heh-rohn keh bee-nee-eh-rah ah-kee)

I will ask you to void.
Le diré que orine.
(Leh dee-reh keh oh-ree-neh)

I will auscultate.
Voy a auscultar/escuchar.
(Boy ah ah-oos-kool-tahr/ehs-koo-chahr)

I will call for a wheel chair.
Llamaré por una silla de ruedas.
(Yah-mah-reh pohr oo-nah see-yah deh roo-eh-dahs)

I will call the radiologist.
Voy a hablarle al radiólogo.
(Boy ah ah-blahr-leh ahl rah-dee-oh-loh-goh)

I will call transportation.
Llamaré al transporte.
(Yah-mah-reh ahl trahns-pohr-teh)

I will check the arm.
Voy a revisar el brazo.
(Boy ah reh-bee-sahr ehl brah-soh)

I will check the ears.
Voy a revisar las orejas.
(Boy ah reh-bee-sahr lahs oh-reh-hahs)

I will check the eyes.
Voy a revisar los ojos.
(Boy ah reh-bee-sahr lohs oh-hohs)

I will check the hand.
Voy a revisar la mano.
(Boy ah reh-bee-sahr lah mah-noh)

I will check the mouth.
Voy a revisar la boca.
(Boy ah reh-bee-sahr lah boh-kah)

I will check the nose.
Voy a revisar la nariz.
(Boy ah reh-bee-sahr lah nah-rees)

I will check the throat.
Voy a revisar la garganta.
(Boy ah reh-bee-sahr lah gahr-gahn-tah)

I will check your abdomen.
Voy a revisar tu abdomen.
(Boy ah reh-bee-sahr too ahb-doh-mehn)

I will check your gums.
Voy a revisar tus encías.
(Boy ah reh-bee-sahr toos ehn-see-ahs)

I will check your head.
Voy a revisar tu cabeza.
(Boy ah reh-bee-sahr too kah-beh-sah)

I will check your liver.
Voy a revisar tu hígado.
(Boy ah reh-bee-sahr too ee-gah-doh)

I will check your teeth.
Voy a revisar tus dientes.
(Boy ah reh-bee-sahr toos dee-ehn-tehs)

I will collect a sample of feces.
Voy a recoger una muestra de excremento.
(Boy ah reh-koh-hehr oo-nah moo-ehs-trah deh ehx-kreh-mehn-toh)

I will examine the anus, strain down.
Voy a examinar el ano, empuja, haz fuerza.
(Boy ah ehx-ah-mee-nahr ehl ah-noh, ehm-poo-hah, ahs foo-ehr-sah)

I will examine the foot.
Voy a examinar el pie.
(Boy ah ehx-ah-mee-nahr ehl pee-eh)

I will examine the genitalia.
Voy a examinar los genitales.
(Boy ah ehx-ah-mee-nahr lohs heh-nee-tah-lehs)

I will examine the leg.
Voy a examinar la pierna.
(Boy ah ehx-ah-mee-nahr lah pee-ehr-nah)

I will examine the rectum.
Voy a examinar el recto.
(Boy ah ehx-ah-mee-nahr ehl rehk-toh)

I will examine the back.
Voy a examinar la espalda.
(Boy ah ehx-ah-mee-nahr lah ehs-pahl-dah)

I will examine your nailbeds.
Voy a examinar la base de tus uñas.
(Boy ah ehx-ah-mee-nahr lah bah-seh deh toos oo-nyahs)

I will give you recommendations for you and the baby.
Le daré recomendaciones para usted y su bebé.
(Leh dah-reh reh-koh-mehn-dah-see-ohn-ehs pah-rah oos-tehd ee soo beh-beh)

I will help you sit.
Le ayudaré a sentarse.
(Leh ah-yoo-dah-reh ah sehn-tahr-seh)

I will inspect your chest.
Voy a revisar tu pecho.
(Boy ah reh-bee-sahr too peh-choh)

I will inspect your skin.
Voy a inspeccionar tu piel.
(Boy ah eens-pehk-see-oh-nahr too pee-ehl)

I will listen first.
Voy a escuchar primero.
(Boy ah ehs-koo-chahr pree-meh-roh)

I will listen to the heart.
Voy a escuchar el corazón.
(Boy ah ehs-koo-chahr ehl koh-rah-sohn)

I will listen to the lungs.
Voy a escuchar los pulmones.
(Boy ah ehs-koo-chahr lohs pool-mohn-ehs)

I will listen to your apical pulse.
Voy a escuchar el latido del corazón.
(Boy ah ehs-koo-chahr ehl lah-tee-doh dehl koh-rah-sohn)

I will not find the street.
No encontraré la calle.
(Noh ehn-kohn-trah-reh lah kah-yeh)

I will observe the jugular vein.
Voy a observar tu vena yugular.
(Boy ah ohb-sehr-bahr too beh-nah yoo-goo-lahr)

I will palpate.
Voy a palpar/tocar.
(Boy ah pahl-pahr/toh-kahr)

I will palpate deeply.
Voy a palpar hondo.
(Boy ah pahl-pahr ohn-doh)

I will palpate it.
Voy a palparla.
(Boy ah pahl-pahr-lah)

I will palpate lightly.
Voy a palpar ligero.
(Boy ah pahl-pahr lee-heh-roh)

I will palpate the abdomen.
Voy a palpar el abdomen.
(Boy ah pahl-pahr ehl ahb-doh-mehn)

I will palpate the axillary nodes.
Voy a palpar los nodos de la axila.
(Boy ah pahl-pahr lohs noh-dohs deh lah ahx-ee-lah)

I will palpate the breast.
Voy a palpar el seno.
(Boy ah pahl-pahr ehl seh-noh)

I will palpate the elbow.
Voy a palpar el codo.
(Boy ah pahl-pahr ehl koh-doh)

I will palpate the groin; strain down.
Voy a palpar las ingles; empuja/empuje.
(Boy ah pahl-pahr lahs een-glehs; ehm-poo-hah/ehm-poo-heh)

I will palpate the hand.
Voy a palpar la mano.
(Boy ah pahl-pahr lah mah-noh)

I will palpate the nodes.
Voy a palpar los nodos.
(Boy ah pahl-pahr lohs noh-dohs)

I will palpate the rectum.
Voy a palpar el recto.
(Boy ah pahl-pahr ehl rehk-toh)

I will palpate the shoulder.
Voy a palpar el hombro.
(Boy ah pahl-pahr ehl ohm-broh)

I will palpate with both hands.
Voy a palpar con las dos manos.
(Boy ah pahl-pahr kohn lahs dohs mah-nohs)

I will palpate your carotid pulse.
Voy a palpar tu pulso de la carótida.
(Boy ah pahl-pahr too pool-soh deh lah kah-roh-tee-dah)

I will palpate your chest.
Voy a palpar tu pecho.
(Boy ah pahl-pahr too peh-choh)

I will palpate your feet and ankles.
Voy a palpar tus pies y tobillos.
(Boy ah pahl-pahr toos pee-ehs ee toh-bee-yohs)

I will palpate your knees.
Voy a palpar tus rodillas.
(Boy ah pahl-pahr toos roh-dee-yahs)

I will percuss.
Voy a percutir.
(Boy ah pehr-koo-teer)

I will percuss your side.
Voy a percutir tu costado.
(Boy ah pehr-koo-teer too kohs-tah-doh)

I will place the trays over the teeth.
Pondré las bandejas sobre los dientes.
(Pohn-dreh lahs bahn-deh-hahs soh-breh lohs dee-ehn-tehs)

I will press on your big toe.
Voy a apretar tu dedo grueso.
(Boy ah ah-preh-tahr too deh-doh groo-eh-soh)

I will put you on the stretcher.
Voy a ponerlo en la camilla.
(Boy ah poh-nehr-loh ehn lah kah-mee-yah)

I will remind you during the day.
Le recordaré durante el día.
(Leh reh-kohr-dah-reh doo-rahn-teh ehl dee-ah)

I will return!
¡Regresaré!
(Reh-greh-sah-reh)

I will return in ten minutes and we can walk down together.
Volveré en diez minutos y podremos caminar juntos.
(Bohl-beh-reh ehn dee-ehs mee-noo-tohs ee poh-dreh-mohs kah-mee-nahr hoon-tohs)

I will return shortly.
Regresaré en seguida.
(Reh-greh-sah-reh ehn seh-ghee-dah)

I will return to ask you more questions.
Regresaré para hacerle más preguntas.
(Reh-greh-sah-reh pah-rah ah-sehr-leh mahs preh-goon-tahs)

I will see the strength of the abdominal muscle.
Voy a ver la fuerza del músculo abdominal.
(Boy ah behr lah foo-ehr-sah dehl moos-koo-loh ahb-doh-mee-nahl)

I will see you, Mrs. García.
Hasta luego, señora García.
(Ahs-tah loo-eh-goh, seh-nyoh-rah Gahr-see-ah)

I will see you tomorrow.
La veré mañana.
(Lah beh-reh mah-nyah-nah)

I will see you tomorrow at nine.
Lo veré mañana a las nueve.
(Loh beh-reh mah-nyah-nah ah lahs noo-eh-beh)

I will show you your room.
Le mostraré su cuarto.
(Leh mohs-trah-reh soo koo-ahr-toh)

I will start by taking vital signs.
Voy a empezar por tomar los signos vitales.
(Boy ah ehm-peh-sahr pohr toh-mahr lohs seeg-nohs bee-tah-lehs)

I will take the radial pulse.
Voy a tomar su pulso radial.
(Boy ah toh-mahr soo pool-soh rah-dee-ahl)

I will take your blood pressure.
Voy a tomar tu presión de sangre.
(Boy ah toh-mahr too preh-see-ohn deh sahn-greh)

I will talk to you every day.
Hablaré con usted todos los días.
(Ah-blah-reh kohn oos-tehd toh-dohs lohs dee-ahs)

I will talk to your mother again.
Hablaré con tu mamá otra vez.
(Ah-blah-reh kohn too mah-mah oh-trah behs)

I will use local anesthetic.
Le pondré/aplicaré anestesia local.
(Leh pohn-dreh/ah-plee-kah-reh ah-nehs-teh-see-ah loh-kahl)

I will use resins.
Usaré resinas.
(Oo-sah-reh reh-see-nahs)

I will wake you up in the morning.
La voy a despertar en la mañana.
(Lah boy ah dehs-pehr-tahr ehn lah mah-nyah-nah)

I wish all of you would leave me alone.
Deseo que todos ustedes me dejen solo.
(Deh-seh-oh keh toh-dohs oos-teh-dehs meh deh-hehn soh-loh)

I would like to talk to you.
Me gustaría hablar contigo/con usted.
(Meh goos-tah-ree-ah ah-blahr kohn-tee-goh/kohn oos-tehd)

If cavities are present, it will help slow the process.
Si tiene cavidades, ayudará a retardar el proceso.
(See tee-ehn-eh kah-bee-dah-dehs, ah-yoo-dahr-ah ah reh-tahr-dahr ehl proh-seh-soh)

If it hurts, tell me.
Si duele, avísame.
(See doo-eh-leh, ah-bee-sah-meh)

If it is a lot, or there is fever . . .
Si es abundante o aparece fiebre . . .
(See ehs ah-boon-dahn-teh oh ah-pah-reh-seh fee-eh-breh)

If it is far, could I drive?
Si está lejos, ¿podría manejar?
(See ehs-tah leh-hohs, poh-dree-ah mah-neh-hahr)

If nurses find expired items in the unit, they return them to the pharmacy for replacement.

Si las enfermeras encuentran artículos con fecha vencida, los regresan a la farmacia donde son reemplazados.
(See lahs ehn-fehr-meh-rahs ehn-koo-ehn-trahn ahr-tee-koo-lohs kohn feh-chah behn-see-dah, lohs reh-greh-sahn ah lah fahr-mah-see-ah dohn-deh sohn reh-ehm-plah-sah-dohs)

If there is no ice in the bucket, call me.
Si no hay hielo en la tina, llámeme.
(See noh ah-ee ee-eh-loh ehn lah tee-nah, yah-meh-meh)

If yes, when is your due date?
Sí es así, ¿cuándo se alivia?
(See ehs ah-see, koo-ahn-doh seh ah-lee-bee-ah)

If you become infected with HIV, what is the risk of getting AIDS?
¿Si ha sido infectado con VIH, cuál es el riesgo de contraer el SIDA?
(See ah see-doh een-fehk-tah-doh kohn VIH, koo-ahl ehs ehl ree-ehs-goh deh kohn-trah-ehr ehl see-dah)

If you do not understand, please let me know.
Si no entiende, dígame por favor.
(See noh ehn-tee-ehn-deh, dee-gah-meh pohr fah-bohr)

If you follow these recommendations . . .
Si usted sigue estos consejos . . .
(See oos-tehd see-geh ehs-tohs kohn-seh-hohs)

If you have been here, I need your card.
Si ha estado aquí, necesito su tarjeta.
(See ah ehs-tah-doh ah-kee, neh-seh-see-toh soo tahr-heh-tah)

If you haven't, please fill out these papers.
Si no, por favor llene estos papeles.
(See noh, pohr fah-bohr yeh-neh ehs-tohs pah-peh-lehs)

If you need more sheets, call the assistant.
Si necesita más sábanas, llame a la asistente.
(See neh-seh-see-tah mahs sah-bah-nahs, yah-meh ah lah ah-sees-tehn-teh)

If you notice fever or any problems in the incision, go to my office immediately.
Si nota fiebre o problemas en la herída, vaya inmediatamente a mi oficina.
(See noh-tah fee-eh-breh oh proh-bleh-mahs ehn lah eh-ree-dah, bah-yah een-meh-dee-ah-tah-mehn-teh ah mee oh-fee-see-nah)

If you react to the medicine . . .
Si reacciona mal al medicamento . . .
(See reh-ahk-see-ohn-ah mahl ahl meh-dee-kah-mehn-toh)

If you see anything wrong, take him to the doctor.
Si nota algo malo, llévelo a su médico.
(See noh-tah ahl-goh mah-loh, yeh-beh-loh ah soo meh-dee-koh)

If you want to watch TV, you have to pay a fee.
Si quiere ver la televisión, tiene que pagar una cuota.
(See kee-eh-reh behr lah teh-leh-bee-see-ohn, tee-eh-neh keh pah-gahr oo-nah koo-oh-tah)

If your behavior changes you must go to a specialist.
Si continúa con cambios en su persona debe acudir con un especialista.
(See kohn-tee-noo-ah kohn kahm-bee-ohs ehn soo pehr-soh-nah deh-beh ah-koo-deer kohn oon ehs-peh-see-ah-lees-tah)

In addition . . .
Además . . .
(Ah-deh-mahs)

In case of a medication error, the doctor is notified.
En caso de error en el medicamento, se notifica al doctor.
(Ehn kah-soh deh eh-rohr ehn ehl meh-dee-kah-mehn-toh, seh noh-tee-fee-kah ahl dohk-tohr)

In case of fire, take the stairs.
En caso de fuego, tome la escalera.
(Ehn kah-soh deh foo-eh-goh, toh-meh lah ehs-kah-leh-rah)

In large part . . .
En gran parte . . .
(Ehn grahn pahr-teh)

In that case, tell me your whole name.
En ese caso, dígame su nombre completo.
(Ehn eh-seh kah-soh, dee-gah-meh soo nohm-breh kohm-pleh-toh)

In the middle of . . .
A mediados de . . .
(Ah meh-dee-ah-dohs deh)

In your case, eat nothing after 8 tonight.
En su caso, no coma nada después de las ocho de la noche.
(Ehn soo kah-soh, noh koh-mah nah-dah dehs-poo-ehs deh lahs oh-choh deh lah noh-cheh)

Include in the label . . .
Incluya en la etiqueta . . .
(Een-kloo-yah ehn lah eh-tee-keh-tah)

Infected persons can transmit the virus.
Las personas infectadas pueden transmitir el virus.
(Lahs pehr-soh-nahs een-fehk-tah-dahs poo-eh-dehn trahns-mee-teer ehl beeroos)

Insert the floss gently between the teeth.
Meta el hilo suavemente en medio de los dientes.
(Meh-tah ehl ee-loh soo-ah-beh-mehn-teh ehn meh-dee-oh deh lohs dee-ehn-tehs)

Intravenous drug abusers
Los que abusan de las drogas intravenosas
(Lohs keh ah-boo-sahn deh lahs droh-gahs een-trah-beh-noh-sahs)

Is he/she with you?
¿El/Ella viene con usted?
(Ehl/Eh-yah bee-eh-neh kohn oos-tehd)

Is he/she at work?
¿Está trabajando?
(Ehs-tah trah-bah-hahn-doh)

Is he/she breast-feeding (taking the breast)?
¿Está tomando pecho?
(Ehs-tah toh-mahn-doh peh-choh)

Is he/she coughing?
¿Está tosiendo?
(Ehs-tah toh-see-ehn-doh)

Is he/she eating well?
¿Está comiendo bien?
(Ehs-tah koh-mee-ehn-doh bee-ehn)

Is he/she hyperactive?
¿Es inquieto(a)/latoso(a)?
(Ehs een-kee-eh-toh[tah]/lah-toh-soh[sah])

Is he/she sleeping well?
¿Está durmiendo bien?
(Ehs-tah door-mee-ehn-doh bee-ehn)

Is he/she taking formula?
¿Tomando fórmula?
(Toh-mahn-doh fohr-moo-lah)

Is he/she urinating well?
¿Orina bien?
(Oh-ree-nah bee-ehn?)

Is it a dry cough?
¿Es tos seca?
(Ehs tohs seh-kah)

Is it a house?
¿Es una casa?
(Ehs oo-nah kah-sah)

Is it far?
¿Está lejos?
(Ehs-tah leh-hohs)

Is it here in town?
¿Está en esta ciudad?
(Ehs-tah ehn ehs-tah see-oo-dahd)

Is it the same color?
¿Es del mismo color?
(Ehs dehl mees-moh koh-lohr)

Is parking available?
¿Hay estacionamiento?
(Ah-ee ehs-tah-see-oh-nah-mee-ehn-toh)

Is someone with you?
¿Hay alguien con usted?
(Ah-ee ahl-gee-ehn kohn oos-tehd)

Is that a lot?
¿Es mucho?
(Ehs moo-choh)

Is that an apartment?
¿Es apartamento?
(Ehs ah-pahr-tah-mehn-toh)

Is that enough?
¿Es mucho/suficiente?
(Ehs moo-choh/soo-fee-see-ehn-teh)

Is that too much?
¿Es mucho/demasiado?
(Ehs moo-choh/deh-mah-see-ah-doh)

Is the pain localized in the same place?
¿El dolor está fijo en el mismo lugar?
(Ehl doh-lohr ehs-tah fee-hoh ehn ehl mees-moh loo-gahr)

Is the pain there all the time, or does it come and go?
¿Está el dolor allí todo el tiempo, o va y viene?
(Ehs-tah ehl doh-lohr ah-yee toh-doh ehl tee-ehm-poh, oh bah ee bee-ehn-eh?)

Is there a danger from donating blood?
¿Qué peligro hay por sangre donada?
(Keh peh-lee-groh ah-ee pohr sahn-greh doh-nah-dah)

Is there a laboratory test for AIDS?
¿Hay pruebas de laboratorio para detectar el SIDA?
(Ah-ee proo-eh-bahs deh lah-boh-rah-toh-ree-oh pah-rah deh-tehk-tahr ehl see-dah)

Is there a policeman?
¿Hay un policía?
(Ah-ee oon poh-lee-see-ah)

Is there any pain?
¿Tiene algún dolor?
(Tee-eh-neh ahl-goon doh-lohr)

Is there anything that worries you?
¿Hay algo que le preocupa?
(Ah-ee ahl-goh keh leh preh-oh-koo-pah)

Is there anything else bothering you?
¿Hay otra cosa que le moleste?
(Ah-ee oh-trah koh-sah keh-leh moh-lehs-teh)

Is there numbness / a tingling sensation / burning in your leg / arm / foot / hand?
¿Está entumecido/adormecido/tiene ardor en su pierna/brazo/pie/mano?
(Ehs-tah ehn-too-meh-see-doh/ah-dohr-meh-see-do/tee-eh-neh ahr-dohr ehn soo pee-ehr-nah/brah-soh/pee-eh/mah-noh)

Is this ______ Hospital?
¿Es este el Hospital ______?
(Ehs ehs-teh ehl ohs-pee-tahl ______)

Is this your first time in the hospital?
¿Es su primera vez en el hospital?
(Ehs soo pree-meh-rah behs ehn ehl ohs-pee-tahl)

Is this your first suicide attempt?
¿Es este su primer intento de suicidio?
(Ehs ehs-teh soo pree-mehr een-tehn-toh deh soo-ee-see-dee-oh)

Is your appetite bad?
¿Tiene mal apetito?
(Tee-eh-neh mahl ah-peh-tee-toh)

Is your family in the city?
¿Está su familia en la ciudad?
(Ehs-tah soo fah-mee-lee-ah ehn lah see-oo-dahd)

Is your water bag broken?
¿Se reventó su bolsa de agua?
(Seh reh-behn-toh soo bohl-sah deh ah-goo-ah)

It is in the middle of the wall.
Está a la mitad de la pared.
(Ehs-tah ah lah mee-tahd deh lah pah-rehd)

It is not very far.
No está muy lejos.
(Noh ehs-tah moo-ee leh-hohs)

It also causes pyorrhea and tooth loss.
Causa pérdida de dientes y piorrea.
(Kah-oo-sah pehr-dee-dah deh dee-ehn-tehs ee pee-oh-reh-ah)

It belongs to the doctor.
Es del doctor.
(Ehs dehl dohk-tohr)

It belongs to the teacher.
Es de la maestra.
(Ehs deh lah mah-ehs-trah)

It can cause drowsiness.
Le puede causar sueño.
(Leh poo-eh-deh kah-oo-sahr soo-eh-nyoh)

It causes dental caries.
Causa caries dental.
(Kah-oo-sah kah-ree-ehs dehn-tahl)

It feels like a board.
Se siente como una tabla.
(Seh see-ehn-teh koh-moh oo-nah tah-blah)

It has the film inside.
Tiene la película adentro.
(Tee-eh-neh lah peh-lee-koo-lah ah-dehn-troh)

It hurts when I let go?
¿Duele cuando dejo ir?
(Doo-eh-leh koo-ahn-doh deh-hoh eer)

It hurts when I press?
¿Duele cuando aplano?
(Doo-eh-leh koo-ahn-doh ah-plah-noh)

It is a procedure used to see how open the veins are throughout the leg.
Es un procedimiento para valorar las venas de su pierna.
(Ehs oon proh-seh-dee-mee-ehn-toh pah-rah bah-loh-rahr lahs beh-nahs deh soo pee-ehr-nah)

It is a six-story building.
Es un edificio de seis pisos
(Ehs oon eh-dee-fee-see-oh deh seh-ees pee-sohs)

It is not as bad when I stay still, but it hurts a lot if I try to move the leg.
No está tan mal cuando estoy quieto, pero me duele mucho si trato de mover la pierna.
(Noh ehs-tah tahn mahl koo-ahn-doh ehs-toh-ee kee-eh-toh, peh-roh meh doo-eh-leh moo-choh see trah-toh deh moh-behr lah pee-ehr-nah)

It is one o'clock.
Es la una.
(Ehs lah oo-nah)

It is open 7:00 A.M. to 12:00 midnight.
Está abierta de 7 de la mañana a doce de la noche/medianoche.
(Ehs-tah ah-bee-ehr-tah deh see-eh-teh deh lah mah-nyah-nah ah doh-seh deh lah noh-cheh/meh-dee-ah-noh-cheh)

It is open Saturday, Sunday, and holidays.
Está abierta los sábados, domingos, y días festivos.
(Ehs-tah ah-bee-ehr-tah lohs sah-bah-dohs, doh-meen-gohs ee dee-ahs fehs-tee-bohs)

It is the next day.
Es el día siguiente.
(Ehs ehl dee-ah see-ghee-ehn-teh)

It is time to go, Roger.
Es tiempo de ir, Roger.
(Ehs tee-ehm-poh deh eer, Roger)

It is time to go to your O.T. appointment.
Es la hora de ir a su cita de terapia ocupacional (OT).
(Ehs lah oh-rah deh eer ah soo see-tah deh teh-rah-pee-ah oh-koo-pah-see-oh-nahl [OT])

It keeps the food warm.
Guarda la comida tibia.
(Goo-ahr-dah lah koh-mee-dah tee-bee-ah)

It looked as if a professional had made it.
Parece como si un profesional lo hubiera hecho.
(Pah-reh-seh koh-moh see oon proh-feh-see-oh-nahl loh oo-bee-eh-rah heh-choh)

It sounds good.
Se oye bien.
(Seh oh-yeh bee-ehn)

It takes 10 minutes.
Se toma diez minutos.
(Seh toh-mah dee-ehs mee-nooh-tohs)

It will also help if you have any teeth that are sensitive.
Ayudará también si los dientes están sensibles.
(Ah-yoo-dah-rah tahm-bee-ehn see lohs dee-ehn-tehs ehs-tahn sehn-see-blehs)

It will take a minute.
Va a tomar un minuto.
(Bah ah toh-mahr oon mee-noo-toh)

It will take ten minutes.
Se tomará diez minutos.
(Seh toh-mah-rah dee-ehs mee-noo-tohs)

Jump with one foot.
Brinca con un pie.
(Breen-kah kohn oon pee-eh)

Keep moving!
¡Siga moviéndose!
(See-gah moh-bee-ehn-doh-seh)

Keep quiet!
¡Estése quieto!/¡No se mueva!
(Ehs-teh-seh kee-eh-toh/Noh seh moo-eh-bah)

Keep the area clean.
Mantenga el área limpia.
(Mahn-tehn-gah ehl ah-reh-ah leem-pee-ah)

Keep the baby awake.
Mantenga al bebé despierto.
(Mahn-tehn-gah ahl beh-beh dehs-pee-ehr-toh)

Keep the leg straight.
Mantenga la pierna derecha.
(Mahn-tehn-gah lah pee-ehr-nah deh-reh-chah)

Keep the siderails up at night.
Mantenga los barandales levantados durante la noche.
(Mahn-tehn-gah lohs bah-rahn-dah-lehs leh-bahn-tah-dohs doo-rahn-teh lah noh-cheh)

Keep your feet together!
¡Ponga los pies juntos!
(Pohn-gah lohs pee-ehs hoon-tohs)

Keep your leg elevated.
Mantenga la pierna elevada.
(Mahn-tehn-gah lah pee-ehr-nah eh-leh-bah-dah)

Kitchen personnel bring the food trays.
Los empleados de la cocina traen las bandejas de comida.
(Lohs ehm-pleh-ah-dohs deh lah koh-see-nah trah-ehn lahs bahn-deh-hahs deh koh-mee-dah)

Kneel down!
¡Póngase de rodillas!
(Pohn-gah-seh deh roh-dee-yahs)

Later on, they will take X-rays.
Más tarde, le van a tomar rayos X.
(Mahs tahr-deh leh bahn ah toh-mahr rah-yohs eh-kees)

Lay down so I can examine you.
Acuéstese para explorarlo.
(Ah-koo-ehs-teh-seh pah-rah ehx-ploh-rahr-loh)

Leave the area uncovered.
Deje el área descubierta.
(Deh-heh ehl ah-reh-ah dehs-koo-bee-ehr-tah)

Lescol for the cholesterol and Naproxin for my aches.
Lescol para el colesterol y Naproxeno para mis dolores.
(Lehs-kohl pah-rah ehl koh-lehs-teh-rohl ee nah-prohx-eh-noh pah-rah mees doh-loh-rehs)

Let it go.
Déjalo ir/Suéltalo.
(Deh-hah-loh eer/Soo-ehl-tah-loh)

Let it out slowly.
Déjalo ir despacio.
(Deh-hah-loh eer dehs-pah-see-oh)

Let me go through.
Déjeme pasar.
(Deh-heh-meh pah-sahr)

Let me know how you feel.
Dígame cómo se siente.
(Dee-gah-meh koh-moh seh see-ehn-teh)

Let me show you the correct way to floss.
Déjeme enseñarle la manera correcta de usar el hilo.
(Deh-heh-meh ehn-seh-nyahr-leh lah mah-neh-rah koh-rehk-tah deh oo-sahr ehl ee-loh)

Let me show you with your toothbrush a way that will help you remove the plaque.
Déjeme enseñarle con su cepillo una manera que le ayudará a quitar la placa.
(Deh-heh-meh ehn-seh-nyahr-leh kohn soo seh-pee-yoh oo-nah mah-neh-rah keh leh ah-yoo-dahr-ah ah kee-tahr lah plah-kah)

Lie down!
¡Acuéstese!
(Ah-koo-ehs-teh-seh)

Lie down, please.
Acuéstese, por favor.
(Ah-koo-ehs-teh-seh, pohr fah-bohr)

Lift the arm!
¡Levante el brazo!
(Leh-bahn-teh ehl brah-soh)

Lift the foot.
Levante el pie.
(Leh-bahn-teh ehl pee-eh)

Lift your hand.
Levante tu mano.
(Leh-bahn-teh too mah-noh)

Lift your head.
Levante tu cabeza.
(Leh-bahn-teh too kah-beh-sah)

Lift your leg.
Levante tu pierna.
(Leh-bahn-teh too pee-ehr-nah)

Lift your right foot.
Levante tu pie derecho.
(Leh-bahn-teh too pee-eh deh-reh-choh)

Lips should not be dry.
Los labios no deben estar secos.
(Lohs lah-bee-ohs noh deh-behn ehs-tahr seh-kohs)

Listen!
¡Oiga!
(Oh-ee-gah)

Listen, please.
Escuchen, por favor.
(Ehs-koo-cheh, pohr fah-bohr)

Look down.
Vea abajo.
(Beh-ah ah-bah-hoh)

Look straight ahead.
Ve directo.
(Beh dee-rehk-toh)

Look straight at the light.
Ve directo a la luz.
(Beh dee-rehk-toh ah lah loos)

Look up; down!
¡Vea arriba; abajo!
(Beh-ah ah-ree-bah; ah-bah-hoh)

Lot number.
Número de lote.
(Noo-meh-roh deh loh-teh)

Lower the foot.
Baje el pie.
(Bah-heh ehl pee-eh)

Lower your head.
Baje la cabeza.
(Bah-heh lah kah-beh-sah)

Lower your legs.
Baje las piernas
(Bah-heh lahs pee-ehr-nahs)

Maintain it like this.
Manténlo así.
(Mahn-tehn-loh ah-see)

Make a fist!
¡Cierre la mano!/¡Haga un puño!
(See-eh-reh lah mah-noh/Ah-gah oon poo-nyoh)

Make some room!
¡Haga lugar!
(Ah-gah loo-gahr)

Make sure that you point the toothbrush toward the gumline.
Asegure que el cepillo apunte hacia la encía.
(Ah-seh-goo-reh keh ehl seh-pee-yoh ah-poon-teh ah-see-ah lah ehn-see-ah)

Make the baby burp.
Haga que el bebé eructe/repita.
(Ah-gah keh ehl beh-beh eh-rook-teh/reh-pee-tah)

May I help you?
¿Puedo ayudarlo?
(Poo-eh-doh ah-yoo-dahr-loh)

Medicaid?
¿Medicaid?
(Meh-dee-kehd)

Moist cough?
¿Tos húmeda?
(Tohs oo-meh-dah)

Monthly, the pharmacy staff inspects the medication area.
Cada mes, los empleados de la farmacia inspeccionan el área de medicamentos.
(Kah-dah mehs lohs ehm-pleh-ah-dohs deh lah fahr-mah-see-ah eens-pehk-see-ohn-ahn ehl ah-reh-ah deh meh-dee-kah-mehn-tohs)

Most have no symptoms.
La mayoría no tiene síntomas.
(Lah mah-yoh-ree-ah noh tee-eh-neh seen-toh-mahs)

Move!
¡Muévase!
(Moo-eh-bah-seh)

Move carefully!
¡Muévase con cuidado!
(Moo-eh-bah-seh kohn koo-ee-dah-doh)

Move it side to side.
Muévela de lado a lado.
(Moo-eh-beh-lah deh lah-doh ah lah-doh)

Move your leg.
Mueve tu pierna.
(Moo-eh-beh too pee-ehr-nah)

Move your leg backward.
Mueve tu pierna para atrás.
(Moo-eh-beh too pee-ehr-nah pah-rah ah-trahs)

Move your leg forward.
Mueve tu pierna para adelante.
(Moo-eh-beh too pee-ehr-nah pah-rah ah-deh-lahn-teh)

Mr. Garza, you probably have appendicitis.
Señor Garza, probablemente tiene apendicitis.
(Seh-nyohr Gahr-sah, proh-bah-bleh-mehn-teh tee-eh-neh ah-pehn-dee-see-tees)

Mr. Garza is sent to the anesthesiologist.
El señor Garza es enviado con el anestesista.
(Ehl seh-nyohr Gahr-sah ehs ehn-bee-ah-doh kohn ehl ah-nehs-teh-sees-tah)

Mr. Garza responds.
El señor Garza responde.
(Ehl seh-nyohr Gahr-sah rehs-pohn-deh)

Mr. Gómez left yesterday.
El señor Gómez salió ayer.
(Ehl seh-nyohr Goh-mehs sah-lee-oh ah-yehr)

Mr. Martínez arrives at the department.
El señor Martínez llega al departamento.
(Ehl seh-nyohr Mahr-tee-nehs yeh-gah ahl deh-pahr-tah-mehn-toh)

Mr. Ríos, how are you?
Señor Ríos, ¿cómo está?
(Seh-nyohr Ree-ohs, koh-moh ehs-tah)

Mrs. García, tomorrow you will be discharged from the hospital.
Señora García, mañana sale usted del hospital.
(Seh-nyoh-rah Gahr-see-ah, mah-nyah-nah sah-leh oos-tehd dehl ohs-pee-tahl)

Mrs. ______, the doctor ordered blood samples.
Señora ______, el doctor ordenó muestras de sangre.
(Seh-nyoh-rah ______, ehl dohk-tohr ohr-deh-noh moo-ehs-trahs deh sahn-greh)

Mrs. ______, I want you to get up and go to urinate.
Señora ______, quiero que se levante y vaya a orinar.
(Seh-nyoh-rah ______, kee-eh-roh keh seh leh-bahn-teh ee bah-yah ah oh-ree-nahr)

Mrs. ______, you need to go to the hospital.
Señora ______, necesita ir al hospital.
(Seh-nyoh-rah ______, neh-seh-see-tah eer ahl ohs-pee-tahl)

Mrs. ______, I need to help you change clothes.
Señora ______, necesito ayudarle a cambiar su ropa.
(Seh-nyoh-rah ______, neh-seh-see-toh ah-yoo-dahr-leh ah kahm-bee-ahr soo roh-pah)

My left leg hurts.
Me duele la pierna izquierda.
(Meh doo-eh-leh lah pee-ehr-nah ees-kee-ehr-dah)

My name is . . .
Mi nombre es . . . /Me llamo . . .
(Mee nohm-breh ehs/Meh yah-moh)

My wife just had a baby.
Mi esposa tuvo un bebé.
(Mee ehs-poh-sah too-boh oon beh-beh)

Name of the drug.
Nombre de la droga/del medicamento.
(Nohm-breh deh lah droh-gah/dehl meh-dee-kah-mehn-toh)

Name of the patient.
Nombre del paciente.
(Nohm-breh dehl pah-see-ehn-teh)

Never?
¿Nunca?
(Noon-kah)

Never mind.
No importa.
(Noh eem-pohr-tah)

No, but there is a test for antibodies.
No, pero hay prueba de anticuerpos.
(Noh, peh-roh ah-ee prooh-eh-bah deh ahn-tee-koo-ehr-pohs)

No, I did not enjoy working on my house.
No, no disfruté el trabajar en mi casa.
(Noh, noh dees-froo-teh ehl trah-bah-hahr ehn mee kah-sah)

No, I just do not want to go. It is not helping me.
No, sólo que no quiero ir. No me está ayudando.
(Noh, soh-loh keh noh kee-eh-roh eer. Noh meh ehs-tah ah-yoo-dahn-doh)

No, I do not speak English.
No, no hablo inglés.
(Noh, noh ah-bloh een-glehs)

No, I do not speak Spanish.
No, no hablo español.
(Noh, noh ah-bloh ehs-pah-nyohl)

No, I don't understand.
No, no comprendo/no entiendo.
(Noh, noh kohm-prehn-doh/noh ehn-tee-ehn-doh)

No, I have not noticed any.
No, no me he dado cuenta de ninguna cosa.
(Noh, noh meh eh dah-doh koo-ehn-tah deh neen-goo-nah koh-sah)

No, it moved to the right side.
No, se recorrió al lado derecho.
(Noh, seh reh-koh-ree-oh ahl lah-doh deh-reh-choh)

No, never.
No, nunca.
(Noh noon-kah)

No, not that I know of.
No, que yo sepa.
(Noh, keh yoh seh-pah)

No problem!
¡No hay problema!
(Noh ah-ee proh-bleh-mah)

No smoking.
No se permite fumar.
(Noh seh pehr-mee-teh foo-mahr)

Nonetheless . . .
Sin embargo . . .
(Seen ehm-bahr-goh)

Normal rectal temperature should be 100.4 degrees Fahrenheit.
La temperatura normal en el recto es de 100.4 grados Fahrenheit.
(Lah tehm-peh-rah-too-rah nohr-mahl ehn ehl rehk-toh ehs deh see-ehn poon-toh koo-ah-troh grah-dohs Fah-rehn-heh-eet)

Not at all.
De ningún modo.
(Deh neen-goon moh-doh)

Not right now, but I will discuss it with my family.
No por ahora, pero lo discutiré con mi familia.
(Noh pohr ah-oh-rah, peh-roh loh dees-koo-tee-reh kohn mee fah-mee-lee-ah)

Nothing seems to make it better or worse.
Nada parece hacerlo peor o mejor.
(Nah-dah pah-reh-seh ah-sehr-loh peh-ohr oh meh-hohr)

Nothing that I have ever known of.
A nada que yo sepa.
(Ah nah-dah keh yoh seh-pah)

Now bend over.
Ahora, agáchate.
(Ah-oh-rah, ah-gah-chah-teh)

Now I am going to give you some fluoride.
Ahora voy a darle fluoruro.
(Ah-oh-rah boy ah dahr-leh floh-roo-roh)

Now I need to X-ray the chest.
Ahora necesito tomar radiografías del pecho.
(Ah-oh-rah neh-seh-see-toh toh-mahr rah-dee-oh-grah-fee-ahs dehl peh-choh)

Now I will examine your abdomen.
Ahora voy a revisar tu abdomen/vientre.
(Ah-oh-rah boy ah reh-bee-sahr too ahb-doh-mehn/bee-ehn-treh)

Now I will examine your skin and chest.
Ahora voy a examinar tu piel y pecho.
(Ah-oh-rah boy ah ehx-ah-mee-nahr too pee-ehl ee peh-choh)

Now raise the left arm.
Ahora levante el brazo izquierdo.
(Ah-oh-rah leh-bahn-teh ehl brah-soh ees-kee-ehr-doh)

Now stand up!
¡Ahora levántate!
(Ah-oh-rah leh-bahn-tah-teh)

Now stand up and walk.
Ahora levántese y camine.
(Ah-oh-rah leh-bahn-teh-seh ee kah-mee-neh)

Now take a deep breath.
Ahora respira hondo/profundo.
(Ah-oh-rah rehs-pee-rah ohn-doh/proh-foon-doh)

Now turn to the screen.
Ahora voltee hacia la placa.
(Ah-oh-rah bohl-teh-eh ah-see-ah lah plah-kah)

Now you can change clothes.
Ahora se puede cambiar de ropa.
(Ah-oh-rah seh poo-eh-deh kahm-bee-ahr deh roh-pah)

Number of:
Número de:
(Noo-meh-roh deh)

Nurses control narcotic records in the unit.
Las enfermeras controlan archivos de narcóticos en el piso.
(Lahs ehn-fehr-meh-rahs kohn-troh-lahn ahr-chee-bohs deh nahr-koh-tee-kohs ehn ehl pee-soh)

Nursing staff take STAT orders to the pharmacy.
Las enfermeras llevan órdenes urgentes a la farmacia.
(Lahs ehm-fehr-meh-rahs yeh-bahn ohr-deh-nehs oor-hehn-tehs ah lah fahr-mah-see-ah)

Of course.
Desde luego.
(Dehs-deh loo-eh-goh)

Often, two times per week.
Seguido, dos veces por semana.
(Seh-gee-doh, dohs beh-sehs pohr seh-mah-nah)

On a scale from 1 [insignificant] to 10 [unbearable] . . .
En una escala del 1 [insignificante] al 10 [intolerable] . . .
(Ehn oo-nah ehs-kah-lah dehl oo-noh [een-seeg-nee-fee-kahn-teh] ahl dee-ehs [een-toh-leh-rah-bleh])

On the one hand . . .
Por un lado . . .
(Pohr oon lah-doh)

Once in a while.
De vez en cuando.
(Deh behs ehn koo-ahn-doh)

One more time.
Una vez más.
(Oo-nah behs mahs)

One tube for a blood count.
Un tubo para una biometría hemática.
(Oon too-boh pah-rah oo-nah bee-oh-meh-tree-ah eh-mah-tee-kah)

Only at parties.
Sólo en las fiestas.
(Soh-loh ehn lahs fee-ehs-tahs)

Only five minutes.
Sólo cinco minutos.
(Soh-loh seen-koh mee-noo-tohs)

Open!
¡Abra!
(Ah-brah)

Open again.
Abre otra vez.
(Ah-breh oh-trah behs)

Open the fingers wide.
Abre los dedos ancho.
(Ah-breh lohs deh-dohs ahn-choh)

Open your books, please.
Abran sus libros, por favor.
(Ah-brahn soos lee-brohs, pohr fah-bohr)

Open your eyes!
¡Abra los ojos!
(Ah-brah lohs oh-hohs)

Open your hand!
¡Abra la mano!
(Ah-brah lah mah-noh)

Open your mouth, please.
Abra la boca, por favor.
(Ah-brah lah boh-kah, pohr fah-bohr)

Oral examination.
Examinación oral.
(Ehx-ah-mee-nah-see-ohn oh-rahl)

Our patient.
Nuestro paciente.
(Noo-ehs-troh pah-see-ehn-teh)

Outpatient prescriptions are filled by the pharmacy.
Las recetas para pacientes de consulta externa se distribuyen por la farmacia.
(Lahs reh-seh-tahs pah-rah pah-see-ehn-tehs deh kohn-sool-tah ehx-tehr-nah seh dees-tree-boo-yehn pohr lah fahr-mah-see-ah)

Over a period . . .
Durante un periodo . . .
(Doo-rahn-teh oon peh-ree-oh-doh)

Over the stool.
Sobre el taburete.
(Soh-breh ehl tah-boo-reh-teh)

Pain?
¿Dolor?
(Doh-lohr)

Pain at the waist?
¿Dolor en la cintura?
(Doh-lor ehn lah seen-too-rah)

Pardon me!
¡Perdóneme!
(Pehr-doh-neh-meh)

Pat his back gently.
Dé palmaditas en la espalda.
(Deh pahl-mah-dee-tahs ehn lah ehs-pahl-dah)

Peanut butter sandwich.
Lonche de crema de cacahuate.
(Lohn-cheh deh kreh-mah deh kah-kah-oo-ah-teh)

Phone for local calls.
Teléfono para llamadas locales.
(Teh-leh-foh-noh pah-rah yah-mah-dahs loh-kahl-ehs)

Place the urine in the brown plastic bottle.
Ponga la orina en la botella de plástico café.
(Pohn-gah lah oh-ree-nah ehn lah boh-teh-yah deh plahs-tee-koh kah-feh)

Place your arms behind your back.
Pon los brazos atrás.
(Pohn lohs brah-sohs ah-trahs)

Place your feet here.
Ponga sus pies aquí.
(Pohn-gah lohs pee-ehs ah-kee)

Place your foot on the opposite knee.
Pon tu pie en la rodilla opuesta.
(Pohn too pee-eh ehn lah roh-dee-yah oh-poo-ehs-tah)

Place your hands behind your head.
Pon tus manos atrás de tu cabeza.
(Pohn toos mah-nohs ah-trahs deh too kah-beh-sah)

Plaque can be prevented by brushing and flossing.
La placa se evita usando hilo dental y cepillo.
(Lah plah-kah seh eh-bee-tah oo-sahn-doh ee-loh dehn-tahl ee seh-pee-yoh)

Plaque gets in between the teeth where the brush cannot reach.
La placa entra en medio de los dientes donde no alcanza el cepillo.
(Lah plah-kah ehn-trah ehn meh-dee-oh deh lohs dee-ehn-tehs dohn-deh noh ahl-kahn-sah ehl seh-pee-yoh)

Plaque is a sticky, colorless layer of bacteria.
La placa es una capa pegajosa sin color y con bacterias.
(Lah plah-kah ehs oo-nah kah-pah peh-gah-hoh-sah seen koh-lohr ee kohn bahk-teh-ree-ahs)

Please!
¡Por favor!
(Pohr fah-bohr)

Please bend your arm for about five minutes.
Por favor, doble el brazo por cinco minutos.
(Pohr fah-bohr, doh-bleh ehl brah-soh pohr seen-koh mee-noo-tohs)

Please breathe normally.
Por favor, respire normal.
(Pohr fah-bohr, rehs-pee-reh nohr-mahl)

Please change clothes.
Por favor, cámbiese de ropa.
(Por fah-bohr, kahm-bee-eh-seh deh roh-pah)

Please come back in a few minutes.
Por favor, regrese en unos minutos.
(Pohr fah-bohr, reh-greh-seh ehn oon-ohs mee-noo-tohs)

Please cross your leg.
Por favor, cruce la pierna.
(Pohr fah-bohr, kroo-seh lah pee-ehr-nah)

Please do not eat anything after midnight.
Por favor, no coma nada después de medianoche.
(Pohr fah-bohr, noh koh-mah nah-dah dehs-poo-ehs deh meh-dee-ah-noh-cheh)

Please don't move.
Por favor, no se mueva.
(Pohr fah-bohr, noh seh moo-eh-bah)

Please keep your appointment.
Por favor, acuda a la cita.
(Pohr fah-bohr, ah-koo-dah ah lah see-tah)

Please lie down.
Por favor, acuéstate.
(Pohr fah-bohr, ah-koo-ehs-tah-teh)

Please open your mouth some more.
Por favor, abra más la boca.
(Pohr fah-bohr, ah-brah mahs lah boh-kah)

Please put this gown on.
Por favor, póngase está bata.
(Pohr fah-bohr, pohn-gah-seh ehs-tah bah-tah)

Please raise this arm.
Por favor, levante este brazo.
(Pohr fah-bohr, leh-bahn-teh ehs-teh brah-soh)

Please repeat slowly.
Por favor, repita despacio.
(Pohr fah-bohr, reh-pee-tah dehs-pah-see-oh)

Please return as needed.
En caso necesario puede regresar.
(Ehn kah-soh neh-seh-sah-ree-oh, poo-eh-deh reh-greh-sahr)

Please return in six months.
Por favor, regrese en seis meses.
(Pohr fah-bohr, reh-greh-seh ehn seh-ees meh-sehs)

Please sign here.
Por favor, firme aquí.
(Pohr fah-bohr, feer-meh ah-kee)

Please sit down.
Siéntese, por favor.
(See-ehn-teh-seh, pohr fah-bohr)

Please sit down in the waiting room.
Por favor, siéntese en la sala de espera.
(Pohr fah-bohr, see-ehn-teh-seh ehn lah sah-lah deh ehs-peh-rah)

Please sit up on the bed.
Por favor, siéntate en la cama.
(Pohr fah-bohr, see-ehn-tah-teh ehn lah kah-mah)

Please stay/remain in bed.
Por favor, quédese en la cama.
(Pohr fah-bohr, keh-deh-seh ehn lah kah-mah)

Please tell the nurse to call me.
Por favor, dígale a la enfermera que me llame.
(Por fah-bohr, dee-gah-leh ah lah ehn-fehr-meh-rah keh meh yah-meh)

Please wait a few minutes.
Por favor, espere unos minutos.
(Poh fah-bohr, ehs-peh-reh oo-nohs mee-noo-tohs)

Please wait 30 minutes.
Por favor, espere treinta minutos.
(Pohr fah-bohr, ehs-peh-reh treh-een-tah mee-noo-tohs)

Point!
¡Apunte!/¡Señale!
(Ah-poon-teh)/Seh-nyah-leh)

Point when it hurts.
Señale cuando duela.
(Seh-nyah-leh koo-ahn-doh doo-eh-lah)

Practice with the brush and make sure you go around all the teeth.
Practique con el cepillo y asegure de cepillar alrededor de todos los dientes.
(Prahk-tee-keh kohn ehl seh-pee-yoh ee ahs-eh-goo-reh deh seh-pee-yahr ahl-reh-deh-dohr deh toh-dohs lohs dee-ehn-tehs)

Press hard!
¡Presione fuerte!
(Preh-see-oh-neh foo-ehr-teh)

Pronounce, please.
Pronuncien, por favor.
(Proh-noon-see-ehn, pohr fah-bohr)

Pull!
¡Jale!
(Hah-leh)

Pull the cord in the bathroom.
Jale el cordón en el baño.
(Hah-leh ehl kohr-dohn ehn ehl bah-nyoh)

Pull the knee to the chest.
Estira la rodilla al pecho.
(Ehs-tee-rah lah roh-dee-yah ahl peh-choh)

Pull up your hips!
¡Levante la cadera!
(Leh-bahn-teh lah kah-deh-rah)

Push!
¡Empuje!
(Ehm-poo-heh)

Push down with your feet against my hands.
Empuje los pies contra mis manos.
(Ehm-poo-heh lohs pee-ehs kohn-trah mees mah-nohs)

Raise your head.
Levanta tu cabeza.
(Leh-bahn-tah too kah-beh-sah)

Rather than . . .
Más bien que . . .
(Mahs bee-ehn keh)

Reactión to transfusions?
¿Reacción a transfusiones?
(Reh-ahk-see-ohn ah tranhs-foo-see-ohn-ehs)

Read, please.
Lea, por favor.
(Leh-ah, pohr fah-bohr)

Relax!
¡Relaje!
(Reh-lah-heh)

Relax, calm down!
¡Relájese, cálmese!
(Reh-lah-heh-seh, kahl-meh-seh)

Relax, it will not hurt!
¡Relájese, no le va a doler!
(Reh-lah-heh-seh, no leh bah ah doh-lehr)

Relax your arm.
Relaje el brazo.
(Reh-lah-heh ehl brah-soh)

Relax your leg.
Relaje la pierna.
(Reh-lah-heh lah pee-ehr-nah)

Relax your muscle.
Relaja tu músculo.
(Reh-lah-hah too moos-koo-loh)

Remember that you are to urinate and put it in the container.
Recuerde que debe orinar y poner la orina en el frasco.
(Reh-koo-ehr-deh keh deh-beh oh-ree-nahr ee poh-nehr lah oh-ree-nah ehn ehl frahs-koh)

Remember that you will do this for 24 hours.
Recuerde que hará esto por veinticuatro horas.
(Reh-koo-ehr-deh keh ah-rah ehs-toh pohr beh-een-tee-koo-ah-troh oh-rahs)

Remember to bring them back.
Acuérdese de devolverlos.
(Ah-koo-ehr-deh-seh deh deh-bohl-behr-lohs)

Repeat, please.
Repitan, por favor.
(Reh-pee-tahn, pohr fah-bohr)

Repeat one, two, three.
Repite uno, dos, tres.
(Reh-pee-teh oo-noh, dohs, trehs)

Repeat the word "99."
Repite la palabra "noventa y nueve."
(Reh-pee-teh lah pah-lah-brah "noh-behn-tah ee noo-eh-beh")

Rest.
Descanse.
(Des-kahn-seh)

Rest now.
Descanse ahora.
(Dehs-kahn-seh ah-oh-rah)

Return in 10 days.
Regrese en diez días.
(Reh-greh-seh ehn dee-ehs dee-ahs)

Right now it is throbbing like a bad toothache.
Ahora está punzando, como un mal dolor de muelas.
(Ah-oh-rah ehs-tah poon-sahn-doh, koh-moh oon mahl doh-lohr deh moo-eh-lahs)

Rinse your mouth.
Enjuague su boca.
(Ehn-hoo-ah-gheh soo boh-kah)

Rotate it.
Rótalo/Dale vuelta.
(Roh-tah-loh/Dah-leh boo-ehl-tah)

Rotate your arm.
Rota tu brazo.
(Roh-tah too brah-soh)

Run!
¡Corra!
(Koh-rah)

Say "aah."
Di "aah."
(Dee "aah")

Say it again.
Dígalo otra vez./Repita.
(Dee-gah-loh oh-trah behs/Reh-pee-tah)

Say your name.
Di tu nombre.
(Dee too nohm-breh)

See you later!
¡Hasta luego!
(Ahs-tah loo-eh-goh)

See your doctor before you refill the prescription.
Vea al doctor antes de surtir la receta.
(Beh-ah ahl dohk-tohr ahn-tehs deh soohr-teer lah reh-seh-tah)

Select your foods after breakfast.
Seleccione las comidas después del desayuno.
(Seh-lehk-see-oh-neh lahs koh-mee-dahs dehs-poo-ehs dehl deh-sah-yoo-noh)

Sexually active homosexual and bisexual males.
Homosexuales activos y hombres bisexuales.
(Oh-moh-sehx-oo-ah-lehs ahk-tee-bohs ee ohm-brehs bee-sehx-oo-ah-lehs)

She assigns a dosage schedule to the order in the computer.
Ella asigna un horario de dosis a la orden en la computadora.
(Eh-yah ah-seeg-nah oon oh-rah-ree-oh deh doh-sees ah lah ohr-dehn ehn lah kohm-poo-tah-doh-rah)

She is content.
Ella está contenta.
(Eh-yah ehs-tah kohn-tehn-tah)

She is happy.
Ella es (está) alegre.
(Eh-yah ehs [ehs-tah] ah-leh-greh)

She is sad.
Ella es (está) triste.
(Eh-yah ehs [ehs-tah] trees-teh)

Shock?
¿Toques?
(Toh-kehs)

Should I drive?
¿Debo de manejar?
(Deh-boh deh mah-neh-hahr)

Show me your tongue!
¡Muéstreme la lengua!
(Moo-ehs-treh-meh lah lehn-goo-ah)

Sign here, please.
Firme aquí, por favor.
(Feer-meh ah-kee, pohr fah-bohr)

Since when?
¿Desde cuándo?
(Dehs-deh koo-ahn-doh)

Sit!
¡Siéntese!
(See-ehn-teh-seh)

Sit down, please.
Siéntese, por favor.
(See-ehn-teh-seh, pohr fah-bohr)

Sit here and wait.
Siéntese aquí y espere.
(See-ehn-teh-seh ah-kee ee ehs-peh-reh)

Sit in the chair.
Siéntese en la silla.
(See-ehn-teh-seh ehn lah see-yah)

Sit upright!
¡Siéntate derecho!
(See-ehn-tah-teh deh-reh-choh)

Sleep at least 6 hours daily.
Duerma por lo menos seis horas diarias.
(Doo-ehr-mah pohr loh meh-nohs seh-ees oh-rahs dee-ah-ree-ahs)

Sleep at least 8 hours.
Duerma al menos ocho horas.
(Doo-ehr-mah ahl meh-nohs oh-choh oh-rahs)

Slowly, please.
Despacio, por favor.
(Dehs-pah-see-oh, pohr fah-bohr)

Smile.
Sonríe.
(Sohn-ree-eh)

So far . . .
Hasta ahora . . .
(Ahs-tah ah-oh-rah)

Social Security?
¿Seguro Social?
(Seh-goo-roh Soh-see-ahl)

Some develop tiredness, fever, loss of appetite, weight loss, diarrhea, night sweats.
Algunos desarrollan cansansio, fiebre, falta de apetito, pérdida de peso, diarrea, sudor nocturno.
(Ahl-goo-nohs deh-sah-roh-yahn kahn-sahn-see-oh, fee-eh-breh, fahl-tah deh ah-peh-tee-toh, pehr-dee-dah deh peh-soh, dee-ah-reh-ah, soo-dohr nohk-toor-noh)

Some people cannot tolerate gas-producing foods and should avoid eating them.
Algunas personas no toleran comidas que producen gas y deben de evitar comerlas.
(Ahl-goo-nahs pehr-soh-nahs noh toh-leh-rahn koh-mee-dahs keh proh-doo-sehn gahs ee deh-behn deh eh-bee-tahr koh-mehr-lahs)

Someone will take you to your room.
Alguien lo llevará a su cuarto.
(Ahl-ghee-ehn loh yeh-bah-rah ah soo koo-ahr-toh)

Sore throat.
Dolor de garganta.
(Doh-lohr deh gahr-gahn-tah)

Sorry, no toothpicks.
Lo siento, no hay palillos.
(Loh see-ehn-toh, noh ah-ee pah-lee-yohs)

Spanish is important.
El español es importante.
(Ehl ehs-pah-nyohl ehs eehm-pohr-tahn-teh)

Speak!
¡Hable!
(Ah-bleh)

Speak slowly, please.
Hable despacio, por favor.
(Ah-bleh dehs-pah-see-oh, pohr fah-bohr)

Squeeze my hand!
¡Apriete mi mano!
(Ah-pree-eh-teh mee mah-noh)

Squeeze the fingers of each of my hands.
Apriete cada uno de los dedos de mis manos.
(Ah-pree-eh-teh kah-dah oo-noh deh lohs deh-dohs deh mees mah-nohs)

Stand straight!
¡Párese derecho!
(Pah-reh-seh deh-reh-choh)

Stand up!
¡Levántate!
(Leh-bahn-tah-teh)

Start at the beginning.
Empiece al principio.
(Ehm-pee-eh-seh ahl preen-see-pee-oh)

Stay as you are.
Quédese cómo está.
(Keh-deh-seh koh-moh ehs-tah)

Stay away!
¡Hazte a un lado!
(Ahs-teh ah uhn lah-doh)

Stay like this for a while.
Quédese así por un rato.
(Keh-deh-seh ah-see pohr oon rah-toh)

Stay sitting.
Quédese sentado.
(Keh-deh-seh sehn-tah-doh)

Stay sitting here.
Quédese sentado aquí.
(Keh-deh-seh sehn-tah-doh ah-kee)

Stay still!
¡Quédese quieto!
(Keh-deh-seh kee-eh-toh)

Sterilize the bottles.
Esterilice las botellas/los biberones.
(Ehs-teh-ree-lee-seh lahs boh-teh-yahs/lohs bee-beh-roh-nehs)

Stick your tongue out.
Saque la lengua.
(Sah-keh lah lehn-goo-ah)

Stop!
¡Párese!/¡Deténte!/¡Deténgase!
(Pah-reh-seh/Deh-tehn-teh/Deh-tehn-gah-seh)

Stop breathing.
No respire.
(Noh rehs-pee-reh)

Straighten the knee.
Endereza la rodilla.
(Ehn-deh-reh-sah lah roh-dee-yah)

Straighten your leg.
Endereza tu pierna.
(Ehn-deh-reh-sah too pee-ehr-nah)

Strain down.
Empuja.
(Ehm-poo-hah)

Studies show that many infected persons remain in good health.
Los estudios muestran que muchas personas infectadas quedan con buena salud.
(Lohs ehs-too-dee-ohs moo-ehs-trahn keh moo-chahs pehr-soh-nahs een-fehk-tah-dahs keh-dahn kohn boo-eh-nah sah-lood)

Such as?
¿Tal cómo?
(Tahl koh-moh)

Swallow!
¡Trague!
(Trah-gheh)

Swollen ankles?
¿Hinchazón en los tobillos?
(Een-chah-sohn ehn lohs toh-bee-yohs)

Take a bath!
¡Báñese!
(Bah-nyeh-seh)

Take a bath every day.
Báñese todos los días.
(Bah-nyeh-seh toh-dohs lohs dee-ahs)

Take a deep breath, hold it.
Respira hondo, deténlo.
(Rehs-pee-rah ohn-doh, deh-tehn-loh)

Take a deep breath; let it go.
Respira hondo; déjalo ir.
(Rehs-pee-rah ohn-doh; deh-hah-loh eer)

Take all the medicine in the prescription.
Tome toda la medicina indicada en la receta.
(Toh-meh toh-dah lah meh-dee-see-nah een-dee-kah-dah ehn lah reh-seh-tah)

Take him for vaccinations at two months.
Llévelo a vacunar a los dos meses.
(Yeh-beh-loh ah bah-koo-nahr ah lohs dohs meh-sehs)

Take it with a full glass of water.
Tómela con un vaso lleno de agua.
(Toh-meh-lah kohn oon bah-soh yeh-noh deh ah-goo-ah)

Take on an empty stomach.
Tómela con el estómago vacío.
(Toh-meh-lah kohn ehl ehs-toh-mah-goh bah-see-oh)

Take one hour before eating.
Tómela una hora antes de comer.
(Toh-meh-lah oo-nah oh-rah ahn-tehs deh koh-mehr)

Take the elevator to the sixth floor.
Tome el elevador al sexto piso.
(Toh-meh ehl eh-leh-bah-dohr ahl sehx-toh pee-soh)

Take the medicine with juice.
Tome la medicina con jugo.
(Toh-meh lah meh-dee-see-nah kohn hoo-goh)

Take the medicine with food.
Tome la medicina con comida.
(Toh-meh lah meh-dee-see-nah kohn koh-mee-dah)

Take the temperature rectally.
Tome la temperatura por el recto.
(Toh-meh lah tehm-peh-rah-too-rah pohr ehl rehk-toh)

Take these pills after dinner.
Tómese estas pastillas después de la cena.
(Toh-meh-seh ehs-tahs pahs-tee-yahs dehs-poo-ehs deh lah seh-nah)

Take this antibiotic to prevent infections and this analgesic for pain.
Tome este antibiótico para evitar infecciones y este analgésico para el dolor.
(Toh-meh ehs-teh ahn-tee-bee-oh-tee-koh pah-rah eh-bee-tahr een-fehk-see-oh-nehs ee ehs-teh ah-nahl-heh-see-koh pah-rah ehl doh-lohr)

Take two aspirins.
Tome dos aspirinas.
(Toh-meh dohs ahs-pee-ree-nahs)

Take your hospital card.
Lleve su tarjeta del hospital.
(Yeh-beh soo tahr-heh-tah dehl ohs-pee-tahl)

Take your medical file.
Lleve su archivo.
(Yeh-beh soo ahr-chee-boh)

Take your shoes off.
Quítate tus zapatos.
(Kee-tah-teh toos sah-pah-tohs)

Take your socks off.
Quítate tus calcetines.
(Kee-tah-teh toos kahl-seh-tee-nehs)

Talk!
¡Hable!
(Ah-bleh)

Telephone number?
¿Número de teléfono?
(Noo-meh-roh deh teh-leh-foh-noh)

Tell me!
¡Dígame!
(Dee-gah-meh)

Tell me, what brought you here?
Dígame, ¿qué lo trajo aquí?
(Dee-gah-meh keh loh trah-hoh ah-kee)

Tell me, where did the pain start?
Dígame, ¿dónde comenzó el dolor?
(Dee-gah-meh dohn-deh koh-mehn-soh ehl doh-lohr)

Tell me, have you ever had a heart attack?
Dígame, ¿ha tenido alguna vez un ataque cardíaco?
(Dee-gah-meh, ah teh-nee-doh ahl-goo-nah behs oon ah-tah-keh kahr-dee-ah-koh)

Tell me if it hurts more when I press or when I let go.
Dígame si duele más al presionar o al retirar la mano.
(Dee-gah-meh see doo-eh-leh mahs ahl preh-see-oh-nahr oh ahl reh-tee-rahr lah mah-noh)

Tell me if there is pain.
Dime si duele.
(Dee-meh see doo-eh-leh)

Tell me if this hurts.
Dime si esto te duele.
(Dee-meh see ehs-toh teh doo-eh-leh)

Tell me what foods.
Dígame qué alimentos.
(Dee-gah-meh keh ah-lee-mehn-tohs)

Tell me when!
¡Dígame cuándo!
(Dee-gah-meh koo-ahn-doh)

Tell me when it feels numb.
Dígame cuándo sienta dormido.
(Dee-gah-meh koo-ahn-doh see-ehn-tah dohr-mee-doh)

Tell me when you feel a contraction!
¡Digame cuándo sienta una contracción!
(Dee-gah-meh koo-ahn-doh see-ehn-tah oo-nah kohn-trahk-see-ohn)

Tell me where it hurts, Mr. Badluck.
Dígame dónde le duele, señor Badluck.
(Dee-gah-meh dohn-deh leh doo-eh-leh, seh-nyohr Badluck)

Tell me why you are here.
Dígame por qué está aquí.
(Dee-gah-meh pohr keh ehs-tah ah-kee)

Tell me your name.
Dígame su nombre.
(Dee-gah-meh soo nohm-breh)

Thank you!
¡Gracias!
(Grah-see-ahs)

Thank you, doctor.
Gracias, doctor.
(Grah-see-ahs, dohk-tohr)

Thank you for talking to me!
¡Gracias por hablar conmigo!
(Grah-see-ahs pohr ah-blahr kohn-mee-goh)

Thank you for the information.
Gracias por la información.
(Grah-see-ahs pohr lah een-fohr-mah-see-ohn)

Thank you very much!
¡Muchas gracias!
(Moo-chahs grah-see-ahs)

That bracelet is hers.
Aquella pulsera es suya.
(Ah-keh-yah pool-seh-rah ehs soo-yah)

That gown is yours.
Aquella bata es suya.
(Ah-keh-yah bah-tah ehs soo-yah)

That is all!
¡Es todo!
(Ehs toh-doh)

That is for sure!
¡Délo por seguro!
(Deh-loh pohr seh-goo-roh)

That is plaque.
Esa es la placa.
(Eh-sah ehs lah plah-kah)

That is why it is important to clean these areas.
Por ello es importante limpiar estas áreas.
(Pohr eh-yoh ehs eem-pohr-tahn-teh leem-pee-ahr ehs-tahs ah-reh-ahs)

The bed has one blanket.
La cama tiene una frazada/colcha.
(Lah kah-mah tee-eh-neh oo-nah frah-sah-dah/kohl-chah)

The bell will sound.
La campana sonará.
(Lah kahm-pah-nah soh-nah-rah)

The bottle will be kept in a bucket with ice.
La botella se mantendrá en una tina con hielo.
(Lah boh-teh-yah seh mahn-tehn-drah ehn oo-nah tee-nah kohn ee-eh-loh)

The building has beige brick.
El edificio tiene ladrillo crema.
(Ehl eh-dee-fee-see-oh tee-eh-neh lah-dree-yoh kreh-mah)

The clerical staff is very important.
Las secretarias son muy importantes.
(Lahs seh-kreh-tah-ree-ahs sohn moo-ee eem-pohr-tahn-tehs)

The clinic is in another building.
La clínica está en otro edificio.
(Lah klee-nee-kah ehs-tah ehn oh-troh eh-dee-fee-see-oh)

The computer says that you have an appointment.
La computadora dice que tiene una cita.
(Lah kohm-poo-tah-doh-rah dee-seh keh tee-eh-neh oo-nah see-tah)

The container will be kept in a bucket with ice.
El frasco se mantendrá en una tina con hielo.
(Ehl frahs-koh seh mahn-tehn-drah ehn oo-nah tee-nah kohn ee-eh-loh)

The cover is hot.
La cubierta está caliente.
(Lah koo-bee-ehr-tah ehs-tah kah-lee-ehn-teh)

The doctor has to prescribe it.
La doctora debe de recetarla.
(Lah dohk-tohr-ah deh-beh deh reh-seh-tahr-lah)

The doctor will give you something for pain.
El doctor le dará algo para el dolor.
(Ehl dohk-tohr leh dah-rah ahl-goh pah-rah ehl doh-lohr)

The doctor will see you in the emergency room.
Lo verá el doctor en el cuarto de emergencia.
(Loh beh-rah ehl dohk-tohr ehn ehl koo-ahr-toh deh eh-mehr-hehn-see-ah)

The doctor will see you there.
El doctor lo verá ahí.
(Ehl dohk-tohr loh beh-rah ah-ee)

The elevators are slow.
Los elevadores son despacios.
(Lohs eh-leh-bah-doh-rehs sohn dehs-pah-see-ohs)

The elevators work twenty-four hours.
Los elevadores funcionan las veinticuatro horas.
(Lohs eh-leh-bah-doh-rehs foon-see-oh-nahn lahs beh-een-tee-koo-ah-troh oh-rahs)

The exam is difficult.
El examen es difícil.
(Ehl ehx-ah-mehn ehs dee-fee-seel)

The following information is included in the label.
La siguiente información se incluye en la etiqueta.
(Lah see-ghee-ehn-teh een-fohr-mah-see-ohn seh een-kloo-yeh ehn lah eh-tee-keh-tah)

The following should be included in your diet every day . . .
Lo siguiente se debe incluir en su dieta todos los días . . .
(Loh see-gee-ehn-teh seh deh-beh een-kloo-eer ehn soo dee-eh-tah toh-dohs lohs dee-ahs)

The fork, spoon, and knife are wrapped in the napkin.
El tenedor, la cuchara y el cuchillo están envueltos en la servilleta.
(Ehl teh-neh-dohr, lah koo-chah-rah ee ehl koo-chee-yoh ehs-tahn ehn-boo-ehl-tohs ehn lah sehr-bee-yeh-tah)

The hours of operation of the inpatient pharmacy are: Monday through Friday, 7:00 A.M. to 1:00 A.M.
El horario de la farmacia para pacientes internados es de: lunes a viernes de las 7 de la mañana a la una de la mañana.
(Ehl oh-rah-ree-oh deh lah fahr-mah-see-ah pah-rah pah-see-ehn-tehs een-tehr-nah-dohs ehs deh: loo-nehs ah bee-ehr-nehs deh lahs see-eh-teh deh lah mah-nyah-nah ah lah oo-nah deh lah mah-nyah-nah)

The inpatient pharmacy is open.
La farmacia para pacientes internados está abierta.
(Lah fahr-mah-see-ah pah-rah pah-see-ehn-tehs een-tehr-nah-dohs ehs-tah ah-bee-ehr-tah)

The kids left their skates on the stairs and I fell over them.
Los niños dejaron los patines en la escalera y me tropecé.
(Lohs nee-nyohs deh-hah-rohn lohs pah-tee-nehs ehn lah ehs-kah-leh-rah ee meh troh-peh-seh)

The line is on the wall.
La línea está en la pared.
(Lah lee-nee-ah ehs-tah ehn lah pah-rehd)

The meals are served at . . .
Los alimentos se sirven a . . .
(Lohs ah-lee-mehn-tohs seh seer-behn ah)

The measurements are difficult.
Las medidas son difíciles.
(Lahs meh-dee-dahs sohn dee-fee-see-lehs).

The name of the street.
El nombre de la calle.
(Ehl nohm-breh deh lah kah-yeh)

The next day, it will be sent to the laboratory.
Al día siguiente, se mandará al laboratorio.
(Ahl dee-ah see-ghee-ehn-teh, seh-mahn-dah-rah ahl lah-boh-rah-toh-ree-oh)

The nurse explains the procedure and hospital routine.
La enfermera le explica el procedimiento y la rutina del hospital.
(Lah ehn-fehr-meh-rah leh ehx-plee-kah ehl proh-seh-dee-mee-ehn-toh ee lah roo-tee-nah dehl ohs-pee-tahl)

The nurse orders the medication from the pharmacy.
La enfermera ordena la medicina de la farmacia.
(Lah ehn-fehr-meh-rah ohr-deh-nah lah meh-dee-see-nah deh lah fahr-mah-see-ah)

The nurse wants to talk to you.
La enfermera quiere hablarle.
(Lah ehn-fehr-meh-rah kee-eh-reh ah-blahr-leh)

The nurse will ask how you feel.
La enfermera le preguntará cómo se siente.
(Lah ehn-fehr-meh-rah leh preh-goon-tah-rah koh-moh seh see-ehn-teh)

The nurse will complete the assessment.
La enfermera completará la evaluación.
(Lah ehn-fehr-meh-rah kohm-pleh-tah-rah lah eh-bah-loo-ah-see-ohn)

The only way we can see plaque is by using a solution that stains the teeth.
La única manera de ver la placa es usar una solución que mancha los dientes.
(Lah oo-nee-kah mah-neh-rah deh behr lah plah-kah ehs oo-sahr oo-nah soh-loo-see-ohn keh mahn-chah lohs dee-ehn-tehs)

The outpatient pharmacy opens daily from 9 A.M. to 6 P.M.
La farmacia de consulta externa abre diariamente de las nueve de la mañana a las seis de la tarde.
(Lah fahr-mah-see-ah deh kohn-sool-tah ehx-tehr-nah ah-breh dee-ah-ree-ah-mehn-teh deh lahs noo-eh-beh deh lah mah-nyah-nah ah lahs seh-ees deh lah tahr-deh)

The pain has gotten worse.
El dolor ha empeorado.
(Ehl doh-lohr ah ehm-peh-ohr-ah-doh)

The pain is constant.
El dolor es constante.
(Ehl doh-lohr ehs kohns-tahn-teh)

The pain is cutting.
El dolor es cortante.
(Ehl doh-lohr ehs kohr-tahn-teh)

The pain is in one place?
¿El dolor es fijo?
(Ehl doh-lohr ehs fee-hoh)

The pain is localized, sharp.
El dolor está fijo, agudo.
(Ehl doh-lohr ehs-tah fee-hoh, ah-goo-doh)

The pain is on the side.
El dolor está en el lado/costado.
(Ehl doh-lohr ehs-tah ehn ehl lah-doh/kohs-tah-doh)

The pain is sharp?
¿El dolor es agudo?
(Ehl doh-lohr ehs ah-goo-doh)

The pain is throbbing.
El dolor es punzante.
(Ehl doh-lohr ehs poon-sahn-teh)

The pain is worse.
El dolor es peor.
(Ehl doh-lohr ehs peh-ohr)

The pain started two hours ago.
El dolor comenzó hace 2 horas.
(Ehl doh-lohr koh-mehn-soh ah-seh dohs oh-rahs)

The pain starts here (beneath the sternum) and goes to my jaw.
El dolor comienza aquí (abajo del esternón) y se va a la mandíbula.
(Ehl doh-lohr koh-mee-ehn-sah ah-kee [ah-bah-hoh dehl ehs-tehr-nohn] ee seh bah ah lah mahn-dee-boo-lah)

The pain starts here and travels down my left arm.
El dolor comienza aquí y se recorre por el brazo izquierdo.
(Ehl doh-lohr koh-mee-ehn-sah ah-kee ee seh reh-koh-reh pohr ehl brah-soh ees-kee-ehr-doh)

The patient asks.
El paciente pregunta.
(Ehl pah-see-ehn-teh preh-goon-tah)

The patient is happy.
El paciente está contento.
(Ehl pah-see-ehn-teh ehs-tah kohn-tehn-toh)

The pharmacist assists with patient education.
El/La farmacéutico(a) asiste con la educación del paciente.
(Ehl/Lah fahr-mah-seh-oo-tee-koh(ah] ah-sees-teh kohn lah eh-doo-kah-see-ohn dehl pah-see-ehn-teh)

The pharmacist interprets the physician's order.
El farmacéutico interpreta la orden del doctor.
(Ehl fahr-mah-seh-oo-tee-koh een-tehr-preh-tah lah ohr-dehn dehl dohk-tohr)

The pharmacy is open Monday through Friday.
La farmacia está abierta de lunes a viernes.
(Lah fahr-mah-see-ah ehs-tah ah-bee-ehr-tah deh loo-nehs ah bee-ehr-nehs)

The pharmacy provides services as an integral part of total patient care.
La farmacia provee servicios como parte integral del cuidado total del paciente.
(Lah fahr-mah-see-ah proh-beh-eh sehr-bee-see-ohs koh-moh pahr-teh een-teh-grahl dehl koo-ee-dah-doh toh-tahl dehl pah-see-ehn-teh)

The pharmacy staff delivers and picks up orders every hour from the floors.
Los empleados de la farmacia recogen y surten órdenes cada hora en los pisos.
(Lohs ehm-pleh-ah-dohs deh lah fahr-mah-see-ah reh-koh-hehn ee soohr-tehn ohr-deh-nehs kah-dah oh-rah ehn lohs pee-sohs)

The plates are plastic.
Los platos son de plástico.
(Lohs plah-tohs sohn deh plahs-tee-koh)

The prescription will be ready at ______.
La receta estará lista a las ______.
(Lah reh-seh-tah ehs-tah-rah lees-tah ah lahs ______)

The procedure is difficult.
El procedimiento es difícil.
(Ehl proh-seh-dee-mee-ehn-toh ehs dee-fee-seel).

The rails lower down.
El barandal se baja.
(Ehl bah-rahn-dahl seh bah-hah)

The rings are mine.
Los anillos son míos.
(Lohs ah-nee-yohs sohn mee-ohs)

The salt and pepper are in these packets.
La sal y la pimienta están en estos paquetes.
(Lah sahl ee lah pee-mee-ehn-tah ehs-tahn ehn ehs-tohs pah-keh-tehs)

The secretary will help.
La secretaria lo ayudará.
(Lah seh-kreh-tah-ree-ah loh ah-yoo-dah-rah)

The stairs are at the end of the hallway.
La escalera está al final del pasillo.
(Lah ehs-kah-leh-rah ehs-tah ahl feen-ahl dehl pah-see-yoh)

The stairs will take you to a walkway.
La escalera lo llevará a un pasillo sobre la calle.
(Lah ehs-kah-leh-rah loh yeh-bah-rah ah oon pah-see-yoh soh-breh lah kah-yeh)

The surgery floor is in the hospital towers.
El piso de cirugía está en las torres del hospital.
(Ehl pee-soh deh see-roo-hee-ah ehs-tah ehn lahs toh-rehs dehl ohs-pee-tahl)

The television has four channels.
El televisor tiene cuatro canales.
(Ehl teh-leh-bee-sohr tee-eh-neh koo-ah-troh kah-nah-lehs)

The water is in the glass/pitcher.
El agua está en el vaso/la jarra.
(Ehl ah-goo-ah ehs-tah ehn ehl bah-soh/lah hah-rah)

Then they will take blood samples.
Luego le van a tomar muestras de sangre.
(Loo-eh-goh leh bahn ah toh-mahr moo-ehs-trahs deh sahn-greh)

Then turn to the left.
Luego dé vuelta a la izquierda.
(Loo-eh-goh deh boo-ehl-tah ah lah ees-kee-ehr-dah)

There are a lot of patients.
Hay muchos pacientes.
(Ah-ee moo-chohs pah-see-ehn-tehs)

There are bathrooms for guests in the corner.
Hay baños para las visitas en la esquina.
(Ah-ee bah-nyohs pah-rah lahs bee-see-tahs ehn lah ehs-kee-nah)

There are many diets available to patients.
Hay muchas dietas para los pacientes.
(Ah-ee moo-chahs dee-eh-tahs pah-rah lohs pah-see-ehn-tehs)

There is a front desk.
Hay un escritorio al frente.
(Ah-ee oon ehs-kree-toh-ree-oh ahl frehn-teh)

There is a shower.
Hay una ducha/regadera.
(Ah-ee oo-nah doo-chah/ reh-gah-deh-rah)

There is a straw.
Hay un popote.
(Ah-ee oon poh-poh-teh)

There is also a bathub / tub.
También hay una bañera/tina.
(Tahm-bee-ehn ah-ee oo-nah bah-nyeh-rah/tee-nah)

There is an educational channel.
Hay un canal educativo.
(Ah-ee oon kah-nahl eh-doo-kah-tee-boh)

There is an emergency light.
Hay una luz para emergencias.
(Ah-ee oo-nah loos pah-rah ehm-ehr-hehn-see-ahs)

There, turn to the left.
Ahí, dé vuelta a la izquierda.
(Ah-ee, deh boo-ehl-tah ah lah ees-kee-ehr-dah)

These books are mine.
Estos libros son míos.
(Ehs-tohs lee-brohs sohn mee-ohs)

These buttons move the bed up / down.
Estos botones mueven la cama arriba/ abajo.
(Ehs-tohs boh-toh-nehs moo-eh-behn lah kah-mah ah-ree-bah/ah-bah-hoh)

These meats can be substituted.
Estas carnes se pueden substituir.
(Ehs-tahs kahr-nehs seh poo-eh-dehn soobs-tee-too-eer)

They are around the corner.
Están alrededor de la esquina.
(Ehs-tahn ahl-reh-deh-dohr deh lah ehs-kee-nah)

They are men.
Ellos son hombres.
(Eh-yohs sohn ohm-brehs)

They are the ones that first greet the patient.
Ellas son las primeras personas que saludan al paciente.
(Eh-yahs sohn lahs pree-meh-rahs pehr-soh-nahs keh sahl-oo-dahn ahl pah-see-ehn-teh)

They can help clean.
Pueden ayudar a limpiar.
(Poo-eh-dehn ah-yoo-dahr ah leem-pee-ahr)

They can't break.
No se pueden quebrar.
(Noh seh poo-eh-dehn keh-brahr)

They will let you talk to your family.
Le permitirán hablar con su familia.
(Leh pehr-mee-tee-rahn ah-blahr kohn soo fah-mee-lee-ah)

This button lowers (raises) the headboard.
Este botón baja (sube) la cabecera de la cama.
(Ehs-teh boh-tohn bah-hah [soo-beh] lah kah-beh-seh-rah deh lah kah-mah)

This chair turns into a bed.
Esta silla se hace cama.
(Ehs-tah see-yah seh ah-seh kah-mah)

This is a handout that deals with the hospital's guidelines.
Este es un folleto que trata de las reglas del hospital.
(Ehs-teh ehs oon foh-yeh-toh keh trah-tah deh lahs reh-glahs dehl ohs pee-tahl)

This is a large place.
Este es un lugar grande.
(Ehs-teh ehs oon loo-gahr grahn-deh)

This is a new formula.
Esta es una fórmula nueva.
(Ehs-tah ehs oo-nah fohr-moo-lah noo-eh-bah)

This is a sedative.
Este es un sedante.
(Ehs-teh ehs oon seh-dahn-teh)

This is an antacid.
Este es un antiácido.
(Ehs-teh ehs oon ahn-tee-ah-see-doh)

This is an employee.
Este es un empleado.
(Ehs-teh ehs oon ehm-pleh-ah-doh)

This is done quickly.
Esto se hace rápido.
(Ehs-toh seh ah-seh rah-pee-doh)

This is my first time here.
Esta es mi primera vez aquí.
(Ehs-tah ehs mee pree-meh-rah behs ah-kee)

This is the call bell/buzzer.
Esta es la campana/el timbre.
(Ehs-tah ehs lah kahm-pah-nah/ehl teem-breh)

This is the clinic.
Esta es la clínica.
(Ehs-tah ehs lah klee-nee-kah)

This is the lobby.
Esta es la sala de espera.
(Ehs-tah ehs lah sah-lah deh ehs-peh-rah)

This is the radio.
Este es el radio.
(Ehs-teh ehs ehl rah-dee-oh)

This is the service area.
Esta es la área de servicio.
(Ehs-tah ehs lah ah-reh-ah deh sehr-bee-see-oh)

This is the tray.
Esta es la bandeja/charola.
(Ehs-tah ehs lah bahn-deh-hah/chah-roh-lah)

This is to help your teeth become stronger.
Esto ayudará a hacer que los dientes sean más fuertes.
(Ehs-toh ah-yoo-dahr-ah ah ah-sehr keh lohs dee-ehn-tehs seh-ahn mahs foo-ehr-tehs)

This is your room.
Este es su cuarto.
(Ehs-teh ehs soo koo-ahr-toh)

This medicine is a pain killer.
Esta medicina quita/alivia el dolor.
(Ehs-tah meh-dee-see-nah kee-tah/ah-lee-bee-ah ehl doh-lohr)

This prescription may be refilled.
Esta receta se puede surtir de nuevo.
(Ehs-tah reh-seh-tah seh poo-eh-deh soohr-teer deh noo-eh-boh)

This prescription may not be refilled.
Esta receta no se puede surtir de nuevo.
(Ehs-tah reh-seh-tah noh seh poo-eh-deh soor-teer deh noo-eh-boh)

This will feel cold.
Esto se sentirá frío.
(Ehs-toh seh sehn-tee-rah free-oh)

This will take you to the end of the hall.
Esto la llevará al fin del pasillo.
(Ehs-toh lah yeh-bah-rah ahl feen dehl pah-see-yoh)

Thought to be/Considering . . .
Considerando . . .
(Kohn-see-deh-rahn-doh)

Three times a day.
Tres veces al día.
(Trehs beh-sehs ahl dee-ah)

Three to five servings of vegetables.
Tres a cinco porciones de vegetables.
(Trehs ah seen-koh pohr-see-oh-nehs deh beh-heh-tah-lehs)

Tighten!
¡Aprieta!
(Ah-pree-eh-tah)

Tighten your muscle!
¡Apriete el músculo!
(Ah-pree-eh-teh ehl moos-koo-loh)

To some extent.
Hasta cierto punto.
(Ahs-tah see-ehr-toh poon-toh)

Today I am here to examine the baby.
Estoy aquí hoy para examinar al bebé.
(Ehs-tohy ah-kee oh-ee pah-rah ehx-ah-mee-nahr ahl beh-beh)

Today is Monday.
Hoy es lunes.
(Oh-ee ehs loo-nehs)

Tomorrow, bring a specimen of your stool in this container.
Mañana, traiga una muestra de su excremento en este frasco.
(Mah-nyah-nah, trah-ee-gah oo-nah moo-ehs-trah deh soo ehx-kreh-mehn-toh ehn ehs-teh frahs-koh)

Tomorrow they will give you a special test.
Mañana le harán un examen especial.
(Mah-nyah-nah leh ah-rahn oon ehx-ah-mehn ehs-peh-see-ahl)

Tonight, eat lightly.
Esta noche coma ligero.
(Ehs-tah noh-cheh koh-mah lee-heh-roh)

Total number of pills.
Número total de pastillas.
(Noo-meh-roh toh-tahl deh pahs-tee-yahs)

Transportation is here.
El transporte está aquí.
(Ehl trahns-pohr-teh ehs-tah ah-kee)

Transportation will take you back to your room.
Transportación lo regresará a su cuarto.
(Trahns-pohr-tah-see-ohn loh reh-greh-sah-rah ah soo koo-ahr-toh)

Try again!
¡Pruebe otra vez!
(Proo-eh-beh oh-trah behs)

Try to calm down.
Trate de calmarse.
(Trah-teh deh kahl-mahr-seh)

Try to have a bowel movement every day.
Procure hacer del baño diariamente.
(Proh-koo-reh ah-sehr dehl bah-nyoh dee-ah-ree-ah-mehn-teh)

Turn!
¡Voltee!
(Bohl-teh-eh)

Turn it to the left.
Voltéalo a la izquierda.
(Bohl-teh-ah-loh ah lah ees-kee-ehr-dah)

Turn it to the right.
Voltéalo a la derecha.
(Bohl-teh-ah-loh ah lah deh-reh-chah)

Turn on your side.
Voltéese de lado.
(Bohl-teh-eh-seh deh lah-doh)

Turn right.
Voltéate a la derecha.
(Bohl-teh-ah-teh ah lah deh-reh-chah)

Turn the forearm.
Voltea el antebrazo.
(Bohl-teh-ah ehl ahn-teh-brah-soh)

Turn to the right.
Voltee a la derecha.
(Bohl-teh-eh ah lah deh-reh-chah)

Turn to your side.
Voltéate de lado.
(Bohl-teh-ah-teh deh lah-doh)

Turn your head to the left.
Voltea la cabeza a la izquierda.
(Bohl-teh-ah lah kah-beh-sah ah lah ees-kee-ehr-dah)

Turn your head to the right.
Voltea la cabeza a la derecha.
(Bohl-teh-ah lah kah-beh-sah ah lah deh-reh-chah)

Twice a day.
Dos veces al día.
(Dohs beh-sehs ahl dee-ah)

Twist your upper extremities.
Tuerce las extremidades superiores.
(Too-ehr-seh lahs ehx-treh-mee-dah-dehs soo-peh-ree-oh-rehs)

Twist your waist.
Tuerce la cintura.
(Too-ehr-seh lah seen-too-rah)

Two to four servings of milk should be included.
Dos a cuatro porciones de leche se debe incluir.
(Dohs ah koo-ah-troh pohr-see-ohn-ehs deh leh-cheh seh deh-beh een-kloo-eer)

Two to four servings of fruit.
Dos a cuatro porciones de fruta.
(Dohs ah koo-ah-troh pohr-see-ohn-ehs deh froo-tah)

Two to three servings daily of meat, fish, or poultry.
Dos a tres porciones diarias de carne, pescado, o aves de corral.
(Dohs ah trehs pohr-see-oh-nehs dee-ah-ree-ahs deh kahr-neh, pehs-kah-doh oh ah-behs deh koh-rahl)

Until now . . .
Hasta ahora . . .
(Ahs-tah ah-oh-rah)

Use dental floss.
Use hilo dental.
(Oo-seh ee-loh dehn-tahl)

Use the house shoes; the floor is cold.
Use las pantunflas/chanclas; el piso está frío.
(Oo-seh lahs pahn-toon-flahs/chahn-klahs; ehl pee-soh ehs-tah free-oh)

Use thumbs and forefingers to guide the floss.
Use el dedo gordo y el índice para guiar el hilo.
(Oo-seh ehl deh-doh gohr-doh ee ehl een-dee-seh pah-rah gee-ahr ehl ee-loh)

Using a circular motion, brush one to two teeth at a time.
Usando movimiento circular, cepille uno o dos dientes a la vez.
(Oo-sahn-doh moh-bee-mee-ehn-toh seer-koo-lahr, seh-pee-yeh oo-noh oh dohs dee-ehn-tehs ah lah behs)

Very good!
¡Muy bien!
(Moo-ee bee-ehn)

Vials, pills, capsules, liquids, and IV fluids are available in the pharmacy.
Botellas, pastillas, cápsulas, líquidos, y sueros se encuentran en la farmacia.
(Boh-teh-yahs, pahs-tee-yahs, kahp-soo-lahs, lee-kee-dohs, ee soo-eh-rohs seh ehn-koo-ehn-trahn ehn lah fahr-mah-see-ah)

Visiting hours are from nine in the morning to nine at night.
Las horas de visita son de las nueve de la mañana a las nueve de la noche.
(Lahs oh-rahs deh bee-see-tah sohn deh lahs noo-eh-beh deh lah mah-nyah-nah ah lahs noo-eh-beh deh lah noh-cheh)

Visiting hours are from two to eight P.M.
Las horas de visita son de las dos a las ocho de la noche.
(Lahs oh-rahs deh bee-see-tah sohn deh lahs dohs ah lahs oh-choh deh lah noh-cheh)

Void a little, then put urine in this cup.
Orine un poco, luego ponga la orina en esta taza.
(Oh-ree-neh oon poh-koh, loo-eh-goh pohn-gah lah oh-ree-nah ehn ehs-tah tah-sah)

Volume, if liquid.
Volumen, si es líquido.
(Boh-loo-mehn, see ehs lee-kee-doh)

Wait!
¡Espere!
(Ehs-peh-reh)

Wait 30 minutes.
Espere treinta minutos.
(Ehs-peh-reh treh-een-tah mee-noo-tohs)

Wait in the lobby.
Espere en el vestíbulo.
(Ehs-peh-reh ehn ehl behs-tee-boo-loh)

Wait several minutes!
¡Espera varios minutos!
(Ehs-peh-rah bah-ree-ohs mee-noo-tohs)

Wait your turn.
Espere su turno.
(Ehs-peh-reh soo toor-noh)

Wake up!
¡Despierte!
(Dehs-pee-ehr-teh)

Walk!
¡Camine!
(Kah-mee-neh)

Walk, please.
Camina, por favor.
(Kah-mee-nah, pohr fah-bohr)

Walk six paces.
Camine seis pasos.
(Kah-mee-neh seh-ees pah-sohs)

Walk straight ahead!
¡Camine derecho!
(Kah-mee-neh deh-reh-choh)

Walk two blocks.
Camine dos cuadras.
(Kah-mee-neh dohs koo-ah-drahs)

Was he/she conscious?
¿Estaba consciente?
(Ehs-tah-bah kohn-see-ehn-teh)

Was he premature?
¿Fue prematuro?
(Foo-eh preh-mah-too-roh)

Was the car burning?
¿Estaba el carro en llamas?
(Ehs-tah-bah ehl kah-roh ehn yah-mahs)

Was the delivery normal?
¿Fue normal el parto?
(Foo-eh nohr-mahl ehl pahr-toh)

Was the victim on the road?
¿Estaba la víctima en el camino?
(Ehs-tah-bah lah beek-tee-mah ehn ehl kah-mee-noh)

Wash fruits and vegetables well.
Lave bien frutas y verduras.
(Lah-beh bee-ehn froo-tahs ee behr-doo-rahs)

Wash hands before eating.
Lave las manos antes de comer.
(Lah-beh lahs mah-nohs ahn-tehs deh koh-mehr)

Wash your face!
¡Lávese la cara!
(Lah-beh-seh lah kah-rah)

Watch for the arrow.
Fíjese en la flecha.
(Fee-heh-seh ehn lah fleh-chah)

Watch his growth and development.
Vigile su crecimiento y desarrollo.
(Bee-hee-leh soo kreh-see-mee-ehn-toh ee deh-sah-roh-yoh)

Watch his navel.
Vigile su ombligo.
(Bee-hee-leh soo ohm-blee-goh)

Watch his urine and his bowel movements.
Vigile su orina y sus excrementos.
(Bee-hee-leh soo oh-ree-nah ee soos ehx-kreh-mehn-tohs)

Watch if he has abnormal movements.
Vigile si presenta movimientos anormales.
(Bee-hee-leh see preh-sehn-tah moh-bee-mee-ehn-tohs ah-nohr-mah-lehs)

Watch if he sleeps quietly.
Vigile si su sueño es tranquilo.
(Bee-hee-leh see soo soo-eh-nyoh ehs trahn-kee-loh)

Watch that his nose is clear.
Vigile que su nariz esté libre.
(Bee-hee-leh keh soo nah reehs ehs-teh lee-breh)

Watch that your wound doesn't get infected.
Vigile que su herida no se infecte.
(Bee-hee-leh keh soo eh-ree-dah noh seh een-fehk-teh)

Watch your bleeding.
Vigile su sangrado.
(Bee-hee-leh soo sahn-grah-doh)

We also have desserts.
También tenemos postres.
(Tahm-bee-ehn teh-neh-mohs pohs-trehs)

We are going in the ambulance.
Vamos en la ambulancia.
(Bah-mohs ehn lah ahm-boo-lahn-see-ah)

We are going to pull . . .
Vamos a jalar . . .
(Bah-mohs ah hah-lahr)

We are going to pull the sheet at the count of three.
Vamos a jalar la sábana al contar tres.
(Bah-mohs ah hah-lahr lah sah-bah-nah ahl kohn-tahr trehs)

We are going to the hospital.
Vamos al hospital.
(Bah-mohs ahl ohs-pee-tahl)

We are going to X-ray.
Vamos a rayos X.
(Bah-mohs ah rah-yohs eh-kees)

We are here.
Estamos aquí.
(Ehs-tah-mohs ah-kee)

We don't serve drinks like Cokes or any canned drinks.
No servimos refrescos cómo Coca-colas o bebidas envasadas.
(Noh sehr-bee-mohs reh-frehs-kohs koh-moh Koh-kah-koh-lahs oh beh-bee-dahs ehn-bah-sah-dahs)

We have cereals.
Tenemos cereales.
(Teh-neh-mohs seh-reh-ah-lehs)

We have meats.
Tenemos carnes.
(Teh-neh-mohs kahr-nehs)

We have to go far.
Tenemos que ir lejos.
(Teh-neh-mohs keh eer leh-hohs)

We inject a radioactive dye into the blood vessels and view the flow of blood through the vessels.
Se inyecta un medio de contraste en los vasos sanguíneos y se valora el flujo de la sangre por las venas.
(Seh een-yehk-tah oon meh-dee-oh deh kohn-trahs-teh ehn lohs bah-sohs sahn-ghee-neh-ohs ee seh bah-lor-ah ehl floo-ho deh lah sahn-greh pohr lahs beh-nahs)

We need to bring you back.
Necesitamos que regrese.
(Neh-seh-see-tah-mohs keh reh-greh-seh)

We need to count.
Tenemos que contar.
(Teh-neh-mohs keh kohn-tahr)

We send the menu to the kitchen.
Mandamos el menú a la cocina.
(Mahn-dah-mohs ehl meh-noo ah lah koh-see-nah)

We serve lunch at noon.
Servimos la comida al mediodía.
(Sehr-bee-mohs lah koh-mee-dah ahl meh-dee-oh-dee-ah)

We will begin with the use of angiography.
Comenzaremos con el estudio de angiografía.
(Koh-mehn-sah-reh-mohs kohn ehl ehs-too-dee-oh deh ahn-gee-oh-grah-fee-ah)

We will start with diagnostic studies to assess how severe your problem might be.
Empezaremos con estudios para evaluar la gravedad de su problema.
(Ehm-peh-sah-reh-mohs kohn ehs-too-dee-ohs pah-rah eh-bah-loo-ahr lah grah-beh-dahd deh soo proh-bleh-mah)

We will X-ray the abdomen again.
Vamos a radiografiar el abdomen otra vez.
(Bah-mohs ah rah-dee-oh-grah-fee-ahr ehl ahb-doh-mehn oh-trah behs)

Wear this bracelet all the time.
Use esta pulsera todo el tiempo.
(Oo-seh ehs-tah pool-seh-rah toh-doh ehl tee-ehm-poh)

Well, it is possible.
Pues, es posible.
(Poo-ehs, ehs poh-see-bleh)

Well, I do have a tingling feeling in my left foot. It must have gone to sleep.
Pues, tengo picazón en el pie izquierdo. Se me durmió.
(Poo-ehs, tehn-goh pee-kah-sohn ehn ehl pee-eh ees-kee-ehr-doh. Seh meh duhr-mee-oh)

Well, I just changed jobs.
Bueno, apenas cambié de trabajo.
(Boo-eh-noh, ah-peh-nahs kahm-bee-eh deh trah-bah-hoh)

Well, you are going home tomorrow, but you must return to my office in eight days so I can remove your sutures.
Bueno, mañana se va a su casa, pero debe regresar a mi oficina en ocho días para retirar los puntos de sutura.
(Boo-eh-noh, mah-nyah-nah seh bah ah soo kah-sah, peh-roh deh-beh reh-greh-sahr ah mee oh-fee-see-nah ehn oh-choh dee-ahs pah-rah reh-tee-rahr lohs poon-tohs deh soo-too-rah)

Were you hit by a car?
¿Le golpeó un carro?
(Leh gohl-peh-oh oon kah-roh)

Were you hospitalized?
¿Lo hospitalizaron?
(Loh ohs-pee-tah-lee-sah-rohn)

Were you knocked down, did you fall, or were you thrown?
¿Se golpeó, se cayó o lo lanzó el impacto?
(Seh gohl-peh-oh, seh kah-yoh oh loh lahn-soh ehl eem-pahk-toh)

Were you thrown forward / backward?
¿Fue lanzado hacia adelante/hacia atrás?
(Foo-eh lahn-sah-doh ah-see-ah ah-deh-lahn-teh/ah-see-ah ah-trahs)

Were you thrown from the car?
¿Fue lanzado fuera del carro?
(Foo-eh lahn-sah-doh foo-eh-rah dehl kah-roh)

What?
¿Qué?
(Keh)

What a beautiful day!
¡Qué día tan hermoso!
(Keh dee-ah tahn ehr-moh-soh)

What are the months of the year?
¿Cuáles son los meses del año?
(Koo-ah-lehs sohn lohs meh-sehs dehl ah-nyoh)

What are the symptoms?
¿Cuáles son los síntomas?
(Koo-ah-lehs sohn lohs seen-toh-mahs)

What brought you to the hospital?
¿Qué lo trajo al hospital?
(Keh loh trah-hoh ahl ohs-pee-tahl)

What can be done to prevent AIDS?
¿Qué se puede hacer para prevenir el SIDA?
(Keh seh poo-eh-deh ah-sehr pah-rah preh-beh-neer ehl see-dah)

What can I help you with?
¿En qué puedo ayudarlo?
(Ehn keh poo-eh-doh ah-yoo-dahr-loh)

What caused the accident?
¿Qué causó el accidente?
(Keh kah-oo-soh ehl ahk-see-dehn-teh)

What caused the pain?
¿Qué causó el dolor?
(Keh kah-oo-soh ehl doh-lohr)

What causes AIDS?
¿Qué causa el SIDA?
(Keh kah-oo-sah ehl see-dah)

What color?
¿De qué color?
(Deh keh koh-lohr)

What day, what month?
¿Qué día, qué mes?
(Keh dee-ah, keh mehs)

What did you do that caused the pain?
¿Qué hacía cuando apareció el dolor?
(Keh ah-see-ah koo-ahn-doh ah-pah-reh-see-oh ehl doh-lohr)

What did you eat?
¿Qué comió?
(Keh koh-mee-oh)

What did you eat for breakfast?
¿Qué comió en el desayuno?
(Keh koh-mee-oh ehn ehl deh-sah-yoo-noh)

What do you do?
¿Qué hace usted?
(Keh ah-seh oos-tehd)

What do you feel?
¿Qué siente?
(Keh see-ehn-teh)

What drugs/medicine do you use?
¿Qué drogas/medicamento usa?
(Keh droh-gahs/meh-dee-kah-mehn-toh oo-sah)

What drugs do you use?
¿Qué drogas usa?
(Keh droh-gahs oo-sah)

What foods do you dislike?
¿Qué alimentos le disgustan?
(Keh ah-lee-mehn-tohs leh dees-goos-tahn)

What foods do you like?
¿Qué alimentos le gustan?
(Keh ah-lee-mehn-tohs leh goos-tahn)

What formula does he take?
¿Qué fórmula toma?
(Keh fohr-moo-lah toh-mah)

What grade are you in?
¿En qué año estás?
(Ehn keh ah-nyoh ehs-tahs)

What happened here?
¿Qué pasa aquí?
(Keh pah-sah ah-kee)

What happened to him?
¿Qué le pasó?
(Keh leh pah-soh)

What happened to you?
¿Qué le pasó?
(Keh leh pah-soh)

What hospital do you go to?
¿A qué hospital va?
(Ah keh ohs-pee-tahl bah)

What house chores do you do?
¿Qué quehaceres haces?
(Keh keh-ah-seh-rehs ah-sehs)

What is . . . ?
¿Qué es . . . ?
(Keh ehs . . .)

What is bothering you the most?
¿Qué es lo qué más le molesta?
(Keh ehs loh keh mahs leh moh-lehs-tah)

What is hurting you?
¿Qué le duele?
(Keh leh doo-eh-leh)

What is that?
¿Qué es eso?
(Keh ehs eh-soh)

What is the address?
¿Cuál es la dirección?
(Koo-ahl ehs lah dee-rehk-see-ohn)

What is the main reason you are here today?
¿Cuál es la razón principal por qué está aquí?
(Koo-ahl ehs lah rah-sohn preen-see-pahl pohr keh ehs-tah ah-kee)

What is the matter?
¿Qué le pasa/sucede?
(Keh leh pah-sah/soo-seh-deh)

What is the name?
¿Cuál es el nombre?
(Koo-ahl ehs ehl nohm-breh)

What is the name of the company?
¿Cómo se llama la compañía?
(Koh-moh seh yah-mah lah kohm-pah-nyee-ah)

What is the name of the insurance?
¿Cuál es el nombre del seguro?
(Koo-ahl ehs ehl nohm-breh dehl seh-goo-roh)

What is the name of the school?
¿Cómo se llama la escuela?
(Koh-moh seh yah-mah lah ehs-koo-eh-lah)

What is the name of the street?
¿Cuál es el nombre de la calle?
(Koo-ahl ehs ehl nohm-breh deh lah kah-yeh)

What is the number of your house?
¿Qué número tiene su casa?
(Keh noo-meh-roh tee-eh-neh soo kah-sah)

What is the pain like?
¿Qué tipo de dolor tiene?
(Keh tee-poh deh doh-lohr tee-eh-neh)

What is the phone number?
¿Cuál es el número de teléfono?
(Koo-ahl ehs ehl noo-meh-roh deh teh-leh-foh-noh)

What is the worst problem?
¿Cuál es su peor problema?
(Koo-ahl ehs soo peh-ohr proh bleh-mah)

What is the year you were born?
¿En qué año nació?
(Ehn keh ah-nyoh nah-see-oh)

What is the zip code?
¿Cuál es el código postal?
(Koo-ahl ehs ehl koh-dee-goh pohs-tahl)

What is this?
¿Qué es esto?
(Keh ehs ehs-toh)

What is wrong?
¿Qué pasa?
(Keh pah-sah)

What is your address?
¿Cuál es su dirección?
(Koo-ahl ehs soo dee-rehk-see ohn)

What is your birthdate? year? month? day?
¿Cuál es la fecha de nacimiento? ¿Año/mes/día?
(Koo-ahl ehs lah feh-chah deh nah-see-mee-ehn-toh/ah-nyoh/mehs/dee-ah)

What is your brother's/sister's name?
¿Cómo se llama su hermano(a)?
(Koh-moh seh yah-mah soo ehr-mah-noh[ah])

What is your husband's/wife's name?
¿Cómo se llama su esposo(a)?
(Koh-moh seh yah-mah soo ehs-poh-soh[ah])

What is your last name?
¿Cómo se apellida?
(Koh-moh seh ah-peh-yee-dah)

What is your name?
¿Cómo se llama usted?
(Koh-moh seh yah-mah oos-tehd)

What is your occupation?
¿Qué clase de trabajo tiene?
(Keh klah-seh deh trah-bah-hoh tee-eh-neh)

What is your religion?
¿Cuál es su religión?
(Koo-ahl ehs soo reh-lee-hee-ohn)

What is your Social Security number?
¿Cuál es su número de Seguro Social?
(Koo-ahl ehs soo noo-meh-roh deh Seh-goo-roh Soh-see-ahl)

What kind?
¿Qué clase?
(Keh klah-seh)

What kind of accident?
¿Qué tipo de accidente?
(Keh tee-poh deh ahk-see-dehn-teh)

What kind of coffee?
¿Qué clase de café?
(Keh klah-seh deh kah-feh)

What kind of drinks?
¿Qué clase de bebidas?
(Keh klah-seh deh beh-bee-dahs)

What kind of grades do you make?
¿Qué calificaciones sacas?
(Keh kah-lee-fee-kah-see-ohn-ehs sah-kahs)

What kind of juices?
¿Qué clase de jugos?
(Keh klah-seh deh hoo-gohs)

What kind of surgery?
¿Qué clase de operaciones?
(Keh klah-seh deh oh-peh-rah-see-ohn-ehs)

What kind of weapons have you used?
¿Qué clase de armas ha usado?
(Keh klah-seh deh ahr-mahs ah oo-sah-doh)

What kind of work do you do?
¿Qué clase de trabajo hace?
(Keh klah-seh deh trah-bah-hoh ah-seh)

What kinds of problems?
¿Qué clase de problemas?
(Keh klah-seh deh proh-bleh-mahs)

What makes the pain better?
¿Qué hace mejorar el dolor?
(Keh ah-seh meh-hoh-rahr ehl doh-lohr)

What medical problem do you have?
¿Qué problema médico tiene?
(Keh proh-bleh-mah meh-dee-koh tee-eh-neh)

What medicines do you take?
¿Qué medicinas toma?
(Keh meh-dee-see-nahs toh-mah)

What other discomfort do you have?
¿Qué otra molestia tiene?
(Keh oh-trah moh-lehs-tee-ah tee-eh-neh)

What problem do you have?
¿Qué problema tiene?
(Keh proh-bleh-mah tee-eh-neh)

What subject do you like best?
¿Qué materia te gusta más?
(Keh mah-teh-ree-ah teh goos-tah mahs)

What symptoms do you have?
¿Qué síntomas tiene?
(Keh seen-toh-mahs tee-eh-neh)

What time is it?
¿Qué hora es?
(Keh oh-rah ehs)

What triggered your depression?
¿Qué precipitó su depresión?
(Keh preh-see-pee-toh soo deh-preh-see-ohn)

What was the color of the urine?
¿Cuál era el color de la orina?
(Koo-ahl eh-rah ehl koh-lohr deh lah oh-ree-nah)

What were you doing?
¿Qué estaba haciendo?
(Keh ehs-tah-bah ah-see-ehn-doh)

What work do you do?
¿Qué trabajo hace usted?
(Keh trah-bah-hoh ah-seh oos-tehd)

What's going on?
¿Qué pasa?
(Keh pah-sah)

What's happening?
¿Qué le pasa?
(Keh leh pah-sah)

Wheat bread and cereals.
Pan de trigo y cereales.
(Pahn deh tree-goh ee seh-reh-ah-lehs)

When?
¿Cuándo?
(Koo-ahn-doh)

When did this happen?
¿Cuándo le pasó esto?
(Koo-ahn-doh leh pah-soh ehs-toh)

When did you notice the skin rash?
¿Cuándo se dió cuenta de la piel rosada?
(Koo-ahn-doh seh dee-oh koo-ehn-tah deh lah pee-ehl roh-sah-dah)

When did you see the dentist last?
¿Cuándo vio al dentista la última vez?
(Koo-ahn-doh bee-oh ahl dehn-tees-tah lah ool-tee-mah behs)

When I tell you . . .
Cuando le diga . . .
(Koo-ahn-doh leh dee-gah)

When I tell you, hold your breath.
Cuando le diga, no respire.
(Koo-ahn-doh leh dee-gah, noh rehs-pee-reh)

When was he born?
¿Cuándo nació?
(Koo-ahn-doh nah-see-oh)

When was the last one?
¿Cuándo fue el último?
(Koo-ahn-doh foo-eh ehl ool-tee-moh)

When was the last time?
¿Cuándo fue la última vez?
(Koo-ahn-doh foo-eh lah ool-tee-mah behs)

When was the last time he had a bowel movement?
¿Cuándo fue la última vez que evacuó/hizo del baño?

(Koo-ahn-doh foo-eh lah ool-tee-mah behs keh eh-bah-koo-oh/ee-soh dehl bah-nyoh)

When was the last time that you took medicine?
¿Cuándo fue la última vez que tomó medicina?
(Koo-ahn-doh foo-eh lah ool-tee-mah behs keh toh-moh meh-dee-see-nah)

When was the last time you ate?
¿Cuándo fue la última vez que comió?
(Koo-ahn-doh foo-eh lah ool-tee-mah behs keh koh-mee-oh)

When was the last time you used the toilet?
¿Cuándo fue la última vez que hizo del baño/obró?
(Koo-ahn-doh foo-eh lah ool-tee-mah behs keh ee-soh dehl bah-nyoh/oh-broh)

When was the last time you were here?
¿Cuándo fue la última vez que estuvo aquí?
(Koo-ahn-doh foo-eh lah ool-tee-mah behs keh ehs-too-boh ah-kee)

When was your last normal period?
¿Cuándo tuvo su última menstruación normal?
(Koo-ahn-doh too-boh soo ool-tee-mah mehns-troo-ah-see-ohn nohr-mahl)

When were you born?
¿En qué año nació?
(Ehn keh ah-nyoh nah-see-oh)

When you get there, turn right.
Cuando llegue ahí, dé vuelta a la derecha.
(Koo-ahn-doh yeh-gheh ah-ee, deh boo-ehl-tah ah lah deh-reh-chah)

When you have pain, do you get nauseated?
Cuando tiene dolor, ¿le dan náuseas?
(Koo-ahn-doh tee-eh-neh doh-lohr, leh dahn nah-oo-seh-ahs)

When you let go.
Al retirar la mano.
(Ahl reh-tee-rahr lah mah-noh)

Where?
¿Dónde?
(Dohn-deh)

Where are they?
¿Dónde están?
(Dohn-deh ehs-tahn)

Where are you from?
¿De dónde es usted?
(Deh dohn-deh ehs oos-tehd)

Where can I reach your mother or father?
¿Dónde puedo localizar a su mamá o su papá?
(Dohn-deh poo-eh-doh loh-kah-lee-sahr ah soo mah-mah oh soo pah-pah)

Where do I need to go?
¿Adónde tengo qué ir?
(Ah-dohn-deh tehn-goh keh eer)

Where do you live?
¿Dónde vive usted?
(Dohn-deh bee-beh oos-tehd)

Where do you work?
¿Dónde trabaja usted?
(Dohn-deh trah-bah-hah oos-tehd)

Where does it hurt?
¿Dónde le duele?
(Dohn-deh leh doo-eh-leh)

Where is it?
¿Dónde está?
(Dohn-deh ehs-tah)

Where is your husband/wife?
¿Dónde está su esposo/esposa?
(Dohn-deh ehs-tah soo ehs-poh-soh/ehs-poh-sah)

Where were you born?
¿Dónde nació usted?
(Dohn-deh nah-see-oh oos-tehd)

Where were you going?
¿Adónde iba?
(Ah-dohn-deh ee-bah)

Where were you hit?
¿Dónde se golpeó?
(Dohn-deh seh gohl-peh-oh)

Which?
¿Cuál?
(Koo-ahl)

Which book do you want?
¿Qué libro quieres?
(Keh lee-broh kee-eh-rehs)

Which kind?
¿Qué clase?
(Keh klah-seh)

Which of the books do you want?
¿Cuál de los libros quieres?
(Koo-ahl deh lohs lee-brohs kee-eh-rehs)

Who?
¿Quién?
(Kee-ehn)

Who? (all)
¿Quiénes?
(Kee-ehn-ehs)

Who can take care of the children?
¿Quién puede cuidar a los niños?
(Kee-ehn poo-eh-deh koo-ee-dahr ah lohs nee-nyohs)

Who can we call in case of an emergency?
¿A quién le llamamos en caso de emergencia?
(Ah kee-ehn leh yah-mah-mohs ehn kah-soh deh eh-mehr-hehn-see-ah)

Who do you talk to?
¿Con quién habla?
(Kohn kee-ehn ah-blah)

Who helps you?
¿Quién te ayuda?
(Kee-ehn teh ah-yoo-dah)

Who helps you at home?
¿Quién le ayuda en casa?
(Kee-ehn leh ah-yoo-dah ehn kah-sah)

Who is at risk of getting AIDS?
¿Quién está en riesgo de contraer el SIDA?
(Kee-ehn ehs-tah ehn ree-ehs-goh deh kohn-trah-ehr ehl see-dah)

Who is going to pay the hospital?
¿Quién va a pagar el hospital?
(Kee-ehn bah ah pah-gahr ehl ohs-pee-tahl)

Who moved him?
¿Quién lo movió?
(Kee-ehn loh moh-bee-oh)

Who saw the accident?
¿Quién vio el accidente?
(Kee-ehn bee-oh ehl ahk-see-dehn-teh)

Who takes care of you at home?
¿Quién lo cuida en casa?
(Kee-ehn loh koo-ee-dah ehn kah-sah)

Who takes you to school?
¿Quién te lleva a la escuela?
(Kee-ehn teh yeh-bah ah lah ehs-koo-eh-lah)

Whose books are these?
¿De quién son estos libros?
(Deh kee-ehn sohn ehs-tohs lee-brohs)

Whose car is it?
¿De quién es el carro?
(Deh kee-ehn ehs ehl kah-roh)

Whose card is it?
¿De quién es la tarjeta?
(Deh kee-ehn ehs lah tahr-heh-tah)

Whose pen is it?
¿De quién es la pluma?
(Deh kee-ehn ehs lah ploo-mah)

Whose X-rays are these?
¿De quién son estos rayos X?
(Deh kee-ehn sohn ehs-tohs rah-yohs eh-kees)

Why?
¿Por qué?
(Pohr keh)

Why are you here?
¿Por qué está aquí?
(Pohr keh ehs-tah ah-kee)

Why do you make me do things I do not want to do?
¿Por qué me haces hacer cosas que no quiero?
(Pohr-keh meh ah-sehs ah-sehr koh-sahs keh noh kee-eh-roh?

Why not?
¿Por qué no?
(Pohr keh noh)

Will it pay for the hospital?
¿Paga por la hospitalización?
(Pah-gah pohr lah ohs-pee-tah-lee-sah-see-ohn)

Will you need to see a social worker?
¿Necesitará ver a la trabajadora social?
(Neh-seh-see-tah-rah behr ah lah trah-bah-hah-doh-rah soh-see-ahl)

Wind 18 inches of floss around one middle finger.
Enrede dieciocho pulgadas de hilo alrededor del tercer dedo.
(Ehn-reh-deh dee-eh-see-oh-choh pool-gah-dahs deh ee-loh ahl-reh-deh-dohr dehl tehr-sehr deh-doh)

Wind the rest around the middle finger of the other hand.
Enrede el resto alrededor del dedo medio de la otra mano.
(Ehn-reh-deh ehl rehs-toh ahl-reh-deh-dohr dehl deh-doh meh-dee-oh deh lah oh-trah mah-noh)

With how many people?
¿Con cuántas personas?
(Kohn koo-ahn-tahs pehr-soh-nahs)

Work phone number?
¿Teléfono del trabajo?
(Teh-leh-foh-noh dehl trah-bah-hoh)

Wrinkle your nose.
Arruga la nariz.
(Ah-roo-gah lah nah-rees)

Write, please.
Escriban, por favor.
(Ehs-kree-bahn, pohr fah-bohr)

Yes, a little.
Sí, un poco.
(See, oon poh-koh)

Yes, go to the end of the hall.
Sí, vaya al final del pasillo.
(See, bah-yah ahl feen-ahl dehl pah-see-yoh)

Yes, I speak English.
Si, yo hablo inglés.
(See, yoh ah-bloh een-glehs)

Yes, I speak Spanish.
Sí , yo hablo español.
(See, yoh ah-bloh ehs-pah-nyohl)

Yes, in the afternoon.
Sí, por la tarde.
(See, pohr lah tahr-deh)

Yes, last week.
Sí, la semana pasada.
(See, lah seh-mah-nah pah-sah-dah)

Yes, my dad.
Sí, mi papá.
(See, mee pah-pah)

Yes, please wait.
Sí, espere, por favor.
(See, ehs-peh-reh, pohr fah-bohr)

Yes, sir.
Sí, señor.
(See, seh-nyohr)

You are giving us permission to treat you.
Nos da usted permiso de tratarla.
(Nohs dah oos-ted pehr-mee-soh deh trah-tahr-lah)

You are giving us permission to treat you here.
Nos da permiso de tratarla aquí.
(Nohs dah pehr-mee-soh deh trah-tahr-lah ah-kee)

You are welcome.
De nada.
(Deh nah-dah)

You can also ask for snacks.
También puede pedir aperitivos.
(Tahm-bee-ehn poo-eh-deh peh-deer ah-peh-ree-tee-bohs)

You can breathe now.
Ya puede respirar.
(Yah poo-eh-deh rehs-pee-rahr)

You can bring your family here.
Puede traer a su familia aquí.
(Poo-eh-deh trah-ehr ah soo fah-mee-lee-ah ah-kee)

You can buy canned drinks in the cafeteria.
Puede comprar bebidas envasadas en la cafetería.
(Poo-eh-deh kohm-prahr beh-bee-dahs ehn-bah-sah-dahs ehn lah kah-feh-teh-ree-ah)

You can call collect.
Puede llamar por cobrar.
(Poo-eh-deh yah-mahr pohr koh-brahr)

You can cross at the walkway.
Puede cruzar por el pasillo sobre la calle.
(Poo-eh-deh kroo-sahr pohr ehl pah-see-yoh soh-breh lah kah-yeh)

You can drink water.
Puede tomar agua.
(Poo-eh-deh toh-mahr ah-goo-ah)

You can eat in your room or in the visitor's lounge.
Puede comer en su cuarto o en el cuarto para visitas.
(Poo-eh-deh koh-mehr ehn soo koo-ahr-toh oh ehn ehl koo-ahr-toh pah-rah bee-see-tahs)

You can feed him/her solid foods.
Puede darle alimentos sólidos.
(Poo-eh-deh dahr-leh ah-lee-mehn-tohs soh-lee-dohs)

You can go back to work in one week.
Puede regresar al trabajo en una semana.
(Poo-eh-deh reh-greh-sahr ahl trah-bah-hoh ehn oo-nah seh-mah-nah)

You can have flowers.
Puede tener flores.
(Poo-eh-deh teh-nehr floh-rehs)

You can make local phone calls.
Puede hacer llamadas locales.
(Poo-eh-deh ah-sehr yah-mah-dahs loh-kah-lehs)

You can order coffee here.
Puede ordenar café aquí.
(Poo-eh-deh ohr-deh-nahr kah-feh ah-kee)

You can order one or two portions.
Puede ordenar una o dos porciones.
(Poo-eh-deh ohr-deh-nahr oo-nah oh dohs pohr-see-oh-nehs)

You can pay on terms.
Puede pagar a plazos.
(Poo-eh-deh pah-gahr ah plah-sohs)

You can put cards on the shelf.
Puede poner tarjetas en el estante.
(Poo-eh-deh poh-nehr tahr-heh-tahs ehn ehl ehs-tahn-teh)

You can raise the feet.
Puede levantar los pies.
(Poo-eh-deh leh-bahn-tahr lohs pee-ehs)

You can raise the head.
Puede levantar la cabeza.
(Poo-eh-deh leh-bahn-tahr lah kah-beh-sah)

You can refill _____ times.
Puede surtir _____ veces.
(Poo-eh-deh soor-teer _____ beh-sehs)

You can smoke in the patio.
Puede fumar en el patio.
(Poo-eh-deh foo-mahr ehn ehl pah-tee-oh)

You can tape pictures to the wall.
Puede pegar retratos en la pared.
(Poo-eh-deh peh-gahr reh-trah-tohs ehn lah pah-rehd)

You can walk on crutches.
Puede caminar con muletas.
(Poo-eh-deh kah-mee-nahr kohn moo-leh-tahs)

You can write an "X."
Puede escribir una "X".
(Poo-eh-deh ehs-kree-beer oo-nah eh-kees)

You cannot hang anything from the ceiling.
No puede colgar nada del techo.
(Noh poo-eh-deh kohl-gahr nah-dah dehl teh-choh)

You cannot hang anything from the door.
No puede colgar nada en la puerta.
(Noh poo-eh-deh kohl-gahr nah-dah ehn lah poo-ehr-tah)

You cannot open the windows.
No puede abrir las ventanas.
(Noh poo-eh-deh ah-breer lahs behn-tah-nahs)

You cannot smoke here.
No puede fumar aquí.
(Noh poo-eh-deh foo-mahr ah-kee)

You cannot smoke in your room.
No puede fumar en el cuarto.
(Noh poo-eh-deh foo-mahr ehn ehl koo-ahr-toh)

You can't miss them!
¡No tiene pierde!
(Noh tee-eh-neh pee-ehr-deh)

You do not know the plan?
¿Usted no sabe el plan?
(Oos-tehd noh sah-beh ehl plahn)

You don't have to pay in full.
No tiene que pagar al contado.
(Noh tee-eh-neh keh pah-gahr ahl kohn-tah-doh)

You enjoyed working on your house yesterday.
Disfrutó el trabajar en su casa ayer.
(Dees-froo-toh ehl trah-bah-hahr ehn soo kah-sah ah-yehr)

You have a private bathroom.
Tiene un baño/inodoro privado.
(Tee-eh-neh oon bah-nyoh/ee noh-doh-roh pree-bah-doh)

You have bruises and white patches.
Tiene moretones y manchas blancas.
(Tee-eh-neh moh-reh-toh-nehs ee mahn-chahs blahn-kahs)

You have to choose three meals a day.
Tiene que escoger tres comidas diarias.
(Tee-eh-neh keh ehs-koh-hehr trehs koh-mee-dahs dee-ah-ree-ahs)

You have to cross the street.
Tiene que cruzar la calle.
(Tee-eh-neh keh kroo-sahr lah kah-yeh)

You have to give permission for treatment.
Tiene que dar permiso para el tratamiento.
(Tee-eh-neh keh dahr pehr-mee-soh pah-rah ehl trah-tah-mee-ehn-toh)

You have to go directly to the floor.
Debe ir al piso directamente.
(Deh-beh eer ahl pee-soh dee-rehk-tah-mehn-teh)

You have to wait your turn.
Tendrá que esperar su turno.
(Tehn-drah keh ehs-peh-rahr soo toor-noh)

You may be here about four hours.
Estará aquí cerca de cuatro horas.
(Ehs-tah-rah ah-kee sehr-kah deh koo-ah-troh oh-rahs)

You must go to the hospital.
Debe ir al hospital.
(Deh-beh eer ahl ohs-pee-tahl)

You must pay a deposit.
Debe pagar un depósito.
(Deh-beh pah-gahr oon deh-poh-see-toh)

You need to be admitted to the hospital.
Necesita internarse al hospital.
(Neh-seh-see-tah een-tehr-nahr-seh ahl ohs-pee-tahl)

You need to brush your teeth better.
Necesita cepillar mejor sus dientes.
(Neh-seh-see-tah seh-pee-yahr meh-hohr soos dee-ehn-tehs)

You need to return.
Necesita regresar.
(Neh-seh-see-tah reh-greh-sahr)

You need to sign this form.
Debe firmar esta forma.
(Deh-beh feer-mahr ehs-tah fohr-mah)

You will be all right!
¡Va a estar bien!
(Bah ah ehs-tahr bee-ehn)

You will feel pain like a pin prick.
Sentirá dolor como una picadura.
(Sehn-tee-rah doh-lohr koh-moh oo-nah pee-kah-doo-rah)

You will get help.
Se le ayudará.
(Seh leh ah-yoo-dah-rah)

You will have to rest at least seven days.
Tendrá que guardar reposo al menos siete días.
(Tehn-drah keh goo-ahr-dahr reh-poh-soh ahl meh-nohs see-eh-teh dee-ahs)

You will have to wait.
Tendrá que esperar.
(Tehn-drah keh ehs-peh-rahr)

You will need a cast.
Necesitará un yeso.
(Neh-seh-see-tah-rah oon yeh-soh)

You will need help.
Va a necesitar ayuda.
(Bah ah neh-seh-see-tahr ah-yoo-dah)

You will need to brush a little better in these areas.
Necesitará cepillarse mejor en estas áreas.
(Neh-seh-see-tah-rah seh-pee-yahr-seh meh-hohr ehn ehs-tahs ah-reh-ahs)

You will pass the cafeteria.
Va a pasar la cafetería.
(Bah ah pah-sahr lah kah-feh-teh-ree-ah)

You will see the sign on the wall.
Verá el letrero en la pared.
(Beh-rah ehl leh-treh-roh ehn lah pah-rehd)

Your appetite is good?
¿Tiene buen apetito?
(Tee-eh-neh boo-ehn ah-peh-tee-toh)

Your clothes go in the closet.
Su ropa va en el closet/ropero/armario.
(Soo roh-pah bah ehn ehl kloh-seht/roh-peh-roh/ahr-mah-ree-oh)

Your diet should be low in fats and hot sauces.
Su dieta debe ser baja en grasas y picantes.
(Soo dee-eh-tah deh-beh sehr bah-hah ehn grah-sahs ee pee-kahn-tehs)

Your family can bring your clothes tomorrow.
Su familia le puede traer su ropa mañana.
(Soo fah-mee-lee-ah leh poo-eh-deh trah-ehr soo roh-pah mah-nyah-nah)

Your family will bring clothes.
Su familia le traerá ropa.
(Soo fah-mee-lee-ah leh trah-eh-rah roh-pah)

Your leg is broken.
Tiene la pierna quebrada.
(Tee-eh-neh lah pee-ehr-nah keh-brah-dah)

Your skin color looks good.
El color de su piel es normal.
(Ehl koh-lohr deh soo pee-ehl ehs nohr-mahl)

Your towels are in the bathroom.
Sus toallas están en el baño.
(Soos too-ah-yahs ehs-tahn ehn ehl bah-nyoh)

Word Index

Words in this index are listed alphabetically according to the English. Verbs are indicated by the English infinitive marker [to]. Nouns are given in the singular form except where a plural is customarily used. Adjectives appear in the masculine singular form. Consult Chapters 34 and 35 for variant (feminine, plural) of nouns and adjectives.

A	**a**	*(ah)*
a, an	**un** (*m.*)/**una** (*f.*)	**(oon/ooh-nah)**
abdomen	**abdomen**	*(ahb-doh-mehn)*
abnormal	**anormal**	*(ah-nohr-mahl)*
about	**acerca de/por**	*(ah-sehr-kah deh/pohr)*
above	**arriba**	*(ah-ree-bah)*
absence	**ausencia**	*(ah-oo-sehn-see-ah)*
abuse	**abuso**	*(ah-boo-soh)*
accent	**acento**	*(ah-sehn-toh)*
[to] accept	**aceptar**	*(ah-sehp-tahr)*
acceptable	**aceptable**	*(ah-sehp-tah-bleh)*
accident	**accidente**	*(ahk-see-dehn-teh)*
according	**según**	*(seh-goon)*
acetic	**acético**	*(ah-seh-tee-koh)*
acne	**acne**	*(ahk-neh)*
acoustic	**acústico**	*(ah-koos-tee-koh)*
acrophobia [height]	**acrofobia**	*(ah-kroh-foh-bee-ah)*
[to] activate	**activar**	*(ahk-tee-bahr)*
addictive	**adicto**	*(ah-deek-toh)*
additive	**aditivo**	*(ah-dee-tee-boh)*
address	**dirección**	*(dee-rehk-see-ohn)*
adenoid	**adenoide**	*(ah-deh-noh-ee-deh)*
adhesive	**adhesivo**	*(ah-deh-see-boh)*
[to] administer	**administrar**	*(ahd-mee-nees-trahr)*
administration	**administración**	*(ahd-mee-nee-strah-see-ohn)*
admitting	**admitiendo**	*(ahd-meh-tee-ehn-doh)*
adrenalism	**adrenalismo**	*(ah-dreh-nah-lees-moh)*
adults	**adultos**	*(ah-dool-tohs)*
[to] advise	**aconsejar**	*(ah-kohn-seh-hahr)*
after	**después de**	*(dehs-poo-ehs deh)*
against	**contra**	*(kohn-trah)*
age	**edad**	*(eh-dahd)*
aggressive	**agresivo**	*(ah-greh-see-boh)*
agoraphobia [open spaces]	**agorafobia**	*(ah-goh-rah-foh-bee-ah)*

[to] agree	**acordar**	*(ah-kohr-dahr)*
air	**aire**	*(ah-ee-reh)*
airway	**vía aérea**	*(bee-ah ah-eh-reh-ah)*
albino	**albino**	*(ahl-bee-noh)*
alcohol	**alcohol**	*(ahl-kohl)*
alert him/her	**avísele**	*(ah-bee-seh-leh)*
alignment	**alineación**	*(ah-lee-neh-ah-see-ohn)*
all	**todo**	*(toh-doh)*
all right	**bien**	*(bee-ehn)*
allergies	**alergias**	*(ah-lehr-hee-ahs)*
allergic	**alérgico**	*(ah-lehr-hee-koh)*
alone	**solo**	*(soh-loh)*
alphabet	**abecedario**	*(ah-beh-seh-dah-ree-oh)*
also	**también**	*(tahm-bee-ehn)*
always	**siempre**	*(see-ehm-preh)*
amber	**ámbar**	*(ahm-bahr)*
ambulance	**ambulancia**	*(ahm-boo-lahn-see-ah)*
amebic	**amébico**	*(ah-meh-bee-koh)*
ammonia	**amonia**	*(ah-moh-nee-ah)*
among	**entre**	*(ehn-treh)*
amputation	**amputación**	*(ahm-poo-tah-see-ohn)*
amputee	**amputado**	*(ahm-poo-tah-doh)*
amygdala	**amígdala**	*(ah-meeg-dah-lah)*
analgesic	**analgésicos**	*(ah-nahl-heh-see-kohs)*
analysis	**análisis**	*(ah-nah-lee-sees)*
[to] analyze	**analizar**	*(ah-nah-lee-sahr)*
anaphylactic shock	**choque anafilático**	*(choh-keh ah-nah-fee-lah-tee-koh)*
anatomic position	**posición anatómica**	*(poh-see-see-ohn ah-nah-toh-mee-kah)*
and	**y**	*(ee)*
anemia	**anemia**	*(ah-neh-mee-ah)*
anemic	**anémico**	*(ah-neh-mee-koh)*
anesthesia	**anestesia**	*(ah-nehs-teh-see-ah)*
aneurysm	**aneurisma**	*(ah-neh-oo-rees-mah)*
anger	**enojo**	*(eh-noh-hoh)*
angina	**angina**	*(ahn-hee-nah)*
angioma	**angioma**	*(ahn-hee-oh-mah)*
angle	**ángulo**	*(ahn-goo-loh)*
angulation	**angulación**	*(ahn-goo-lah-see-ohn)*
ant	**hormiga**	*(ohr-mee-gah)*
antacid	**antiácidos**	*(ahn-tee-ah-see-dohs)*
anthropophobia [people]	**antropofobia**	*(ahn-troh-poh-foh-bee-ah)*
antianxiety	**ansiolíticos**	*(ahn-see-oh-lee-tee-kohs)*
antiarrhythmic	**antiarritmias**	*(ahn-tee-ah-reet-mee-ahs)*
antibiotic	**antibiótico**	*(ahn-tee-bee-oh-tee-koh)*
anticoagulant	**anticoagulante**	*(ahn-tee-koh-ah-goo-lahn-teh)*
anticonvulsant	**anticonvulsivo**	*(ahn-tee-kohn-bool-see-boh)*
antidiarrheal	**antidiarrea**	*(ahn-tee-dee-ah-reh-ah)*
antiemetic	**antiemético**	*(ahn-tee-eh-meh-tee-koh)*
antiepileptic	**antiepiléptico**	*(ahn-tee-eh-pee-lehp-tee-koh)*
antiestreptolysin	**antiestreptolicinas**	*(ahn-tee-ehs-trehp-toh-lee-see-nahs)*
antihistamine	**antihistamínico**	*(ahn-tee-ees-tah-mee-nee-koh)*

antiviral	**antivirus/antivirales**	*(ahn-tee-bee-roos/ahn-tee-bee-rah-lehs)*
anxiety	**ansiedad**	*(ahn-see-eh-dahd)*
anxious	**ansioso**	*(ahn-see-oh-soh)*
any	**alguno**	*(ahl-goo-noh)*
aorta	**aorta**	*(ah-ohr-tah)*
apothecary	**apotecarios**	*(ah-poh-teh-kah-ree-ohs)*
appendicitis	**apendicitis**	*(ah-pehn-dee-see-tees)*
appendix	**apéndice**	*(ah-pehn-dee-seh)*
appetizers	**bocadillos**	*(boh-kah-dee-yohs)*
appetizing	**apetitosas**	*(ah-peh-tee-toh-sahs)*
apple	**manzana**	*(mahn-sah-nah)*
[to] appreciate	**apreciar**	*(ah-preh-see-ahr)*
approaches	**se dirige**	*(seh dee-ree-heh)*
April	**abril**	*(ah-breel)*
are dispensed	**son distribuidos**	*(sohn dees-tree-boo-ee-dohs)*
are not	**no son**	*(noh sohn)*
around	**alrededor de**	*(ahl-reh-deh-dohr deh)*
arrest	**arresto**	*(ah-rehs-toh)*
[to] arrive	**llegar**	*(yeh-gahr)*
arrow	**flecha**	*(fleh-chah)*
arteriogram	**arteriograma**	*(ahr-teh-ree-oh-grah-mah)*
arteriosclerosis	**arterioesclerosis**	*(ahr-teh-ree-oh-ehs-kleh-roh-sees)*
arthritis	**artritis**	*(ahr-tree-tees)*
articles	**artículos**	*(ahr-tee-koo-lohs)*
artificial eye	**ojo artificial**	*(oh-hoh ahr-tee-fee-see-ahl)*
as	**por/como**	*(pohr/koh-moh)*
[to] ask [a question]	**preguntar**	*(preh-goon-tahr)*
asparagus	**espárragos**	*(ehs-pah-rah-gohs)*
aspirin	**aspirina**	*(ahs-pee-ree-nah)*
[to] assess	**asesorar**	*(ah-seh-soh-rahr)*
assessment	**avalúo**	*(ah-bah-loo-oh)*
assist them	**ayúdeles**	*(ah-yoo-deh-lehs)*
asthma	**asma**	*(ahs-mah)*
at the	**al (*m.*)/a la (*f.*)**	*(ahl/ah lah)*
at	**a**	*(ah)*
attention	**atención**	*(ah-tehn-see-ohn)*
August	**agosto**	*(ah-gohs-toh)*
aunt	**tía**	*(tee-ah)*
[to] auscultate	**auscultar**	*(ah-oos-kool-tahr)*
author	**autor**	*(ah-oo-tohr)*
[to] authorize	**autorizar**	*(ah-oo-toh-ree-sahr)*
available	**disponible**	*(dees-poh-nee-bleh)*
avenue	**avenida**	*(ah-beh-nee-dah)*
avocados	**aguacates**	*(ah-goo-ah-kah-tehs)*
[to] avoid	**evitar**	*(eh-bee-tahr)*
B	**b**	*(beh)*
baby	**bebé**	*(beh-beh)*
baby tooth	**diente de leche**	*(dee-ehn-teh deh leh-cheh)*
bacon	**tocino**	*(toh-see-noh)*
bacteria	**bacteria**	*(bahk-teh-ree-ah)*

bad	**mal**	*(mahl)*
baked	**asado**	*(ah-sah-doh)*
baked chicken	**pollo asado**	*(poh-yoh ah-sah-doh)*
baked potatoes	**papas asadas**	*(pah-pahs ah-sah-dahs)*
balanced	**balanceada**	*(bah-lahn-seh-ah-dah)*
banana	**plátano**	*(plah-tah-noh)*
barbaric	**bárbaro**	*(bahr-bah-roh)*
barbiturates	**barbitúricos**	*(bahr-bee-too-ree-kohs)*
basin	**lavabo**	*(lah-bah-doh)*
[to] bathe	**bañar**	*(bah-nyahr)*
bathroom	**cuarto de baño**	*(koo-ahr-toh deh bah-nyoh)*
[to] be	**estar/ser**	*(ehs-tahr/sehr)*
[to] be able to	**poder**	*(poh-dehr)*
[to] be afraid	**temer**	*(teh-mehr)*
[to] be available	**encontrar**	*(ehn-kohn-trahr)*
[to] be born	**nacer**	*(nah-sehr)*
[to] be supportive	**apoyar**	*(ah-poh-yahr)*
beans	**frijoles**	*(free-hoh-lehs)*
[to] beat	**golpear**	*(gohl-peh-ahr)*
because	**porque**	*(pohr-keh)*
[to] become ill	**enfermarse**	*(ehn-fehr-mahr-seh)*
bed	**cama**	*(kah-mah)*
bed rail	**barandal**	*(bah-rahn-dahl)*
bedpan	**bacín**	*(bah-seen)*
bedroom	**recámara/habitación**	*(reh-kah-mah-rah/ah-bee-tah-see-ohn)*
bedspread	**colcha**	*(kohl-chah)*
beef	**carne de res**	*(kahr-neh deh rehs)*
beet	**betabel**	*(beh-tah-behl)*
before	**antes de**	*(ahn-tehs deh)*
beginning	**principio**	*(preen-see-pee-oh)*
behavior	**conducta**	*(kohn-dook-tah)*
behind	**detrás de**	*(deh-trahs deh)*
[to] believe	**creer**	*(kreh-ehr)*
bell(s)	**campana[s]**	*(kahm-pah-nah[s])*
below	**abajo**	*(ah-bah-hoh)*
[to] bend	**doblar**	*(doh-blahr)*
beneath	**debajo de**	*(deh-bah-hoh deh)*
benign	**benigno**	*(beh-neeg-noh)*
bereavement	**desamparo**	*(dehs-ahm-pah-roh)*
besides	**además de**	*(ah-deh-mahs deh)*
better	**mejor**	*(meh-hohr)*
between	**entre**	*(ehn-treh)*
big	**grande**	*(grahn-deh)*
birth control	**control de fertilidad**	*(kohn-trohl deh fehr-tee-lee-dahd)*
birthmark	**lunar**	*(loo-nahr)*
biscuits	**bisquetes**	*(bees-keh-tehs)*
bit	**poco**	*(poh-koh)*
Bite!	**¡Muerda!**	*(Moo-ehr-dah)*
black	**negro**	*(neh-groh)*
blanket	**frazada/covertor**	*(frah-sah-dah/koh-behr-tohr)*
[to] bleed	**sangrar**	*(sahn-grahr)*

bleeding	**sangrado**	*(sahn-grah-doh)*
blocks	**cuadras**	*(koo-ah-drahs)*
blonde	**rubio**	*(roo-bee-oh)*
blood	**sangre**	*(sahn-greh)*
blood bank	**banco de sangre**	*(bahn-koh deh sahn-greh)*
blood count	**biometría hemática**	*(bee-oh-meh-tree-ah eh-mah-tee-kah)*
blood flow	**circulación sanguínea**	*(seer-koo-lah-see-ohn sahn-gee-nee-ah)*
blood stream	**arroyo de la sangre**	*(ah-roh-yoh deh lah sahn-greh)*
blouse	**blusa**	*(bloo-sah)*
blue	**azul**	*(ah-sool)*
bluish	**azulosa**	*(ah-soo-loh-sah)*
body	**cuerpo**	*(koo-ehr-poh)*
[to] boil	**hervir**	*(ehr-beer)*
boiled	**cocidas**	*(koh-see-dahs)*
book	**libro**	*(lee-broh)*
[to] bore	**aburrir**	*(ah-boo-reer)*
boredom	**fastidio**	*(fahs-tee-dee-oh)*
boric acid	**ácido bórico**	*(ah-see-doh boh-ree-koh)*
bottle	**botella**	*(boh-teh-yah)*
bowel	**intestino**	*(een-tehs-tee-noh)*
boy(s)	**muchacho/niño**	*(moo-chah-choh/nee-nyoh)*
braces	**abrazaderas**	*(ah-brah-sah-deh-rahs)*
bradycardia	**bradicardia**	*(brah-dee-kahr-dee-ah)*
brand names	**marcas de productos**	*(mahr-kahs deh proh-dook-tohs)*
bread(s)	**pan(es)**	*(pahn[-ehs])*
breaded	**empanizado**	*(ehm-pah-nee-sah-doh)*
[to] break	**romper**	*(rohm-pehr)*
breakfast	**desayuno**	*(deh-sah-yoo-noh)*
breast	**pechuga**	*(peh-choo-gah)*
[to] breathe	**respirar**	*(rehs-pee-rahr)*
[to] bring	**traer**	*(trah-ehr)*
[to] bring near	**acercar**	*(ah-sehr-kahr)*
broiled	**hervidos**	*(hehr-bee-dohs)*
broiled fish	**pescado al horno**	*(pehs-kah-doh ahl ohr-noh)*
broken bone	**hueso roto**	*(oo-eh-soh roh-toh)*
bronchitis	**bronquitis**	*(brohn-kee-tees)*
brother	**hermano**	*(ehr-mah-noh)*
brother-in-law	**cuñado**	*(koo-nyah-doh)*
brown (*color*)	**café**	*(kah-feh)*
brown (*skin tone*)	**moreno**	*(moh-reh-noh)*
bruises	**moretones**	*(moh-reh-toh-nehs)*
[to] build	**construir**	*(kohns-troo-eer)*
building	**edificio**	*(eh-dee-fee-see-oh)*
burns	**quemaduras**	*(keh-mah-doo-rahs)*
[to] burp	**repetir/eructar**	*(reh-peh-teer/eh-rook-tahr)*
burritos	**burritos**	*(boo-ree-tohs)*
butter	**mantequilla**	*(mahn-teh-kee-yah)*
button	**botón**	*(boh-tohn)*
buzzing	**zumbido**	*(soom-bee-doh)*
by	**por**	*(pohr)*
by mouth	**por la boca**	*(pohr lah boh-kah)*

C	c	*(seh)*
cabbage	**col/repollo**	*(kohl/reh-poh-yoh)*
cafe	**café**	*(kah-feh)*
cafeteria	**cafetería**	*(kah-feh-teh-ree-ah)*
caffeine	**cafeína**	*(kah-feh-ee-nah)*
cake	**pastel**	*(pahs-tehl)*
[to] call [for]	**llamar**	*(yah-mahr)*
call-bell	**campana/timbre**	*(kahm-pah-nah/teem-breh)*
callus	**callo**	*(kah-yoh)*
calm	**calma**	*(kahl-mah)*
can	**poder**	*(poh-dehr)*
cancer	**cáncer**	*(kahn-sehr)*
candy	**dulces**	*(dool-sehs)*
canes	**bastones**	*(bahs-toh-nehs)*
canteloupe	**melón**	*(meh-lohn)*
capsule	**cápsula**	*(kahp-soo-lah)*
carbonated drinks	**bebidas gaseosas**	*(beh-bee-dahs gah-seh-oh-sahs)*
card	**tarjeta**	*(tahr-heh-tah)*
cardiac	**cardíaco**	*(kahr-dee-ah-koh)*
cardiopulmonary	**cardiopulmonar**	*(kahr-dee-oh-pool-moh-nahr)*
care	**cuidado**	*(koo-ee-dah-doh)*
caries	**caries**	*(kah-ree-ehs)*
carotid	**carótida**	*(kah-roh-tee-dah)*
carrots	**zanahorias**	*(sah-nah-oh-ree-ahs)*
[to] carry	**llevar**	*(yeh-bahr)*
cash	**dinero**	*(dee-neh-roh)*
casts	**lanzamientos**	*(lahn-sah-mee-ehn-tohs)*
cataract	**catarata**	*(kah-tah-rah-tah)*
categories	**categorías**	*(kah-teh-goh-ree-ahs)*
cause	**causa**	*(kah-oo-sah)*
cavity	**cavidad**	*(kah-bee-dahd)*
ceiling	**techo**	*(teh-choh)*
celery	**apio**	*(ah-pee-oh)*
cell	**célula**	*(seh-loo-lah)*
cement	**cemento**	*(seh-mehn-toh)*
centimeter	**centímetro**	*(sehn-tee-meh-troh)*
cereal (cooked)	**cereal cocido**	*(seh-reh-ahl koh-see-doh)*
cereal (dry)	**cereal seco**	*(seh-reh-ahl seh-koh)*
chair	**silla**	*(see-yah)*
chancre	**chancro**	*(chahn-kroh)*
[to] change	**cambiar**	*(kahm-bee-ahr)*
change (*coins*)	**cambio**	*(kahm-bee-oh)*
channel	**canal**	*(kah-nahl)*
chaplain	**capellán**	*(kah-peh-yahn)*
chapter	**capítulo**	*(kah-pee-too-loh)*
characteristics	**características**	*(kahr-ahk-teh-rees-tee-kahs)*
[to] chat	**charlar**	*(chahr-lahr)*
cheek	**mejilla**	*(meh-hee-yah)*
chemotherapy	**quimioterapia**	*(kee-mee-oh-teh-rah-pee-ah)*
cherries	**cerezas**	*(seh-reh-sahs)*
chest	**pecho**	*(peh-choh)*
chest pain	**dolor en el pecho**	*(doh-lohr ehn ehl peh-choh)*

chest X-ray	**radiografía de tórax**	*(rah-dee-oh-grah-fee-ah deh toh-rahx)*
chicken	**pollo**	*(poh-yoh)*
child	**niño/niña**	*(nee-nyoh/nee-nyah)*
children	**niños/hijos**	*(nee-nyohs/ee-hohs)*
chocolate	**chocolate**	*(choh-koh-lah-teh)*
[to] choke	**ahogar**	*(ah-oh-gahr)*
cholesterol	**colesterol**	*(koh-lehs-teh-rohl)*
[to] choose	**escoger**	*(ehs-koh-hehr)*
chops	**chuletas**	*(choo-leh-tahs)*
cianotic	**cianótico**	*(see-ah-noh-tee-koh)*
cirrhosis	**cirrosis**	*(see-roh-sees)*
classification	**clasificación**	*(klah-see-fee-kah-see-ohn)*
classified	**clasificado**	*(klah-see-fee-kah-doh)*
[to] classify	**clasificar**	*(klah-see-fee-kahr)*
claustrophobia [closed spaces]	**claustrofobia**	*(klah-oos-troh-foh-bee-ah)*
[to] clean	**limpiar**	*(leem-pee-ahr)*
clear	**claro**	*(klah-roh)*
clinic	**clínica**	*(klee-nee-kah)*
clinical	**clínico**	*(klee-nee-koh)*
[to] close	**cerrar**	*(seh-rahr)*
closed reduction	**reducción cerrada**	*(reh-dook-see-ohn seh-rah-dah)*
clothes	**ropa**	*(roh-pah)*
coagulated	**coagulado**	*(koh-ah-goo-lah-doh)*
coagulation	**coagulación**	*(koh-ah-goo-lah-see-ohn)*
coat	**abrigo**	*(ah-bree-goh)*
cocaine	**cocaína**	*(koh-kah-ee-nah)*
coffee	**café**	*(kah-feh)*
cognitive	**cognoscitivo**	*(kohg-noh-see-tee-boh)*
cold	**frío**	*(free-oh)*
colic	**cólico**	*(koh-lee-koh)*
[to] collect	**coleccionar**	*(koh-lehk-see-ohn-ahr)*
Colles' fracture	**fractura de Colles**	*(frahk-too-rah deh Koh-yehs)*
colonel	**coronel**	*(koh-rohn-ehl)*
coma	**coma**	*(koh-mah)*
comatose	**comatoso**	*(koh-mah-toh-soh)*
comb	**peine**	*(peh-ee-neh)*
[to] come	**venir**	*(beh-neer)*
commands	**mandatos**	*(mahn-dah-tohs)*
comminuted fractures	**fracturas conminutas**	*(frahk-too-rahs kohn-mee-noo-tahs)*
common	**común**	*(koh-moon)*
common-law wife	**concubina**	*(kohn-koo-bee-nah)*
[to] communicate	**comunicar**	*(koh-moo-nee-kahr)*
communication	**comunicación**	*(koh-moo-nee-kah-see-ohn)*
community	**comunidad**	*(koh-moo-nee-dahd)*
comparison	**comparación**	*(kohm-pah-rah-see-ohn)*
[to] complain	**quejar**	*(keh-hahr)*
complete blood count	**biometría hemática**	*(bee-oh-meh-tree-ah eh-mah-tee-kah)*
complete dentures	**dentadura completa**	*(dehn-tah-doo-rah kohm-pleh-tah)*
complication	**complicación**	*(kohm-plee-kah-see-ohn)*

compound fractures	**fracturas compuestas**	*(frahk-too-rahs kohm-poo-ehs-tahs)*
compromise	**compromiso**	*(kohm-proh-mee-soh)*
concepts	**conceptos**	*(kohn-sehp-tohs)*
condiments	**condimentos**	*(kohn-dee-mehn-tohs)*
[to] conduct	**conducir**	*(kohn-doo-seer)*
[to] confirm	**confirmar**	*(kohn-feer-mahr)*
[to] confuse	**confundir**	*(kohn-foon-deer)*
consciousness	**conocimiento**	*(koh-noh-see-mee-ehn-toh)*
[to] conserve	**conservar**	*(kohn-sehr-bahr)*
constipation	**constipación**	*(kohns-tee-pah-see-ohn)*
consultant	**consultante**	*(kohn-sool-tahn-teh)*
content	**contenido**	*(kohn-teh-nee-doh)*
continued	**continuado**	*(kohn-tee-noo-ah-doh)*
continuity	**continuidad**	*(kohn-tee-noo-ee-dahd)*
contraceptives	**contraceptivos**	*(kohn-trah-sehp-tee-bohs)*
contractions	**contracciones**	*(kohn-trahk-see-ohn-ehs)*
contrast	**contraste**	*(kohn-trahs-teh)*
[to] control	**controlar**	*(kohn-troh-lahr)*
convenient	**conveniente**	*(kohn-beh-nee-ehn-teh)*
[to] cook	**cocinar**	*(koh-see-nahr)*
cookies	**galletas**	*(gah-yeh-tahs)*
coping	**sobrellevando**	*(soh-breh-yeh-bahn-doh)*
copper	**cobre**	*(koh-breh)*
corn	**maíz/elote**	*(mah-ees/eh-loh-teh)*
corn bread	**pan de maíz**	*(pahn deh mah-ees)*
corn flakes	**hojitas de maíz**	*(oh-hee-tahs deh mah-ees)*
corner	**esquina**	*(ehs-kee-nah)*
cortisone	**cortisona**	*(kohr-tee-sohn-ah)*
cosmetics	**cosméticos**	*(kohs-meh-tee-kohs)*
cottage cheese	**requesón**	*(reh-keh-sohn)*
cough	**tos**	*(tohs)*
cousin	**primo/prima**	*(pree-moh/pree-mah)*
cousins	**primos**	*(pree-mohs)*
[to] cover	**cubrir**	*(koo-breer)*
crab	**cangrejo**	*(kahn-greh-hoh)*
crackers	**galletas saladas**	*(gah-yeh-tahs sah-lah-dahs)*
cream	**crema**	*(kreh-mah)*
cream of wheat	**crema de trigo**	*(kreh-mah deh tree-goh)*
crisis	**crisis**	*(kree-sees)*
[to] cross	**cruzar**	*(kroo-sahr)*
crowns	**coronas**	*(koh-roh-nahs)*
crutches	**muletas**	*(moo-leh-tahs)*
[to] cry	**llorar**	*(yoh-rahr)*
crystal	**cristal**	*(krees-tahl)*
cubic	**cúbico**	*(koo-bee-koh)*
cubic centimeter	**centímetro cúbico**	*(sehn-tee-meh-troh koo-bee-koh)*
cucumbers	**pepinos**	*(peh-pee-nohs)*
cup	**taza**	*(tah-sah)*
[to] cure	**curar**	*(koo-rahr)*
custard	**flan**	*(flahn)*
customary	**acostumbra**	*(ah-kohs-toom-brah)*

[to] cut	**cortar**	*(kohr-tahr)*
[to] cut down	**reducir**	*(reh-doos-keer)*
D	**d**	*(deh)*
dad	**papá**	*(pah-pah)*
dark	**negro**	*(neh-groh)*
daughter	**hija**	*(ee-hah)*
days	**días**	*(dee-ahs)*
[to] deal with	**tratar**	*(trah-tahr)*
debris	**restos**	*(rehs-tohs)*
decaffeinated	**descafeinado**	*(dehs-kah-feh-ee-nah-doh)*
December	**diciembre**	*(dee-see-ehm-breh)*
decent	**decente**	*(deh-sehn-teh)*
[to] decide that	**decidir que**	*(deh-see-deer keh)*
decongestants	**descongestionantes**	*(dehs-kohn-hehs-tee-oh-nahn-tehs)*
defense	**defensa**	*(deh-fehn-sah)*
deficiency	**deficiencia**	*(deh-fee-see-ehn-see-ah)*
dehydrated	**deshidratado**	*(deh-see-drah-tah-doh)*
dehydration	**deshidratación**	*(deh-see-drah-tah-see-ohn)*
delirious	**delirio**	*(deh-lee-ree-oh)*
demented	**demente**	*(deh-mehn-teh)*
dementia	**demencia**	*(deh-mehn-see-ah)*
dental	**dental**	*(dehn-tahl)*
dental floss	**hilo dental**	*(ee-loh dehn-tahl)*
dental plaque	**sarro**	*(sah-roh)*
dental surgeon	**cirujano dentista**	*(see-roo-hah-noh dehn-tees-tah)*
dentifrice	**dentífrico**	*(dehn-tee-free-koh)*
dentist	**dentista**	*(dehn-tees-tah)*
dentures	**dentadura postiza**	*(dehn-tah-doo-rah pohs-tee-sah)*
[to] deny	**negar**	*(neh-gahr)*
department	**departamento**	*(deh-pahr-tah-mehn-toh)*
dependence	**dependencia**	*(deh-pehn-dehn-see-ah)*
dependent	**dependiente**	*(deh-pehn-dee-ehn-teh)*
depressed	**deprimido**	*(deh-pree-mee-doh)*
[to] deserve	**merecer**	*(meh-reh-sehr)*
desserts	**postres**	*(pohs-trehs)*
[to] destroy	**destruir**	*(dehs-troo-eer)*
[to] detect	**descubrir**	*(dehs-koo-breer)*
detection	**detección**	*(deh-tehk-see-ohn)*
[to] determine	**determinar**	*(deh-tehr-mee-nahr)*
development	**desarrollo**	*(deh-sah-roh-yoh)*
diabetes	**diabetes**	*(dee-ah-beh-tehs)*
diabetic	**diabético**	*(dee-ah-beh-tee-koh)*
diagnosis	**diagnóstico**	*(dee-ahg-nohs-tee-koh)*
diagnostic	**diagnóstico**	*(dee-ahg-nohs-tee-koh)*
diagnostic tests	**pruebas de diagnóstico**	*(proo-eh-bahs deh dee-ahg-nohs-tee-koh)*
diamonds	**diamantes**	*(deh-ah-mahn-tehs)*
diaper	**pañal**	*(pah-nyahl)*
diarrhea	**diarrea**	*(dee-ah-reh-ah)*
[to] die	**morir**	*(moh-reer)*
diet(s)	**dieta(s)**	*(dee-eh-tah[s])*

English	Spanish	Pronunciation
different	**diferente**	*(dee-feh-rehn-teh)*
difficulty	**dificultad**	*(dee-fee-kool-tahd)*
digitalis	**digitálicos**	*(dee-hee-tah-lee-kohs)*
diluent	**diluente**	*(dee-loo-ehn-teh)*
dinner	**cena**	*(seh-nah)*
direct	**directo**	*(dee-rehk-toh)*
directions	**direcciones**	*(dee-rehk-see-ohn-ehs)*
[to] disappear	**desaparecer**	*(deh-sah-pah-reh-sehr)*
disclosing solution	**solución reveladora**	*(soh-loo-see-ohn reh-beh-lah-doh-rah)*
discomfort	**molestia**	*(moh-lehs-tee-ah)*
[to] discover	**descubrir**	*(dehs-koo-breer)*
dish	**plato**	*(plah-toh)*
disorder	**desorden**	*(deh-sohr-dehn)*
division	**división**	*(dee-bee-see-ohn)*
dizzy	**mareado**	*(mah-reh-ah-doh)*
dizzy spell	**desmayo/mareo**	*(dehs-mah-yoh/mah-reh-oh)*
[to] do	**hacer**	*(ah-sehr)*
doctor (*f.*)	**doctora/médica**	*(dohk-tohr-ah/meh-dee-kah)*
doctor (*m.*)	**doctor/médico**	*(dohk-tohr/meh-dee-koh)*
doctor's office	**oficina/consultorio**	*(oh-fee-see-nah/kohn-sool-toh-ree-oh)*
door	**puerta**	*(poo-ehr-tah)*
dose	**dosis**	*(doh-sees)*
[to] draw (*a picture*)	**dibujar**	*(dee-boo-hahr)*
[to] draw (pull/ take out)	**sacar/tirar**	*(sah-kahr/tee-rahr)*
dream	**sueño**	*(soo-eh-nyoh)*
dress	**vestido**	*(behs-tee-doh)*
[to] dress	**vestir**	*(behs-teer)*
[to] drink	**beber/tomar**	*(beh-behr/toh-mahr)*
drop	**gota**	*(goh-tah)*
drugs	**drogas**	*(droh-gahs)*
dry	**seco**	*(seh-koh)*
duck	**pato**	*(pah-toh)*
during	**durante**	*(doo-rahn-teh)*
E	**e**	*(eh)*
each	**cada**	*(kah-dah)*
early	**temprano**	*(tehm-prah-noh)*
east	**este**	*(ehs-teh)*
[to] eat	**comer**	*(koh-mehr)*
[to] eat breakfast	**desayunar**	*(deh-sah-yoo-nahr)*
ecchymosis	**equimosis**	*(eh-kee-moh-sees)*
eczema	**eczema**	*(ehk-seh-mah)*
egg	**huevo**	*(oo-eh-boh)*
egg yolk	**yema de huevo**	*(yeh-mah deh oo-eh-bohs)*
eggplant	**berenjena**	*(beh-rehn-heh-nah)*
eight	**ocho**	*(oh-choh)*
eight A.M.	**las ocho**	*(lahs oh-choh)*
eight hundred	**ochocientos**	*(oh-choh-see-ehn-tohs)*
eight P.M.	**las veinte horas**	*(lahs beh-een-teh oh-rahs)*
eighteen	**dieciocho**	*(dee-eh-see-oh-choh)*
eighth	**octavo**	*(ohk-tah-boh)*

eighty	**ochenta**	*(oh-chehn-tah)*
either . . . or	**o . . . o**	*(oh . . . oh)*
elderly	**anciano**	*(ahn-see-ah-noh)*
electrocardiogram	**electrocardiograma**	*(eh-lehk-troh-kahr-dee-oh-grah-mah)*
elevator	**elevador**	*(eh-leh-bah-dohr)*
eleven	**once**	*(ohn-seh)*
eleven A.M.	**las once**	*(lahs ohn-seh)*
eleven P.M.	**las veintitrés horas**	*(lahs beh-een-tee-trehs oh-rahs)*
embolism	**embolismo**	*(ehm-bohl-ees-moh)*
[to] embrace	**abrazar**	*(ah-brah-sahr)*
emerald	**esmeralda**	*(ehs-meh-rahl-dah)*
emergency	**emergencia**	*(eh-mehr-hehn-see-ah)*
emergency room	**cuarto de emergencia**	*(koo-ahr-toh deh eh-mehr-hehn-see-ah)*
emetic	**emético**	*(eh-meh-tee-koh)*
[to] employ	**emplear**	*(ehm-pleh-ahr)*
enamel	**esmalte**	*(ehs-mahl-teh)*
enchiladas	**enchiladas**	*(ehn-chee-lah-dahs)*
end: at the end	**al final**	*(ahl fee-nahl)*
endoscopic	**endoscópico**	*(ehn-dohs-koh-pee-koh)*
endoscopy	**endoscopía**	*(ehn-dohs-koh-pee-ah)*
enema	**enema/sonda**	*(eh-neh-mah/sohn-dah)*
English	**inglés**	*(een-glehs)*
enteritis	**enteritis**	*(ehn-teh-ree-tees)*
environment	**ambiente familiar**	*(ahm-bee-ehn-teh fah-mee-lee-ahr)*
epigastrium	**epigastrio**	*(eh-pee-gahs-tree-oh)*
epilepsy	**epilepsia**	*(eh-pee-lehp-see-ah)*
error	**error**	*(eh-rohr)*
especially	**especialmente**	*(ehs-peh-see-ahl-mehn-teh)*
essence	**esencia**	*(eh-sehn-see-ah)*
essential	**esencial**	*(eh-sehn-see-ahl)*
etiology	**etiología**	*(eh-tee-oh-loh-hee-ah)*
euphoric	**eufórico**	*(eh-oo-foh-ree-koh)*
[to] evaluate	**evaluar**	*(eh-bah-loo-ahr)*
evaluation	**evaluación**	*(eh-bah-loo-ah-see-ohn)*
every	**cada uno/todos**	*(kah-dah oo-noh/toh-dohs)*
every time	**cada vez**	*(kah-dah behs)*
everything	**todo**	*(toh-doh)*
examinations	**exámenes**	*(ehx-ah-meh-nehs)*
[to] examine	**examinar**	*(ehx-ah-mee-nahr)*
excrement	**excremento**	*(ehx-kreh-mehn-toh)*
Excuse me!	**¡Perdón!**	*(Pehr-dohn)*
exercise	**ejercicio**	*(eh-hehr-see-see-oh)*
exit sign	**salida**	*(sah-lee-dah)*
[to] explain	**explicar**	*(ehx-plee-kahr)*
explains	**explica**	*(ehx-plee-kah)*
expression	**expresión**	*(ehx-preh-see-ohn)*
external	**externo**	*(ehx-tehr-noh)*
[to] extract	**extraer/sacar**	*(ehx-trah-ehr/sah-kahr)*
extraction	**extracción**	*(ehx-trahk-see-ohn)*
exudate	**exudado**	*(ehx-oo-dah-doh)*
eyetooth	**diente canino/colmillo**	*(dee-ehn-teh kah-nee-noh/kohl-mee-yoh)*

F	**f**	*(eh-feh)*
facial	**facial**	*(fah-see-ahl)*
factors	**factores**	*(fahk-toh-rehs)*
[to] fail	**fallar**	*(fah-yahr)*
fajitas	**fajitas**	*(fah-hee-tahs)*
fall (*autumn*)	**otoño**	*(oh-toh-nyoh)*
false	**falso**	*(fahl-soh)*
familiar	**familiar**	*(fah-mee-lee-ahr)*
family	**familia**	*(fah-mee-lee-ah)*
far	**lejos**	*(leh-hohs)*
fasting	**en ayunas**	*(ehn ah-yoo-nahs)*
fat	**gordura/obeso**	*(gohr-doo-rah/oh-beh-soh)*
fatal	**fatal**	*(fah-tahl)*
father	**padre**	*(pah-dreh)*
father-in-law	**suegro**	*(soo-eh-groh)*
fats	**grasas**	*(grah-sahs)*
February	**febrero**	*(feh-breh-roh)*
[to] feel	**sentir**	*(sehn-teer)*
fever	**fiebre**	*(fee-eh-breh)*
few	**pocos**	*(poh-kohs)*
fibroid	**fibroide**	*(fee-broh-ee-deh)*
fifteen	**quince**	*(keen-seh)*
fifth	**quinto**	*(keen-toh)*
fifty	**cincuenta**	*(seen-koo-ehn-tah)*
[to] fill [*a tooth*]	**empastar/rellenar**	*(ehm-pahs-tahr/reh-yeh-nahr)*
[to] fill [*out*]	**llenar**	*(yeh-nahr)*
[to] find	**descubrir/hallar**	*(dehs-koo-breer/ah-yahr)*
[to] find out	**descubrir**	*(dehs-koo-breer)*
findings	**hallazgos**	*(ah-yahs-gohs)*
[to] finish	**acabar**	*(ah-kah-bahr)*
fire	**fuego/lumbre**	*(foo-eh-goh/loom-breh)*
fire escape	**escape de fuego**	*(ehs-kah-peh deh foo-eh-goh)*
first	**primero**	*(pree-meh-roh)*
fish	**pescado**	*(pehs-kah-doh)*
fistula	**fístula**	*(fees-too-lah)*
five	**cinco**	*(seen-koh)*
five A.M.	**las cinco**	*(lahs seen-koh)*
five hundred	**quinientos**	*(kee-nee-ehn-tohs)*
five P.M.	**las diecisiete horas**	*(lahs dee-eh-see-see-eh-teh oh-rahs)*
[to] fix	**componer**	*(kohm-poh-nehr)*
fixation	**fijación**	*(fee-hah-see-ohn)*
fixed bridge	**puente fijo**	*(poo-ehn-teh fee-hoh)*
flat	**indiferente**	*(een-dee-feh-rehn-teh)*
flexibility	**flexibilidad**	*(flehx-ee-bee-lee-dahd)*
floor	**piso**	*(pee-soh)*
flower vase	**florero**	*(floh-reh-roh)*
fluid	**fluído**	*(floo-ee-doh)*
fluoride	**fluoruro**	*(floh-roo-roh)*
[to] fly	**volar**	*(boh-lahr)*
[to] follow	**seguir**	*(seh-geer)*
following	**siguiente**	*(see-gee-ehn-teh)*
foods	**comidas**	*(koh-mee-dahs)*

for	**de/por/para**	*(deh/pohr/pah-rah)*
fork	**tenedor**	*(teh-neh-dohr)*
form	**forma**	*(fohr-mah)*
formula	**fórmula**	*(fohr-moo-lah)*
forty	**cuarenta**	*(koo-ah-rehn-tah)*
four A.M.	**las cuatro**	*(lahs koo-ah-troh)*
four	**cuatro**	*(koo-ah-troh)*
four hundred	**cuatrocientos**	*(koo-ah-troh-see-ehn-tohs)*
four P.M.	**las dieciséis horas**	*(lahs dee-eh-see-seh-ees oh-rahs)*
four thousand	**cuatro mil**	*(koo-ah-troh meel)*
fourteen	**catorce**	*(kah-tohr-seh)*
fourth	**cuarto**	*(koo-ahr-toh)*
fractures	**fracturas**	*(frahk-too-rahs)*
fragments	**fragmentos**	*(frahg-mehn-tohs)*
freckles	**pecas**	*(peh-kahs)*
fremitus	**frémito**	*(freh-mee-toh)*
french fries	**papas fritas**	*(pah-pahs free-tahs)*
fresh	**fresco**	*(frehs-koh)*
Friday	**viernes**	*(bee-ehr-nehs)*
fried	**frito**	*(free-toh)*
fried chicken	**pollo frito**	*(poh-yoh free-toh)*
friend	**amigo/amiga**	*(ah-mee-goh/ah-mee-gah)*
friendship	**amistad**	*(ah-mees-tahd)*
from	**de**	*(deh)*
frontal	**frontal**	*(frohn-tahl)*
frozen	**helado/congelado**	*(eh-lah-doh/kohn-heh-lah-doh)*
fruit	**fruta**	*(froo-tah)*
fuchsia	**fiucha**	*(fee-oo-chah)*
function	**función**	*(foon-see-ohn)*
fundamental	**fundamental**	*(foon-dah-mehn-tahl)*
fungus	**hongos**	*(ohn-gohs)*
G	**g**	*(jeh)*
[to] gain	**ganar**	*(gah-nahr)*
gallbladder	**vesícula biliar/hiel**	*(beh-see-koo-lah bee-lee-ahr/ee-ehl)*
gallon	**galón**	*(gah-lohn)*
gangrene	**gangrena**	*(gahn-greh-nah)*
gastroenteritis	**gastroenteritis**	*(gahs-troh-ehn-teh-ree-tees)*
gel / gelatin	**gelatina**	*(geh-lah-tee-nah)*
general	**general**	*(heh-neh-rahl)*
general chemistry	**química sanguínea**	*(kee-mee-kah sahn-gee-neh-ah)*
generic	**genérico**	*(heh-neh-ree-koh)*
genial	**genial**	*(heh-nee-ahl)*
get	**consiga**	*(kohn-see-gah)*
[to] get acquainted	**darse a conocer**	*(dahr-seh ah koh-noh-sehr)*
[to] get better	**mejorar**	*(meh-hoh-rahr)*
[to] get up	**levantar**	*(leh-bahn-tahr)*
gingivitis	**gingivitis**	*(heen-hee-bee-tees)*
girl	**niña/muchacha**	*(nee-nyah/moo-chah-chah)*
[to] give	**dar**	*(dahr)*
glass (*for drinking*)	**vaso**	*(bah-soh)*
glass (*the material*)	**vidrio**	*(bee-dree-oh)*

[eye] glasses	**anteojos/lentes**	*(ahn-teh-oh-hohs/lehn-tehs)*
glaucoma	**glaucoma**	*(glah-oo-koh-mah)*
globule	**glóbulo**	*(gloh-boo-loh)*
gloves	**guantes**	*(goo-ahn-tehs)*
glycosuria	**glucosuria**	*(gloo-koh-soo-ree-ah)*
[to] go	**ir**	*(eer)*
[to] go by	**pasar**	*(pah-sahr)*
[to] go out	**salir**	*(sah-leer)*
[to] go to bed	**acostarse**	*(ah-kohs-tahr-seh)*
goals	**metas**	*(meh-tahs)*
godfather	**padrino**	*(pah-dree-noh)*
godmother	**madrina**	*(mah-dree-nah)*
godparents	**padrinos**	*(pah-dree-nohs)*
gold tooth	**diente de oro**	*(dee-ehn-teh deh oh-roh)*
golden	**dorado**	*(doh-rah-doh)*
good	**bueno**	*(boo-eh-noh)*
gout	**gota**	*(goh-tah)*
gown	**bata**	*(bah-tah)*
grains	**granos**	*(grah-nohs)*
grams	**gramos**	*(grah-mohs)*
grandchildren	**nietos**	*(nee-eh-tohs)*
grandfather	**abuelo**	*(ah-boo-eh-loh)*
grandmother	**abuela**	*(ah-boo-eh-lah)*
grandparents	**abuelos**	*(ah-boo-eh-lohs)*
grape(s)	**uva(s)**	*(oo-bah[s])*
grapefruit	**toronja**	*(toh-rohn-hah)*
grave	**grave**	*(grah-beh)*
gray	**gris**	*(grees)*
grayish	**grisáseo**	*(gree-sah-seh-oh)*
grayish-white	**canoso**	*(kah-noh-soh)*
great grandparents	**bisabuelos**	*(bee-sah-boo-eh-lohs)*
green	**verde**	*(behr-deh)*
green beans	**ejotes/habichuelas**	*(eh-hoh-tehs/ah-bee-choo-eh-lahs)*
[to] greet	**saludar**	*(sah-loo-dahr)*
greetings	**saludos**	*(sah-loo-dohs)*
[to] grieve	**afligir**	*(ah-flee-heer)*
growth	**crecimiento**	*(kreh-see-mee-ehn-toh)*
guide	**guía**	*(gee-ah)*
guilt	**culpa**	*(kool-pah)*
gumboil	**flemón/absceso**	*(fleh-mohn/ahb-seh-soh)*
gynecologist	**ginecólogo**	*(hee-neh-koh-loh-goh)*
H	**h**	*(ah-cheh)*
hairbrush	**cepillo de pelo**	*(seh-pee-yoh deh peh-loh)*
hallway	**pasillo**	*(pah-see-yoh)*
ham	**jamón**	*(hah-mohn)*
hamburger	**hamburguesa**	*(ahm-boor-geh-sah)*
hand	**mano**	*(mah-noh)*
handshake	**apretón de manos**	*(ah-preh-tohn deh mah-nohs)*
handy	**conveniente**	*(kohn-beh-nee-ehn-teh)*
[to] hang	**colgar**	*(kohl-gahr)*
hard-boiled	**duros**	*(doo-rohs)*

has	**tiene**	*(tee-eh-neh)*
[to] have (possess)	**tener**	*(teh-nehr)*
[to] have (auxiliary verb)	**haber**	*(ah-behr)*
hazel	**castaño**	*(kahs-tah-nyoh)*
he	**él**	*(ehl)*
head	**cabeza**	*(kah-beh-sah)*
headache	**dolor de cabeza**	*(doh-lohr deh kah-beh-sah)*
[to] heal	**sanar**	*(sah-nahr)*
healing	**curación**	*(koo-rah-see-ohn)*
health	**salud**	*(sah-lood)*
[to] hear	**oír**	*(oh-eer)*
hear me	**oírme**	*(oh-eer-meh)*
hearing aid	**aparato para oír**	*(ah-pah-rah-toh pah-rah oh-eer)*
heart	**corazón**	*(koh-rah-sohn)*
heat	**calor**	*(kah-lohr)*
hello	**hola**	*(oh-lah)*
help	**ayuda**	*(ah-yoo-dah)*
helpful	**útil**	*(oo-teel)*
hematology	**hematología**	*(eh-mah-toh-loh-hee-ah)*
hematoma	**hematoma**	*(eh-mah-toh-mah)*
hemorrhage	**hemorragia**	*(eh-moh-rah-hee-ah)*
hemolysis	**hemólisis**	*(eh-moh-lee-sees)*
hepatitis	**hepatitis**	*(eh-pah-tee-tees)*
her	**ella**	*(eh-yah)*
here	**aquí**	*(ah-kee)*
hernia	**hernia**	*(ehr-nee-ah)*
[to] hesitate	**vacilar**	*(bah-see-lahr)*
high	**alto**	*(ahl-toh)*
him	**él**	*(ehl)*
hip	**cadera**	*(kah-deh-rah)*
hip fracture	**fractura de cadera**	*(frahk-too-rah deh kah-deh-rah)*
his	**su**	*(soo)*
Hispanic	**hispano**	*(ees-pah-noh)*
history	**historia**	*(ees-toh-ree-ah)*
[to] hit	**pegar**	*(peh-gahr)*
home	**casa/hogar**	*(kah-sah/oh-gahr)*
hope	**esperanza**	*(ehs-peh-rahn-sah)*
hose/stockings	**medias**	*(meh-dee-ahs)*
hospital	**hospital**	*(ohs-pee-tahl)*
hospital policy	**reglas del hospital**	*(reh-glahs dehl ohs-pee-tahl)*
hostility	**hostilidad**	*(ohs-tee-lee-dahd)*
hot	**caliente**	*(kah-lee-ehn-teh)*
hot dog	**emparedado de salchicha**	*(ehm-pah-reh-dah-doh deh sahl-chee-chah)*
hot sauce	**salsa picante**	*(sahl-sah pee-kahn-teh)*
hour	**hora**	*(oh-rah)*
house	**casa**	*(kah-sah)*
household (measure)	**casera**	*(kah-seh-rah)*
how?	**¿cómo?**	*(koh-moh)*
how many?	**¿cuántos?**	*(koo-ahn-tohs)*

however	**pero**	*(peh-roh)*
humanistic	**humanístico**	*(oo-mahn-ees-tee-koh)*
[to] hunt	**cazar**	*(kah-sahr)*
[to] hurt	**doler**	*(doh-lehr)*
husband	**esposo**	*(ehs-poh-soh)*
hydrophobia [water]	**hidrofobia**	*(ee-droh-foh-bee-ah)*
hygienist	**higienista**	*(ee-hee-eh-nees-tah)*
hypertension	**hipertensión**	*(ee-pehr-tehn-see-ohn)*
hyperthermia	**hipertermia**	*(ee-pehr-tehr-mee-ah)*
hypoglycemia	**hipoglucemia**	*(ee-poh-gloo-seh-mee-ah)*
I	**i**	*(ee)*
I	**yo**	*(yoh)*
ice	**hielo**	*(ee-eh-loh)*
ice cream	**nieve/helado/ mantecado**	*(nee-eh-beh/eh-lah-doh/mahn-teh-kah-doh)*
icteric	**ictérico**	*(eek-teh-ree-koh)*
idea	**idea**	*(ee-deh-ah)*
identified	**identificado**	*(ee-dehn-tee-fee-kah-doh)*
if	**si**	*(see)*
[to] ignore	**ignorar**	*(eeg-noh-rahr)*
illness	**enfermedad**	*(ehn-fehr-meh-dahd)*
image	**imagen**	*(ee-mah-hehn)*
immature bone	**hueso inmaduro**	*(oo-eh-soh een-mah-doo-roh)*
implant	**implante**	*(eem-plahn-teh)*
implementation	**implementación**	*(eem-pleh-mehn-tah-see-ohn)*
implications	**implicaciones**	*(eem-plee-kah-see-ohn-ehs)*
important	**importante**	*(eem-pohr-tahn-teh)*
impression	**impresión**	*(eem-preh-see-ohn)*
in	**en**	*(ehn)*
in front of	**enfrente de/delante de**	*(ehn-frehn-teh deh/deh-lahn-teh deh)*
in the morning	**en la mañana**	*(ehn lah mah-nyah-nah)*
incidence	**incidencia**	*(een-see-dehn-see-ah)*
incision	**incisión**	*(een-see-see-ohn)*
independence	**independencia**	*(een-deh-pehn-dehn-see-ah)*
index card	**tarjeta**	*(tahr-heh-tah)*
indications	**indicaciones**	*(een-dee-kah-see-oh-nehs)*
indigestion	**indigestión**	*(een-dee-gehs-tee-ohn)*
[to] induce	**inducir**	*(een-doo-seer)*
infancy	**infancia**	*(een-fahn-see-ah)*
infection	**infección**	*(een-fehk-see-ohn)*
inflammation	**inflamación**	*(een-flah-mah-see-ohn)*
[to] inform	**informar**	*(een-fohr-mahr)*
inhalant	**inhalante**	*(een-ah-lahn-teh)*
injection	**inyección**	*(een-yehk-see-ohn)*
insect	**insecto**	*(een-sehk-toh)*
instant	**instantáneo**	*(eens-tahn-tah-neh-oh)*
instructions	**instrucciones**	*(eens-trook-see-ohn-ehs)*
instrument	**instrumento**	*(eens-troo-mehn-toh)*
insulin	**insulina**	*(een-soo-lee-nah)*

insurance	**seguro**	*(seh-goo-roh)*
integral	**integral**	*(een-teh-grahl)*
interaction	**interacción**	*(een-tehr-ahk-see-ohn)*
interest	**interés**	*(een-teh-rehs)*
internal	**interior**	*(een-teh-ree-ohr)*
interpersonal	**interpersonal**	*(een-tehr-pehr-soh-nahl)*
[to] interpret	**interpretar**	*(een-tehr-preh-tahr)*
interrogation	**interrogación**	*(een-teh-roh-gah-see-ohn)*
interventions	**intervenciones**	*(een-tehr-behn-see-oh-nehs)*
intimate	**íntimo**	*(een-tee-moh)*
intramuscular	**intramuscular**	*(een-trah-moos-koo-lahr)*
intravenous	**intravenoso**	*(een-trah-beh-noh-soh)*
iodine	**yodo**	*(yoh-doh)*
[to] irradiate	**irradiar**	*(ee-rah-dee-ahr)*
irritable	**irritable**	*(ee-ree-tah-bleh)*
is / it is	**es/está**	*(ehs/ehs-tah)*
it (neutral)	**lo/la**	*(loh/lah)*
J	**j**	*(hoh-tah)*
jacket	**chaqueta**	*(chah-keh-tah)*
jam	**confitura**	*(kohn-fee-too-rah)*
January	**enero**	*(eh-neh-roh)*
jelly	**jalea**	*(hah-leh-ah)*
jewelry	**joyas**	*(hoh-yahs)*
[to] joke	**bromear**	*(broh-meh-ahr)*
jugular	**yugular**	*(yoo-goo-lahr)*
juice	**jugo**	*(hoo-goh)*
juicy	**jugoso**	*(hoo-goh-soh)*
July	**julio**	*(hoo-lee-oh)*
[to] jump	**saltar**	*(sahl-tahr)*
June	**junio**	*(hoo-nee-oh)*
just	**justo/solo**	*(hoos-toh/soh-loh)*
juvenile	**juvenil**	*(hoo-beh-neel)*
K	**k**	*(kah)*
[to] keep	**guardar/mantener**	*(goo-ahr-dahr/mahn-teh-nehr)*
ketoacidosis	**cetoacidosis**	*(seh-toh-ah-see-doh-sees)*
key (*adjective*)	**clave**	*(klah-beh)*
[to] kid	**bromear**	*(broh-meh-ahr)*
kilogram	**kilogramo/kilo**	*(kee-loh-grah-moh/kee-loh)*
[to] kiss	**besar**	*(beh-sahr)*
kitchen	**cocina**	*(koh-see-nah)*
kleptomania	**cleptomanía**	*(klehp-toh-mah-nee-ah)*
knife	**cuchillo**	*(koo-chee-yoh)*
[to] knock	**golpear**	*(gohl-peh-ahr)*
[to] know	**conocer/saber**	*(koh-noh-sehr/sah-behr)*
L	**l**	*(eh-leh)*
laboratory	**laboratorio**	*(lah-boh-rah-toh-ree-oh)*
lamb	**cordero**	*(kohr-deh-roh)*
lamp	**lámpara**	*(lahm-pah-rah)*
lancet	**lanceta**	*(lahn-seh-tah)*

language	**lengua/idioma**	*(lehn-goo-ah/ee-dee-oh-mah)*
laparoscopy	**laparoscopia**	*(lah-pah-rahs-koh-pee-ah)*
laryngitis	**laringitis**	*(lah-reen-hee-tees)*
last	**último**	*(ool-tee-moh)*
last name	**apellido**	*(ah-peh-yee-doh)*
laurel	**laurel**	*(lah-oo-rehl)*
lavage	**lavabo**	*(lah-bah-boh)*
laxative	**laxante/purgante**	*(lahx-ahn-teh/poor-gahn-teh)*
lead	**plomo**	*(ploh-moh)*
[to] leave	**dejar**	*(deh-hahr)*
left	**izquierdo**	*(ees-kee-ehr-doh)*
leg	**pierna**	*(pee-ehr-nah)*
lemon	**limón**	*(lee-mohn)*
lesions	**lesiones**	*(leh-see-oh-nehs)*
less	**menos**	*(meh-nohs)*
[to] let go	**soltar**	*(sohl-tahr)*
lettuce	**lechuga**	*(leh-choo-gah)*
leukocytes	**leucocitos**	*(leh-oo-koh-see-tohs)*
level	**nivel**	*(nee-behl)*
[to] lie down	**acostar**	*(ah-kohs-tahr)*
[to] lift	**levantar/elevar**	*(leh-bahn-tahr/eh-leh-bahr)*
ligament	**ligamento**	*(lee-gah-mehn-toh)*
light	**luz**	*(loos)*
light touch	**caricia**	*(kah-ree-see-ah)*
like	**como**	*(koh-moh)*
lima beans	**habas**	*(ah-bahs)*
lime	**lima/limón**	*(lee-mah/lee-mohn)*
limitations	**limitaciones**	*(lee-mee-tah-see-ohn-ehs)*
linen	**lino**	*(lee-noh)*
lingual	**lingual**	*(leen-goo-ahl)*
lipoatrophy	**lipotrofia**	*(lee-poh-troh-fee-ah)*
lipstick	**lápiz de labios**	*(lah-pees deh lah-bee-ohs)*
liquid	**líquido**	*(lee-kee-doh)*
list	**lista**	*(lees-tah)*
[to] listen	**escuchar**	*(ehs-koo-chahr)*
liter	**litro**	*(lee-troh)*
lithium	**litio**	*(lee-tee-oh)*
little (*quantity*)	**poco**	*(poh-koh)*
[to] live	**vivir**	*(bee-beer)*
liver	**hígado**	*(ee-gah-doh)*
living room	**sala**	*(sah-lah)*
lobby	**sala de espera/ vestíbulo**	*(sah-lah deh ehs-peh-rah/behs-tee-boo-loh)*
loneliness	**soledad**	*(soh-leh-dahd)*
loose clothes	**ropa cómoda**	*(roh-pah koh-moh-dah)*
[to] lose	**perder**	*(pehr-dehr)*
loss	**pérdida**	*(pehr-dee-dah)*
lotion	**loción**	*(loh-see-ohn)*
love	**amor**	*(ah-mohr)*
low	**bajo**	*(bah-hoh)*
low cholesterol (use)	**poco colesterol**	*(poh-koh koh-lehs-teh-rohl)*
low sodium (use)	**poca sal**	*(poh-kah sahl)*

low-fat (*diet*)	**de poca grasa**	*(deh poh-kah grah-sah)*
low-cholesterol (*diet*)	**de colesterol bajo**	*(deh koh-lehs-teh-rohl bah-hoh)*
low-sodium (*diet*)	**baja en sal**	*(bah-hah ehn sahl)*
[to] lower	**rebajar/bajar**	*(reh-bah-hahr/bah-hahr)*
lubricant	**lubricante**	*(loo-bree-kahn-teh)*
lunch	**comida**	*(koh-mee-dah)*
lungs	**pulmones**	*(pool-moh-nehs)*
lupus	**lupos**	*(loo-pohs)*
M	**m**	*(eh-meh)*
macaroni	**macarrones**	*(mah-kah-roh-nehs)*
machine	**máquina**	*(mah-kee-nah)*
magnetic	**magnético**	*(mahg-neh-tee-koh)*
major complications	**complicaciones mayores**	*(kohm-plee-kah-see-oh-nehs mah-yoh-rehs)*
[to] make	**hacer**	*(ah-sehr)*
malignant	**maligno**	*(mah-leeg-noh)*
man	**hombre**	*(ohm-breh)*
management	**manejo**	*(mah-neh-hoh)*
manifestation	**manifestación**	*(mah-nee-fehs-tah-see-ohn)*
manipulation	**manipulación**	*(mah-nee-poo-lah-see-ohn)*
manual	**manual**	*(mah-noo-ahl)*
many	**muchos/muchas**	*(moo-chohs/moo-chahs)*
March	**marzo**	*(mahr-soh)*
marrow	**médula**	*(meh-doo-lah)*
[to] marry	**casar**	*(kah-sahr)*
martyr	**mártir**	*(mahr-teer)*
mashed	**majadas**	*(mah-hah-dahs)*
mashed potatoes	**puré de papas**	*(poo-reh deh pah-pahs)*
material	**material**	*(mah-teh-ree-ahl)*
mathematics	**matemáticas**	*(mah-teh-mah-tee-kahs)*
mature bone	**hueso maduro**	*(oo-eh-soh mah-doo-roh)*
May	**mayo**	*(mah-yoh)*
may help you	**le puede ayudar**	*(leh poo-eh-deh ah-yoo-dahr)*
may not be	**no se pueden**	*(noh seh poo-eh-dehn)*
mayonnaise	**mayonesa**	*(mah-yoh-neh-sah)*
me	**mí**	*(mee)*
meals	**comidas**	*(koh-mee-dahs)*
measures	**medidas**	*(meh-dee-dahs)*
meat	**carne**	*(kahr-neh)*
mechanisms	**mecanismos**	*(meh-kah-nees-mohs)*
medical	**médico**	*(meh-dee-koh)*
medical treatment	**tratamiento médico**	*(trah-tah-mee-ehn-toh meh-dee-koh)*
medication	**medicamento**	*(meh-dee-kah-mehn-toh)*
medicine	**medicina**	*(meh-dee-see-nah)*
medulla	**médula**	*(meh-doo-lah)*
melon	**melón**	*(meh-lohn)*
member	**miembro**	*(mee-ehm-broh)*
[to] memorize	**memorizar**	*(meh-moh-ree-sahr)*
memory	**memoria**	*(meh-moh-ree-ah)*
meningitis	**meningitis**	*(meh-neen-hee-tees)*

mental retardation	**retraso mental**	*(reh-trah-soh mehn-tahl)*
menu	**menú**	*(meh-noo)*
meter	**metro**	*(meh-troh)*
methodology	**metodología**	*(meh-toh-doh-loh-hee-ah)*
metric	**métrico**	*(meh-tree-koh)*
[to] migrate	**emigrar**	*(eh-mee-grahr)*
mikophobia [germs]	**micofobia**	*(mee-koh-foh-bee-ah)*
milk	**leche**	*(leh-cheh)*
milligram	**miligramo**	*(mee-lee-grah-moh)*
milliliter	**mililitro**	*(mee-lee-lee-troh)*
minerals	**minerales**	*(mee-neh-rah-lees)*
minimum	**mínimo**	*(mee-nee-moh)*
mirror	**espejo**	*(ehs-peh-hoh)*
miscellaneous	**misceláneo**	*(mee-seh-lah-neh-oh)*
Miss	**señorita**	*(seh-nyoh-ree-tah)*
mistrust	**desconfianza**	*(dehs-kohn-fee-ahn-sah)*
model	**modelo**	*(moh-deh-loh)*
modern	**moderno**	*(moh-dehr-noh)*
modifiers	**modificadores**	*(moh-dee-fee-kah-doh-rehs)*
molar	**muela**	*(moo-eh-lah)*
mole	**verruga**	*(beh-roo-gah)*
mom	**mamá**	*(mah-mah)*
Monday	**lunes**	*(loo-nehs)*
month	**mes**	*(mehs)*
moral	**moral**	*(moh-rahl)*
more	**mucho/más**	*(moo-choh/mahs)*
morphine	**morfina**	*(mohr-fee-nah)*
mother	**madre**	*(mah-dreh)*
mother-in-law	**suegra**	*(soo-eh-grah)*
mouth	**boca**	*(boh-kah)*
movable bridge	**puente móvil**	*(poo-ehn-teh moh-beel)*
[to] move	**mover**	*(moh-behr)*
Mr.	**señor**	*(seh-nyohr)*
Mrs.	**señora**	*(seh-nyoh-rah)*
mustard	**mostaza**	*(mohs-tah-sah)*
mysophobia [dirt]	**misofobia**	*(mee-soh-foh-bee-ah)*
N	**n**	*(eh-neh)*
[to] name	**nombrar**	*(nohm-brahr)*
name	**nombre**	*(nohm-breh)*
napkin	**servilleta**	*(sehr-bee-yeh-tah)*
narcotics	**narcóticos**	*(nahr-koh-tee-kohs)*
nasal	**nasal**	*(nah-sahl)*
nausea	**náusea**	*(nah-oo-seh-ah)*
navel	**ombligo**	*(ohm-blee-goh)*
near	**cerca de**	*(sehr-kah deh)*
[to] need	**necesitar**	*(neh-seh-see-tahr)*
needle	**aguja**	*(ah-goo-hah)*
needs	**necesidades**	*(neh-seh-see-dah-dehs)*
neither	**tampoco**	*(tahm-poh-koh)*
neither . . . nor	**ni . . . ni**	*(nee . . . nee)*

neonatal	**neonatal**	*(neh-oh-nah-tahl)*
nephew	**sobrino**	*(soh-bree-noh)*
nephropathy	**nefropatía**	*(neh-froh-pah-tee-ah)*
nervous	**nervioso**	*(nehr-bee-oh-soh)*
neuropathy	**neuropatía**	*(neh-oo-roh-pah-tee-ah)*
neurotic	**neurótico**	*(neh-oo-roh-tee-koh)*
neutral	**neutral**	*(neh-oo-trahl)*
never	**jamás/nunca**	*(hah-mahs/noon-kah)*
next	**siguiente**	*(see-gee-ehn-teh)*
nicotine	**nicotina**	*(nee-koh-tee-nah)*
niece	**sobrina**	*(soh-bree-nah)*
nightgown / gown	**camisa de dormir/bata**	*(kah-mee-sah deh dohr-meer)/(bah-tah)*
night table	**mesa de noche**	*(meh-sah deh noh-cheh)*
nine	**nueve**	*(noo-eh-beh)*
nine A.M.	**las nueve**	*(lahs noo-eh-beh)*
nine hundred	**novecientos**	*(noh-beh-see-ehn-tohs*
nine P.M.	**las veintiuna horas**	*(lahs beh-een-tee-oo-nah oh-rahs)*
nineteen	**diecinueve**	*(dee-eh-see-noo-eh-beh)*
ninety	**noventa**	*(noh-behn-tah)*
ninth	**noveno**	*(noh-beh-noh)*
nitroglycerin	**nitroglicerina**	*(nee-troh-glee-seh-ree-nah)*
no	**no**	*(noh)*
no one	**nadie**	*(nah-dee-eh)*
no salt	**sín sal**	*(seen sahl)*
no smoking	**no se permite fumar**	*(noh seh pehr-mee-teh foo-mahr)*
nobody	**nadie**	*(nah-dee-eh)*
none	**ninguno**	*(neen-goo-noh)*
normal	**normal**	*(nohr-mahl)*
north	**norte**	*(nohr-teh)*
nose	**nariz**	*(nah-rees)*
not	**no**	*(noh)*
not any	**ninguno**	*(neen-goo-noh)*
not translated	**no se traducen**	*(noh seh trah-doo-sehn)*
note	**note**	*(noh-teh)*
nothing	**nada**	*(nah-dah)*
noun	**nombre**	*(nohm-breh)*
November	**noviembre**	*(noh-bee-ehm-breh)*
novocaine	**novocaína**	*(noh-boh-kah-ee-nah)*
now	**ahora**	*(ah-oh-rah)*
nuclear medicine	**medicina nuclear**	*(meh-dee-see-nah noo-kleh-ahr)*
nuctophobia [darkness]	**nuctofobia**	*(nook-toh-foh-bee-ah)*
number	**número**	*(noo-meh-roh)*
nurse	**enfermero/enfermera**	*(ehn-fehr-meh-roh/ehn-fehr-meh-rah)*
nurses' station	**estación de enfermeras**	*(ehs-tah-see-ohn deh ehn-fehr-meh-rahs)*
nutrition	**nutrición**	*(noo-tree-see-ohn)*
O	**o**	*(oh)*
oatmeal	**avena**	*(ah-beh-nah)*
obesity	**obesidad**	*(oh-beh-see-dahd)*

[to] observe	**observar**	*(ohb-sehr-bahr)*
obsession	**obsesión**	*(ohb-seh-see-ohn)*
obstruction	**obstrucción**	*(ohbs-trook-see-ohn)*
occasion	**ocasión**	*(oh-kah-see-ohn)*
occasionally	**ocasionalmente**	*(oh-kah-see-ohn-ahl-mehn-teh)*
occipital	**occipital**	*(ohk-see-pee-tahl)*
[to] occur	**ocurrir**	*(oh-koo-reer)*
October	**octubre**	*(ohk-too-breh)*
odontalgia	**odontalgia**	*(oh-dohn-tahl-hee-ah)*
of	**de**	*(deh)*
of each other	**uno de otro**	*(oo-noh deh oh-troh)*
office	**oficina**	*(oh-fee-see-nah)*
oil	**aceite**	*(ah-seh-ee-teh)*
ointment	**ungüento**	*(oon-goo-ehn-toh)*
older	**mayor**	*(mah-yohr)*
olive	**aceituna**	*(ah-seh-ee-too-nah)*
on	**en**	*(ehn)*
oncology	**oncología**	*(ohn-koh-loh-hee-ah)*
one	**un/uno**	*(oon/oo-noh)*
one A.M.	**la una**	*(lah oo-nah)*
one fourth	**un cuarto**	*(oon koo-ahr-toh)*
one half	**un medio**	*(oon meh-dee-oh)*
one hundred	**cien**	*(see-ehn)*
one P.M.	**las trece horas**	*(lahs treh-seh oh-rahs)*
one third	**un tercio**	*(oon tehr-see-oh)*
one thousand	**mil**	*(meel)*
onion	**cebolla**	*(seh-boh-yah)*
only	**solamente**	*(sohl-lah-mehn-teh)*
opaque	**opaco**	*(oh-pah-koh)*
[to] open	**abrir**	*(ah-breer)*
open reduction	**reducción abierta**	*(reh-dook-see-ohn ah-bee-ehr-tah)*
[to] operate	**operar**	*(oh-peh-rahr)*
operating room	**quirófano**	*(kee-roh-fah-noh)*
ophthalmic	**oftálmico**	*(ohf-tahl-mee-koh)*
opinion	**opinión**	*(oh-pee-nee-ohn)*
opportunity	**oportunidad**	*(oh-pohr-too-nee-dahd)*
optic	**óptico**	*(ohp-tee-koh)*
or	**o**	*(oh)*
oral	**oral**	*(oh-rahl)*
orange	**naranja**	*(nah-rahn-hah)*
orangy	**anaranjado**	*(ah-nah-rahn-hah-doh)*
[to] order (ask for)	**solicitar**	*(sohl-ee-see-tahr)*
orders	**órdenes**	*(ohr-deh-nehs)*
organ	**órgano**	*(ohr-gah-noh)*
other	**otro**	*(oh-troh)*
otic	**ótico**	*(oh-tee-koh)*
ounce	**onza**	*(ohn-sah)*
outside of	**fuera de**	*(foo-eh-rah deh)*
ovary	**ovario**	*(oh-bah-ree-oh)*
over	**sobre**	*(soh-breh)*
over-easy (*eggs*)	**volteados**	*(bohl-teh-ah-dohs)*
oxygen	**oxígeno**	*(ohx-ee-heh-noh)*

P	**p**	*(peh)*
pacemaker	**marcapasos**	*(mahr-kah-pah-sohs)*
package	**paquete**	*(pah-keh-teh)*
pain	**dolor**	*(doh-lohr)*
[to] paint	**pintar**	*(peen-tahr)*
pajama	**pijama**	*(pee-hah-mah)*
palate	**paladar**	*(pah-lah-dahr)*
pale	**pálido**	*(pah-lee-doh)*
palmar	**palmar**	*(pahl-mahr)*
[to] palpate	**palpar**	*(pahl-pahr)*
palpation	**palpación**	*(pahl-pah-see-ohn)*
palpitation	**palpitación**	*(pahl-pee-tah-see-ohn)*
pancake	**panqueque/hojuela**	*(pahn-keh-keh/oh-hoo-eh-lah)*
pancreas	**páncreas**	*(pahn-kreh-ahs)*
pancreatitis	**pancreatitis**	*(pahn-kreh-ah-tee-tees)*
panic	**pánico**	*(pahn-nee-koh)*
pans	**vasijas**	*(bah-see-hahs)*
pants / slacks	**pantalones**	*(pahn-tah-loh-nehs)*
paralisis	**parálisis**	*(pah-rah-lee-sees)*
paralytic	**paralítico**	*(pah-rah-lee-tee-koh)*
parents	**padres**	*(pah-drehs)*
part	**parte**	*(pahr-teh)*
partial denture	**dentadura parcial**	*(dehn-tah-doo-rah pahr-see-ahl)*
pat	**palmadita**	*(pahl-mah-dee-tah)*
patch	**parche**	*(pahr-cheh)*
pathogen	**patogénico**	*(pah-toh-heh-nee-koh)*
pathological	**patológico**	*(pah-toh-loh-hee-koh)*
pathology	**patología**	*(pah-toh-loh-hee-ah)*
pathophysiology	**fisiopatología**	*(fee-see-oh-pah-toh-loh-hee-ah)*
patient	**paciente**	*(pah-see-ehn-teh)*
[to] pay	**pagar**	*(pah-gahr)*
peas	**chícharos**	*(chee-chah-rohs)*
peaches	**duraznos**	*(doo-rahs-nohs)*
pears	**peras**	*(peh-rahs)*
pecan / nut	**nuez**	*(noo-ehs)*
pelvic fracture	**fractura pélvica**	*(frahk-too-rah pehl-bee-kah)*
pelvis	**pelvis**	*(pehl-bees)*
pencil	**lápiz**	*(lah-pees)*
penis	**pene**	*(peh-neh)*
people	**gente**	*(hehn-teh)*
pepper	**pimienta**	*(pee-mee-ehn-tah)*
perfume	**perfume**	*(pehr-foo-meh)*
permission	**permiso**	*(pehr-mee-soh)*
person	**persona**	*(pehr-soh-nah)*
personal	**personal**	*(pehr-soh-nahl)*
personality	**personalidad**	*(pehr-soh-nah-lee-dahd)*
pharmacy	**farmacia**	*(fahr-mah-see-ah)*
phases	**fases**	*(fah-sehs)*
philosophy	**filosofía**	*(fee-loh-soh-fee-ah)*
phone	**teléfono**	*(teh-leh-foh-noh)*
phrases	**frases**	*(frah-sehs)*

physician (*f.*)	**médica/doctora**	*(meh-dee-kah/dohk-toh-rah)*
physician (*m.*)	**médico/doctor**	*(meh-dee-koh/dohk-tohr)*
physicians (*f.*)	**médicas/doctoras**	*(meh-dee-kahs/dohk-toh-rahs)*
physicians (*m.*)	**médicos/doctores**	*(meh-dee-kohs/dohk-toh-rehs)*
physique	**físico**	*(fee-see-koh)*
pickle	**pepino**	*(peh-pee-noh)*
pie	**pastel**	*(pahs-tehl)*
piece	**pieza**	*(pee-ehs-ah)*
pill	**píldora**	*(peel-doh-rah)*
pillow	**almohada**	*(ahl-moh-ah-dah)*
pillowcase	**funda**	*(foon-dah)*
pin prick	**picadura**	*(pee-kah-doo-rah)*
pineapple	**piña**	*(pee-nyah)*
pink	**rosa**	*(roh-sah)*
pinkish	**rosado**	*(roh-sah-doh)*
pinto beans	**frijoles pintos**	*(free-hoh-lehs peen-tohs)*
pity	**lástima**	*(lahs-tee-mah)*
pizza	**pizza**	*(pee-sah)*
place (destination)	**lugar**	*(loo-gahr)*
[to] place (put on)	**poner**	*(poh-nehr)*
placing it	**colocándolo**	*(koh-loh-kahn-doh-loh)*
plan	**plan**	*(plahn)*
planning	**planificación**	*(plah-nee-fee-kah-see-ohn)*
plants	**plantas**	*(plahn-tahs)*
plate	**plato**	*(plah-toh)*
[to] play	**jugar**	*(hoo-gahr)*
please	**por favor**	*(pohr fah-bohr)*
plum	**ciruelo**	*(see-roo-eh-loh)*
plural	**plural**	*(ploo-rahl)*
pneumonia	**pulmonía/neumonía**	*(pool-moh-nee-ah/neh-oo-moh-nee-ah)*
[to] point	**señalar/apuntar**	*(seh-nyah-lahr/ah-poon-tahr)*
poisons	**venenos**	*(beh-neh-nohs)*
polydipsia	**polidipsia**	*(poh-lee-deep-see-ah)*
polyphagia	**polifagia**	*(poh-lee-fah-hee-ah)*
polyuria	**poliuria**	*(poh-lee-oo-ree-ah)*
porcelain	**porcelana**	*(pohr-seh-lah-nah)*
pork	**puerco**	*(poo-ehr-koh)*
postoperative	**postoperatorio**	*(pohst-oh-peh-rah-toh-ree-oh)*
potatoes	**papas**	*(pah-pahs)*
potential	**posibles**	*(poh-see-blehs)*
pots	**trastes**	*(trahs-tehs)*
pound	**libra**	*(lee-brah)*
practice	**práctica**	*(prahk-tee-kah)*
pregnant	**embarazada**	*(ehm-bah-rah-sah-dah)*
preoperative	**preoperatorio**	*(preh-oh-peh-rah-toh-ree-oh)*
preparation	**preparación**	*(preh-pah-rah-see-ohn)*
[to] prepare	**preparar**	*(preh-pah-rahr)*
prescribed	**recetado**	*(reh-seh-tah-doh)*
prescription	**receta**	*(reh-seh-tah)*
[to] present	**presentar**	*(preh-sehn-tahr)*
present day	**moderno**	*(moh-dehr-noh)*
pressure	**presión**	*(preh-see-ohn)*

prevention	**prevención**	*(preh-behn-see-ohn)*
preventive	**preventivo**	*(preh-behn-tee-boh)*
priest	**sacerdote/cura**	*(sah-sehr-doh-teh/koo-rah)*
prison	**cárcel/prisión**	*(kahr-sehl/pree-see-ohn)*
probable	**probable**	*(proh-bah-bleh)*
problem	**problema**	*(proh-bleh-mah)*
procedure	**procedimiento**	*(proh-seh-dee-mee-ehn-toh)*
progression	**progresión**	*(proh-greh-see-ohn)*
prolonged stress	**tensión prolongada**	*(tehn-see-ohn proh-lohn-gah-dah)*
[to] promise	**prometer**	*(proh-meh-tehr)*
pronounce	**pronuncia**	*(pro-noon-see-ah)*
pronouns	**pronombres**	*(proh-nohm-brehs)*
pronunciation	**pronunciación**	*(proh-noon-see-ah-see-ohn)*
[to] protect	**proteger**	*(proh-teh-hehr)*
[to] provide	**proveer**	*(proh-beh-ehr)*
[to] provoke	**provocar**	*(proh-boh-kahr)*
prune	**ciruelo**	*(see-roo-eh-loh)*
pruritic	**prurítico**	*(proo-ree-tee-koh)*
psoriasis	**soriasis**	*(soh-ree-ah-sees)*
pubic	**púbico**	*(poo-bee-koh)*
public	**público**	*(poo-blee-koh)*
[to] pull	**jalar**	*(hah-lahr)*
pulmonary hypertension	**hipertensión pulmonar**	*(ee-pehr-tehn-see-ohn pool-moh-nahr)*
pulse	**pulso**	*(pool-soh)*
puncture	**pinchazo/picadura**	*(peen-chah-soh/pee-kah-doo-rah)*
pure	**puro**	*(poo-roh)*
pureed	**puré**	*(poo-reh)*
purpose	**propósito**	*(proh-poh-see-toh)*
pyorrhea	**piorrea**	*(pee-oh-reh-ah)*
Q	**q**	*(koo)*
quart	**cuarto**	*(koo-ahr-toh)*
question	**pregunta**	*(preh-goon-tah)*
R	**r**	*(eh-reh)*
racial	**racial**	*(rah-see-ahl)*
radio	**radio**	*(rah-dee-oh)*
radioactive	**radioactivo**	*(rah-dee-oh-ahk-tee-boh)*
radiologic	**radiológico**	*(rah-dee-oh-loh-hee-koh)*
radiotherapy	**radioterapia**	*(rah-dee-oh-teh-rah-pee-ah)*
railroad	**tren**	*(trehn)*
[to] raise	**levantar**	*(leh-bahn-tahr)*
raisins	**pasas**	*(pah-sahs)*
rare	**raro**	*(rah-roh)*
raw	**crudo**	*(kroo-doh)*
razor	**navaja**	*(nah-bah-hah)*
[to] reach	**alcanzar**	*(ahl-kahn-sahr)*
[to] read	**leer**	*(leh-ehr)*
[to] realign	**realinear**	*(reh-ah-lee-nee-ahr)*
reason	**razón**	*(rah-sohn)*
[to] reassure	**asegurar**	*(ah-seh-goo-rahr)*

[to] receive	**recibir**	*(reh-see-beer)*
receptionist	**recepcionista**	*(reh-sehp-see-ohn-ees-tah)*
[to] recognize	**reconocer**	*(reh-koh-noh-sehr)*
recommendations	**recomendaciones**	*(reh-koh-men-dah-see-ohn-es)*
recovery	**recuperación**	*(reh-koo-peh-rah-see-ohn)*
recovery room	**cuarto de recuperación**	*(koo-ahr-toh deh reh-koo-peh-rah-see-ohn)*
rectal	**rectal**	*(rehk-tahl)*
rectum	**recto**	*(rehk-toh)*
recuperating	**recuperando**	*(reh-koo-peh-rahn-doh)*
red	**rojo**	*(roh-hoh)*
red spots	**manchas rojas**	*(mahn-chahs roh-hahs)*
red meat	**carne roja**	*(kahr-neh roh-hah)*
[to] reduce	**reducir**	*(reh-doo-seer)*
reduction	**reducción**	*(reh-dook-see-ohn)*
refried	**refrito**	*(reh-free-toh)*
regular	**regular**	*(reh-goo-lahr)*
rehabilitation	**rehabilitación**	*(reh-ah-bee-lee-tah-see-ohn)*
relation	**relación**	*(reh-lah-see-ohn)*
[to] remain	**quedar**	*(keh-dahr)*
[to] remember	**acordar/recordar**	*(ah-kohr-dahr/reh-kohr-dahr)*
[to] repell	**repeler**	*(reh-peh-lehr)*
replantation	**reimplantación**	*(reh-eehm-plahn-tah-see-ohn)*
reports	**reportes**	*(reh-pohr-tehs)*
requirement	**requerimiento**	*(reh-keh-ree-mee-ehn-toh)*
residue	**residuo**	*(reh-see-doo-oh)*
resin	**resina**	*(reh-see-nah)*
resonance	**resonancia**	*(reh-sohn-ahn-see-ah)*
respect	**respeto**	*(rehs-peh-toh)*
respiratory arrest	**paro respiratorio**	*(pah-roh rehs-pee-rah-toh-ree-oh)*
[to] respond	**responder**	*(rehs-pohn-dehr)*
response	**contestación**	*(kohn-tehs-tah-see-ohn)*
rest	**reposo**	*(reh-poh-soh)*
restless	**inquieto**	*(een-kee-eh-toh)*
restroom	**cuarto de baño**	*(koo-ahr-toh deh bah-nyoh)*
retinopathy	**retinopatía**	*(reh-tee-noh-pah-tee-ah)*
[to] return	**volver/regresar**	*(bohl-behr/reh-greh-sahr)*
[to] revise	**revisar**	*(reh-bee-sahr)*
rheumatic	**reumático**	*(reh-oo-mah-tee-koh)*
rheumatic fever	**fiebre reumática**	*(fee-eh-breh reh-oo-mah-tee-kah)*
ribs	**costillas**	*(kohs-tee-yahs)*
rice	**arroz**	*(ah-rohs)*
right	**derecho**	*(deh-reh-choh)*
rigidity	**rigidez**	*(ree-hee-dehs)*
risk	**riesgo**	*(ree-ehs-goh)*
road	**camino**	*(kah-mee-noh)*
roast beef	**rosbif**	*(rohs-beef)*
roast	**rostizado**	*(rohs-tee-sah-doh)*
rolls	**panecillos**	*(pah-neh-see-yohs)*
room	**cuarto**	*(koo-ahr-toh)*
roseola	**roseola**	*(roh-seh-oh-lah)*
rotation	**rotación**	*(roh-tah-see-ohn)*

route	**ruta**	*(roo-tah)*
routine	**rutina**	*(roo-tee-nah)*
[to] rub	**frotar/restregar**	*(froh-tahr/rehs-treh-gahr)*
rubella	**rubéola**	*(roo-beh-oh-lah)*
S	**s**	*(eh-seh)*
saccharin	**sacarina**	*(sah-kah-ree-nah)*
salad	**ensalada**	*(ehn-sah-lah-dah)*
saliva	**saliva**	*(sah-lee-bah)*
salt	**sal**	*(sahl)*
sample	**muestra**	*(moo-ehs-trah)*
sanitary	**sanitario**	*(sah-nee-tah-ree-oh)*
Saturday	**sábado**	*(sah-bah-doh)*
saucer	**platillo**	*(plah-tee-yoh)*
sausage	**chorizo/salchicha**	*(choh-ree-soh/sahl-chee-chah)*
science	**ciencia**	*(see-ehn-see-ah)*
scleral	**escleral**	*(ehs-kleh-rahl)*
scorpion	**alacrán**	*(ah-lah-krahn)*
scrambled (*eggs*)	**revueltos**	*(reh-boo-ehl-tohs)*
scratch	**raspón**	*(rahs-pohn)*
[to] scream	**gritar**	*(gree-tahr)*
sealant	**placa protectora**	*(plah-kah proh-tehk-toh-rah)*
season	**estación**	*(ehs-tah-see-ohn)*
sebaceous	**sebáceo**	*(seh-bah-seh-oh)*
second	**segundo**	*(seh-goon-doh)*
[to] secrete	**secretar**	*(seh-kreh-tahr)*
sedative	**sedativo/sedante**	*(seh-dah-tee-boh/seh-dahn-teh)*
[to] see	**ver**	*(behr)*
[to] select	**seleccionar**	*(seh-lehk-see-oh-nahr)*
selected	**selecto**	*(seh-lehk-toh)*
selection	**selección**	*(seh-lehk-see-ohn)*
[to] sell	**vender**	*(behn-dehr)*
semi-solid	**semi-sólido**	*(seh-mee-soh-lee-doh)*
sensitive	**sensitivo**	*(sehn-see-tee-boh)*
sentence	**oración**	*(oh-rah-see-ohn)*
[to] separate	**separar**	*(seh-pah-rahr)*
September	**septiembre**	*(sehp-tee-ehm-breh)*
series	**serie**	*(seh-ree-eh)*
serology	**serología**	*(seh-roh-loh-hee-ah)*
[to] serve	**servir**	*(sehr-beer)*
served: are served	**se sirven**	*(seh seer-behn)*
services	**servicios**	*(sehr-bee-see-ohs)*
setting	**área**	*(ah-reh-ah)*
seven	**siete**	*(see-eh-teh)*
seven A.M.	**las siete**	*(lahs see-eh-teh)*
seven hundred	**setecientos**	*(seh-teh-see-ehn-tohs)*
seven P.M.	**las diecinueve horas**	*(lahs dee-eh-see-noo-eh-beh oh-rahs)*
seventeen	**diecisiete**	*(dee-eh-see-see-eh-teh)*
seventh	**séptimo**	*(sehp-tee-moh)*
seventy	**setenta**	*(seh-tehn-tah)*
several	**varios**	*(bah-ree-ohs)*
sex	**sexo**	*(sehx-oh)*

sexual	**sexual**	*(sehx-oo-ahl)*
[to] shake	**temblar**	*(tehm-blahr)*
she	**ella**	*(eh-yah)*
sheet	**sábana**	*(sah-bah-nah)*
shirt	**camisa**	*(kah-mee-sah)*
shoes	**zapatos**	*(sah-pah-tohs)*
shortening	**manteca**	*(mahn-teh-kah)*
should	**debe**	*(deh-beh)*
shower	**baño/regadera**	*(bah-nyoh/reh-gah-deh-rah)*
shrimp	**camarones**	*(kah-mah-roh-nehs)*
sign (*information*)	**letrero**	*(leh-treh-roh)*
signs (*directions*)	**señales**	*(seh-nyah-lehs)*
signature	**firma**	*(feer-mah)*
similar	**similar**	*(see-mee-lahr)*
simple	**sencillo**	*(sehn-see-yoh)*
since	**desde/como**	*(dehs-deh/koh-moh)*
single	**solo**	*(soh-loh)*
singular	**singular**	*(seen-goo-lahr)*
sistemic	**sistémico**	*(sees-teh-mee-koh)*
sister	**hermana**	*(ehr-mah-nah)*
sister-in-law	**cuñada**	*(koo-nyah-dah)*
[to] sit	**sentar**	*(sehn-tahr)*
Sit!	**¡Siéntese!**	*(See-ehn-teh-seh)*
sites	**sitios**	*(see-tee-ohs)*
situation	**situación**	*(see-too-ah-see-ohn)*
six	**seis**	*(seh-ees)*
six A.M.	**las seis**	*(lahs seh-ees)*
six hundred	**seisientos**	*(seh-ees-ee-ehn-tohs)*
six P.M.	**las dieciocho horas**	*(lahs dee-eh-see-oh-choh oh-rahs)*
sixteen	**dieciseis**	*(dee-ehs-ee-seh-ees)*
sixth	**sexto**	*(sehx-toh)*
sixty	**sesenta**	*(seh-sehn-tah)*
skirt	**falda**	*(fahl-dah)*
[to] sleep	**dormir**	*(dohr-meer)*
small	**pequeño/chico**	*(peh-keh-nyoh/chee-koh)*
smile	**sonrisa**	*(sohn-ree-sah)*
[to] smoke	**fumar**	*(fooh-mahr)*
so	**así que**	*(ah-see keh)*
social	**social**	*(soh-see-ahl)*
social worker	**trabajador(a) social**	*(trah-bah-hah-dohr[-doh-rah] soh-see-ahl)*
sociocultural	**sociocultural**	*(soh-see-oh-kool-too-rahl)*
socks	**calcetines/calcetas**	*(kahl-seh-tee-nehs/kahl-seh-tahs)*
sofa	**sofá**	*(soh-fah)*
soft	**suave**	*(soo-ah-beh)*
soldier	**soldado**	*(sohl-dah-doh)*
solid	**sólido**	*(soh-lee-doh)*
solution	**solución**	*(soh-loo-see-ohn)*
solvent	**solvente**	*(sohl-behn-teh)*
somatic	**somático**	*(soh-mah-tee-koh)*
somatization	**somatización**	*(soh-mah-tee-sah-see-ohn)*
some	**algunos/unos**	*(ahl-goo-nohs/oo-nohs)*

some hearts	**unos corazones**	*(oo-nohs koh-rah-soh-nehs)*
some tables	**unas mesas**	*(oo-nahs meh-sahs)*
somebody, someone	**alguien**	*(ahl-gee-ehn)*
something	**algo**	*(ahl-goh)*
sometimes	**a veces/algunas veces**	*(ah beh-sehs/ahl-goo-nahs beh-sehs)*
son	**hijo**	*(ee-hoh)*
soup	**caldo/sopa**	*(kahl-doh/soh-pah)*
south	**sur**	*(soor)*
spaghetti	**espaguetis**	*(ehs-pah-geh-tees)*
Spanish	**español**	*(ehs-pah-nyohl)*
[to] speak	**hablar**	*(ah-blahr)*
special	**especial**	*(ehs-peh-see-ahl)*
specimen	**muestra**	*(moo-ehs-trah)*
spices	**especias**	*(ehs-peh-see-ahs)*
spicy	**condimentado**	*(kohn-dee-mehn-tah-doh)*
spinach	**espinaca**	*(ehs-pee-nah-kah)*
spinal	**espinal**	*(ehs-pee-nahl)*
spirit	**espíritu**	*(ehs-pee-ree-too)*
[to] spread (extend)	**extender**	*(ehx-tehn-dehr)*
[to] spread (topical)	**untar**	*(oohn-tahr)*
spring	**primavera**	*(pree-mah-beh-rah)*
stairs	**escalera**	*(ehs-kah-leh-rah)*
[to] start	**comenzar**	*(koh-mehn-sahr)*
STAT	**STAT**	*(ehs-taht)*
steak	**bistec**	*(bees-tehk)*
[to] step	**pisar**	*(pee-sahr)*
stepdaughter	**hijastra**	*(ee-hahs-trah)*
stepfather	**padrastro**	*(pah-drahs-troh)*
stepmother	**madrastra**	*(mah-drahs-trah)*
stepson	**hijastro**	*(ee-hahs-troh)*
sterile	**estéril**	*(ehs-teh-reel)*
sternum	**esternón**	*(ehs-tehr-nohn)*
stethoscope	**estetoscopio**	*(ehs-teh-tohs-koh-pee-oh)*
stockings	**medias**	*(meh-dee-ahs)*
stomach	**estómago**	*(ehs-toh-mah-goh)*
[to] stop	**parar**	*(pah-rahr)*
straight	**derecho**	*(deh-reh-choh)*
straw	**popote**	*(poh-poh-teh)*
strawberry	**fresa**	*(freh-sah)*
street	**calle**	*(kah-yeh)*
stroke	**ataque de apoplejía**	*(ah-tah-keh deh ah-poh-pleh-hee-ah)*
studies	**estudios**	*(ehs-too-dee-ohs)*
stupor	**estupor**	*(ehs-too-pohr)*
subaxillary	**subaxilar**	*(soob-ahx-ee-lahr)*
subcutaneous	**subcutáneo**	*(soob-koo-tah-neh-oh)*
sublingual	**sublingual**	*(soob-leen-goo-ahl)*
subnormal	**subnormal**	*(soob-nohr-mahl)*
substernal	**substernal**	*(soobs-tehr-nahl)*
substitutes	**substitutos**	*(soobs-tee-too-tohs)*
successful	**con éxito**	*(kohn ehx-ee-toh)*
[to] suffer	**sufrir**	*(soo-freer)*

sugar	**azúcar**	*(ah-soo-kahr)*
suit	**traje**	*(trah-heh)*
summer	**verano**	*(beh-rah-noh)*
Sunday	**domingo**	*(doh-meen-goh)*
supper	**cena**	*(seh-nah)*
suppository	**supositorio**	*(soo-poh-see-toh-ree-oh)*
surgeon	**cirujano**	*(see-roo-hah-noh)*
surgery	**cirugía**	*(see-roo-hee-ah)*
surgical	**quirúrgico**	*(kee-roor-hee-koh)*
surroundings	**alrededor**	*(ahl-reh-deh-dohr)*
[to] suspend	**suspender**	*(soos-pehn-dehr)*
sutures	**suturas/puntos**	*(soo-too-rahs/poon-tohs)*
sweater	**chamarra/suéter**	*(chah-mah-rah/soo-eh-tehr)*
swelling	**hinchado**	*(een-chah-doh)*
swollen ankles	**tobillos hinchados**	*(toh-bee-yohs een-chah-dohs)*
symbol	**símbolo**	*(seem-boh-loh)*
symptoms	**síntomas**	*(seen-toh-mahs)*
syncope	**síncope**	*(seen-koh-peh)*
syndrome	**síndrome**	*(seen-droh-meh)*
syringe	**jeringa**	*(heh-reen-gah)*
syrup	**jarabe/zumo**	*(hah-rah-beh/soo-moh)*
systemic	**sistemático**	*(sees-teh-mah-tee-koh)*
systole	**sístole**	*(sees-toh-leh)*
T	**t**	*(teh)*
table	**mesa**	*(meh-sah)*
tablespoon	**cuchara**	*(koo-chah-rah)*
tablet	**tableta**	*(tah-bleh-tah)*
tacos	**tacos**	*(tah-kohs)*
[to] take	**tomar/llevar**	*(toh-mahr/yeh-bahr)*
[to] take out	**sacar**	*(sah-kahr)*
[to] talk	**hablar**	*(ah-blahr)*
[to] talk to	**hablar con**	*(ah-blahr kohn)*
tamales	**tamales**	*(tah-mah-lehs)*
taste	**gusto**	*(goos-toh)*
tea	**té**	*(teh)*
teaspoon	**cucharita**	*(koo-chah-ree-tah)*
technician	**técnico**	*(tehk-nee-koh)*
television set	**televisor**	*(teh-leh-bee-sohr)*
[to] tell	**decir**	*(deh-seer)*
temperature	**temperatura**	*(tehm-peh-rah-too-rah)*
temporal	**temporal**	*(tehm-poh-rahl)*
ten	**diez**	*(dee-ehs)*
ten A.M.	**las diez**	*(lahs dee-ehs)*
ten P.M.	**las veintidós horas**	*(lahs beh-een-tee-dohs oh-rahs)*
tense	**tenso**	*(tehn-soh)*
tension	**tensión**	*(tehn-see-ohn)*
tenth	**décimo**	*(deh-see-moh)*
terminal	**terminal**	*(tehr-mee-nahl)*
terms	**términos**	*(tehr-mee-nohs)*
tests	**pruebas**	*(proo-eh-bahs)*
tetanus	**tétanos**	*(teh-tah-nohs)*

than	**que**	*(keh)*
thanatophobia [death]	**tanatofobia**	*(tah-nah-toh-foh-bee-ah)*
thank you	**gracias**	*(grah-see-ahs)*
that (far away)	**aquel/aquella**	*(ah-kehl/ah-keh-yah)*
that (there)	**eso/esa**	*(eh-soh/eh-sah)*
that have	**que tienen**	*(keh tee-eh-nehn)*
the	**el/la**	*(ehl/lah)*
their	**su/sus**	*(soo/soos)*
them	**ustedes**	*(oos-teh-dehs)*
theories	**teorías**	*(teh-oh-ree-ahs)*
therapeutic measures	**medidas terapéuticas**	*(meh-dee-dahs teh-rah-peh-oo-tee-kahs)*
therapy	**terapia**	*(teh-rah-pee-ah)*
there is/are	**hay**	*(ah-ee)*
therefore	**poreso**	*(pohr-eh-soh)*
thermometer	**termómetro**	*(tehr-moh-meh-troh)*
these	**estos/estas**	*(ehs-tohs/ehs-tahs)*
they	**ellos/ellas**	*(eh-yohs/eh-yahs)*
third	**tercero**	*(tehr-seh-roh)*
thirteen	**trece**	*(treh-seh)*
thirty	**treinta**	*(treh-een-tah)*
this (here)	**esto/esta**	*(ehs-toh/ehs-tah)*
three	**tres**	*(trehs)*
three A.M.	**las tres**	*(lahs trehs)*
three fourths	**tres cuartos**	*(trehs koo-ahr-tohs)*
three hundred	**trescientos**	*(trehs-see-ehn-tohs)*
three P.M.	**las quince horas**	*(lahs keen-seh oh-rahs)*
three thousand	**tres mil**	*(trehs meel)*
throat culture	**exudado faríngeo**	*(ehx-oo-dah-doh fah-reen-heh-oh)*
thrombus	**coágulo/trombo**	*(koh-ah-goo-loh/trohm-boh)*
Thursday	**jueves**	*(hoo-eh-behs)*
thyroid	**tiroide**	*(tee-roh-ee-deh)*
tie (necktie)	**corbata**	*(kohr-bah-tah)*
time	**tiempo**	*(tee-ehm-poh)*
tissue (*body*)	**tejido**	*(teh-hee-doh)*
tissue (*paper*)	**tisú**	*(tee-sooh)*
tissue damage	**daño del tejido**	*(dah-nyoh dehl teh-hee-doh)*
to	**a**	*(ah)*
toast	**pan tostado**	*(pahn tohs-tah-doh)*
toilet	**escusado**	*(ehs-koo-sah-doh)*
tolerant	**tolerante**	*(toh-leh-rahn-teh)*
tomato	**tomate**	*(toh-mah-teh)*
tomorrow	**mañana**	*(mah-nyah-nah)*
tonsillitis	**tonsilitis/amigdalitis**	*(tohn-see-lee-tees/ah-meeg-dah-lee-tees)*
too much	**demasiado**	*(deh-mah-see-ah-doh)*
tooth	**diente**	*(dee-ehn-teh)*
toothache	**dolor de muelas**	*(doh-lohr deh moo-eh-lahs)*
toothbrush	**cepillo de dientes**	*(seh-pee-yoh deh dee-ehn-tehs)*
toothpaste	**pasta de dientes**	*(pahs-tah deh dee-ehn-tehs)*
toothpick	**palillo**	*(pah-lee-yoh)*

topical	**topical/tópico**	*(toh-pee-kahl/toh-pee-koh)*
torso	**torso**	*(tohr-soh)*
total	**total**	*(toh-tahl)*
toward	**hacia**	*(ah-see-ah)*
towel	**toalla**	*(too-ah-yah)*
tower	**torre**	*(toh-reh)*
traction	**tracción**	*(trak-see-ohn)*
[to] translate	**traducir/interpretar**	*(trah-doo-seer/een-tehr-preh-tahr)*
transparent	**transparente**	*(trahns-pah-rehn-teh)*
traumatic	**traumático**	*(trah-oo-mah-tee-koh)*
treatment	**tratamiento**	*(trah-tah-mee-ehn-toh)*
tree	**árbol**	*(ahr-bohl)*
trust	**confianza**	*(kohn-fee-ahn-sah)*
[to] try	**intentar/tratar**	*(een-tehn-tahr/trah-tahr)*
tubes	**tubos**	*(too-bohs)*
tuberculosis	**tuberculosis**	*(too-behr-koo-loh-sees)*
Tuesday	**martes**	*(mahr-tehs)*
tumor	**tumor**	*(too-mohr)*
tuna	**atún**	*(ah-toon)*
turkey	**pavo/guajolote**	*(pah-boh/goo-ah-hoh-loh-teh)*
[to] turn	**voltear/girar**	*(bohl-teh-ahr/hee-rahr)*
[to] turn off	**apagar**	*(ah-pah-gahr)*
twelve	**doce**	*(doh-seh)*
twelve midnight	**las veinticuatro horas**	*(lahs beh-een-tee-koo-ah-troh oh-rahs)*
twelve noon	**las doce**	*(lahs doh-seh)*
twenty	**veinte**	*(beh-een-teh)*
twenty-four	**veinticuatro**	*(beh-een-tee-koo-ah-troh)*
two	**dos**	*(dohs)*
two A.M.	**las dos**	*(lahs dohs)*
two hundred	**doscientos**	*(doh-see-ehn-tohs)*
two P.M.	**las catorce horas**	*(lahs kah-tohr-seh oh-rahs)*
two thousand	**dos mil**	*(dohs meel)*
two thousand two	**dos mil dos**	*(dohs meel dohs)*
type	**tipo**	*(tee-poh)*
types of fractures	**tipos de fracturas**	*(tee-pohs deh frak-too-rahs)*
U	**u**	*(oo)*
ulcer	**úlcera**	*(ool-seh-rah)*
ulnar	**ulnar**	*(ool-nahr)*
ultrasound	**ultrasonido**	*(ool-trah-soh-nee-doh)*
uncle	**tío**	*(tee-oh)*
under	**debajo de**	*(deh-bah-hoh deh)*
underwear	**ropa interior**	*(roh-pah een-teh-ree-ohr)*
union	**unión**	*(oo-nee-ohn)*
universal	**universal**	*(oo-nee-behr-sahl)*
until	**hasta**	*(ahs-tah)*
urea	**urea**	*(oo-reh-ah)*
uremia	**uremia**	*(oo-reh-mee-ah)*
ureteritis	**uretritis**	*(oo-reh-tree-tees)*
urinal	**pato**	*(pah-toh)*
urine	**orina**	*(oh-ree-nah)*
urticaria	**urticaria**	*(oor-tee-kah-ree-ah)*

[to] use	**usar**	*(oo-sahr)*
used	**usado**	*(oo-sah-doh)*
useful	**útil**	*(oo-teel)*
uterus	**útero**	*(oo-teh-roh)*
[to] utilize	**utilizar**	*(oo-tee-lee-sahr)*
uvula	**úvula**	*(oo-boo-lah)*
V	**v**	*(beh)*
vaccinations	**vacunas**	*(bah-koo-nahs)*
vaginal	**vaginal**	*(bah-hee-nahl)*
vaginitis	**vaginitis**	*(bah-hee-nee-tees)*
vagus	**vago**	*(bah-goh)*
valve	**válvula**	*(bahl-boo-lah)*
vanilla	**vainilla**	*(bah-ee-nee-yah)*
vapor	**vapor**	*(bah-pohr)*
varices	**varices**	*(bah-ree-sehs)*
varicocele	**varicocele**	*(bah-ree-koh-seh-leh)*
variety	**variedad**	*(bah-ree-eh-dahd)*
vegetables	**vegetales**	*(beh-heh-tah-lehs)*
vein	**vena**	*(beh-nah)*
venereal	**venéreo**	*(beh-neh-reh-oh)*
ventilation	**ventilación**	*(behn-tee-lah-see-ohn)*
verbs	**verbos**	*(behr-bohs)*
vertebrate	**vertebrado**	*(behr-teh-brah-doh)*
vertigo	**vértigo**	*(behr-tee-goh)*
vestibule	**vestíbulo**	*(behs-tee-boo-loh)*
veterinary	**veterinaria**	*(beh-teh-ree-nah-ree-ah)*
victims	**víctimas**	*(beek-tee-mahs)*
vinegar	**vinagre**	*(bee-nah-greh)*
violet	**violeta**	*(bee-oh-leh-tah)*
virgin	**virgen**	*(beer-hehn)*
visible	**visible**	*(bee-see-bleh)*
vision	**visión**	*(bee-see-ohn)*
[to] visit	**visitar**	*(bee-see-tahr)*
visiting hours	**horas de visita**	*(oh-rahs deh bee-see-tah)*
vital	**vital**	*(bee-tahl)*
vital signs	**signos vitales**	*(seeg-nohs bee-tah-lehs)*
vitamins	**vitaminas**	*(bee-tah-mee-nahs)*
voice	**voz**	*(bohs)*
volume	**volumen**	*(boh-loo-mehn)*
[to] vomit	**vomitar**	*(boh-mee-tahr)*
vomiting	**vomitando**	*(boh-mee-tahn-doh)*
W	**w**	*(doh-bleh beh)*
[to] wait	**esperar**	*(ehs-peh-rahr)*
[to] wake	**despertar**	*(dehs-pehr-tahr)*
Wake up!	**¡Despierte!**	*(Dehs-pee-ehr-teh)*
[to] walk	**caminar**	*(kah-mee-nahr)*
walker	**andadera**	*(ahn-dah-deh-rah)*
wall	**pared**	*(pah-rehd)*
[to] want	**querer**	*(keh-rehr)*
warning	**advertencia**	*(ahd-behr-tehn-see-ah)*

[to] wash	**lavar**	*(lah-bahr)*
watch	**reloj**	*(reh-lohj)*
watchman	**velador**	*(beh-lah-dohr)*
water	**agua**	*(ah-goo-ah)*
water jug	**jarra**	*(hah-rah)*
watermelon	**sandía**	*(sahn-dee-ah)*
we	**nosotros/nosotras**	*(noh-soh-trohs/noh-soh-trahs)*
Wednesday	**miércoles**	*(mee-ehr-koh-lehs)*
week	**semana**	*(seh-mah-nah)*
went out	**salió**	*(sah-lee-oh)*
west	**oeste**	*(oh-ehs-teh)*
what? / which?	**¿cuál?/¿qué?**	*(koo-ahl/keh)*
wheat	**trigo**	*(tree-goh)*
when?	**¿cuándo?**	*(koo-ahn-doh)*
where?	**¿dónde?**	*(dohn-deh)*
white	**blanco**	*(blahn-koh)*
white cells	**glóbulos blancos**	*(gloh-boo-lohs blahn-kohs)*
white spots	**manchas blancas**	*(mahn-chahs blahn-kahs)*
who?	**¿quién?**	*(kee-ehn)*
whole	**entero**	*(ehn-teh-roh)*
whole milk	**leche entera**	*(leh-cheh ehn-teh-rah)*
why?	**¿por qué?**	*(pohr keh)*
wife	**esposa**	*(ehs-poh-sah)*
will have	**tendrá**	*(tehn-drah)*
will help you	**le ayudará**	*(leh ah-yoo-dah-rah)*
will remember	**recordará**	*(reh-kohr-dah-rah)*
will talk	**hablará**	*(ah-blah-rah)*
window	**ventana**	*(behn-tah-nah)*
window (pane)	**ventana de vidrio**	*(behn-tah-nah deh bee-dree-oh)*
wings	**alas**	*(ah-lahs)*
winter	**invierno**	*(een-bee-ehr-noh)*
[to] wish	**desear**	*(deh-seh-ahr)*
with	**con**	*(kohn)*
within	**dentro de**	*(dehn-troh deh)*
without	**sin**	*(seen)*
woman	**mujer**	*(moo-hehr)*
words	**palabras**	*(pah-lah-brahs)*
[to] work	**trabajar**	*(trah-bah-hahr)*
worker	**trabajador**	*(trah-bah-hah-dohr)*
wound	**herida**	*(eh-ree-dah)*
[to] write	**escribir**	*(ehs-kree-beer)*
writing	**escribiendo**	*(ehs-kree-bee-ehn-doh)*
X	**ex**	*(eh-kees)*
X-ray room	**cuarto de rayos X**	*(koo-ahr-toh deh rah-yohs eh-kees)*
X-rays	**rayos X**	*(rah-yohs eh-kees)*
xiphoid	**xifoide**	*(see-foh-ee-deh)*
Y	**y**	*(ee-gree-eh-gah)*
year	**año**	*(ah-nyoh)*
yellow	**amarillo**	*(ah-mah-ree-yoh)*
yes	**sí**	*(see)*

yogurt	**yogur**	*(yoh-goor)*
you (*familiar*)	**tú**	*(too)*
you (*formal*)	**usted**	*(oos-tehd)*
you can	**puede**	*(poo-eh-deh)*
you know	**sabe**	*(sah-beh)*
you need	**necesita**	*(neh-seh-see-tah)*
you sign	**firme**	*(feer-meh)*
young man/ woman	**joven**	*(hoh-behn)*
young people	**jóvenes**	*(hoh-beh-nehs)*
your	**su/sus**	*(soo/soos)*
yourself	**su**	*(soo)*
yourselves	**ellos/ellas**	*(eh-yohs/eh-yahs)*
Z	**z**	*(seh-tah)*
zone	**zona**	*(soh-nah)*
zoology	**zoología**	*(soh-oh-loh-hee-ah)*
zoophobia [animals]	**zoofobia**	*(soh-oh-foh-bee-ah)*
zygomatic	**cigomático**	*(see-goh-mah-tee-koh)*